Contemporary Cardiology

Series Editor

Peter P. Toth
Ciccarone Center for the Prevention of Cardiovascular Disease
Johns Hopkins University School of Medicine, Baltimore, MD, USA

For more than a decade, cardiologists have relied on the Contemporary Cardiology series to provide them with forefront medical references on all aspects of cardiology. Each title is carefully crafted by world-renown cardiologists who comprehensively cover the most important topics in this rapidly advancing field. With more than 75 titles in print covering everything from diabetes and cardiovascular disease to the management of acute coronary syndromes, the Contemporary Cardiology series has become the leading reference source for the practice of cardiac care.

Thorsten M. Leucker • Gary Gerstenblith
Editors

Cardiovascular Disease in the Elderly

Second Edition

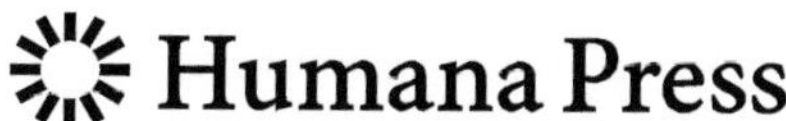 Humana Press

Editors
Thorsten M. Leucker
School of Medicine
Johns Hopkins University
Baltimore, MD, USA

Gary Gerstenblith
School of Medicine
Johns Hopkins University
Baltimore, MD, USA

ISSN 2196-8969   ISSN 2196-8977   (electronic)
Contemporary Cardiology
ISBN 978-3-031-16596-2   ISBN 978-3-031-16594-8   (eBook)
https://doi.org/10.1007/978-3-031-16594-8

This Humana imprint is published by the registered company Springer Nature Switzerland AG
The registered company address is: Gewerbestrasse 11, 6330 Cham, Switzerland

Preface

We are in the middle of an explosive growth of the elderly population in the United States and worldwide, and the most rapid growth is occurring in the subgroup of our population 85 years of age and older. Accompanying this demographic shift is a significant rise in the number of older patients with cardiovascular diseases (CVD) such as hypertension, valvular heart disease, coronary artery disease, rhythm abnormalities, and heart failure. Today, patients over the age of 65 years account for most of all deaths related to CVD.

With this shift of demographics and the multitude of new treatments available to treat CVD, healthcare providers are increasingly called on to make decisions as to whether or not to recommend these therapies to their patients. However, it often remains uncertain whether or not diagnostic and therapeutic interventions employed in the younger patient population can be extrapolated to the elderly because of marked differences in physiology, expected life span, complication rates, and increased comorbidities. Therefore, it is of the utmost importance that physicians at the forefront of treating elderly patients with CVD, including primary care providers, geriatricians, and cardiologists, but also surgeons and anesthesiologists are familiar with the age-associated changes in cardiovascular physiology, structure, and the impact of comorbid conditions to accurately assess and successfully treat older adults at risk for CVD or with established CVD.

The first edition of *Cardiovascular Disease in the Elderly* was published almost two decades ago, and much has evolved since then. In this second edition, existing chapters have been updated, and new chapters of interest have been added. Specifically, this second edition focuses on the unique aspects of primary and secondary prevention of CVD in the elderly, accurate assessment of vascular function using novel imaging approaches, as well as the distinctive factors to consider when administering pharmacotherapy in the older patient population. Furthermore, all important aspects of cardiovascular care are covered in detail in the remaining chapters, providing evidence-based approaches guided by the latest clinical evidence. The chapters are written and updated by leading experts in their fields who have studied extensively, and in many cases conducted the studies on which, current recommendations are based.

Baltimore, MD, USA   Thorsten M. Leucker
Baltimore, MD, USA   Gary Gerstenblith

Contents

Contributors

David Blitzer Division of Cardiac, Thoracic, and Vascular Surgery, Columbia University Vagelos College of Physicians and Surgeons, New York, NY, USA

Hugh Calkins Division of Cardiology, Department of Medicine, Johns Hopkins University, School of Medicine, Baltimore, MD, USA

Matthews Chacko Division of Cardiovascular Medicine, Vanderbilt University Medical Center, Nashville, TN, USA

Andrew Cluckey Division of Cardiovascular Medicine, Vanderbilt University Medical Center, Nashville, TN, USA

Marie Therese Cooney St Vincent's University Hospital, Dublin, Ireland

School of Medicine, University College Dublin, Dublin, Ireland

Matthew J. Czarny Division of Cardiology, Johns Hopkins University School of Medicine, Baltimore, MD, USA

Cherie N. Dahm Division of Cardiovascular Medicine, Vanderbilt University Medical Center, Nashville, TN, USA

Abdulla A. Damluji The Inova Center of Outcomes Research, Inova Heart and Vascular Institute, Falls Church, VA, USA

Milind Y. Desai Section of Cardiovascular Imaging, Heart, Vascular and Thoracic Institute, Cleveland Clinic, Cleveland, OH, USA

Gary Gerstenblith Division of Cardiology, Department of Medicine, Johns Hopkins University School of Medicine, Baltimore, MD, USA

Joseph Goldenberg Divison of Cardiology, School of Medicine, Johns Hopkins University, Baltimore, MD, USA

Sheraz Hussain Geriatrics and Palliative Care Medicine, University of Chicago, Chicago, IL, USA

Thorsten M. Leucker Division of Cardiology, Department of Medicine, Johns Hopkins University School of Medicine, Baltimore, MD, USA

John W. McEvoy University Hospital Galway and SAOLTA University Health Care Group, Galway, Ireland

National University of Ireland School of Medicine, Galway, Ireland

National Institute for Prevention and Cardiovascular Health, National University of Ireland Galway, Galway, Ireland

Ella Murphy University Hospital Galway and SAOLTA University Health Care Group, Galway, Ireland

National University of Ireland School of Medicine, Galway, Ireland

National Institute for Prevention and Cardiovascular Health, National University of Ireland Galway, Galway, Ireland

Brent G. Petty Pharmacy & Therapeutics Committee, Johns Hopkins University School of Medicine, Baltimore, MD, USA

Faisal Rahman Division of Cardiology, Johns Hopkins University School of Medicine, Baltimore, MD, USA

Jon R. Resar Division of Cardiology, Johns Hopkins University School of Medicine, Baltimore, MD, USA

Amit Rout University of Louisville School of Medicine, Louisville, KY, USA

Ryan Wallace Division of Cardiology, Department of Medicine, Johns Hopkins University, School of Medicine, Baltimore, MD, USA

Tom Kai Ming Wang Section of Cardiovascular Imaging, Heart, Vascular and Thoracic Institute, Cleveland Clinic, Cleveland, OH, USA

David D. Yuh Division of Cardiac Surgery, Department of Surgery, Stamford Health, Stamford, CT, USA

Atherosclerotic Cardiovascular Disease Prevention in the Older Adult: Part 1

Ella Murphy, Marie Therese Cooney, and John W. McEvoy

1 Introduction

While we have made remarkable advances in cardiovascular disease (CVD) prevention over the past century, CVD remains the leading cause of death globally, and the absolute numbers of incident CVD events have been increasing with the advancing age of populations around the world [1]. CVD is also a major cause of disability, functional decline, loss of independence, hospitalisations, and reduction in quality of life among older adults [2, 3]. Therefore, with an ageing population, prevention of CVD in this cohort is a major global health priority. Despite this, older patients, particularly those over the age of 75 years, have been significantly underrepresented in most major cardiovascular trials. Concurrently, with increasing life expectancy, multimorbidity has become an endemic phenomenon in the older patient cohort, yet it is precisely the older patients with more complex comorbidities, significant physical or cognitive disabilities, frailty, or those in nursing homes or assisted living, that have been excluded from virtually all trials. As a result, much of our data for these patients has been extrapolated from younger, healthier patients [4]. While there is increasing recognition that older patients may require a different approach, current

E. Murphy · J. W. McEvoy (✉)
University Hospital Galway and SAOLTA University Health Care Group, Galway, Ireland

National University of Ireland School of Medicine, Galway, Ireland

National Institute for Prevention and Cardiovascular Health, National University of Ireland Galway, Galway, Ireland
e-mail: johnwilliam.mcevoy@nuigalway.ie

M. T. Cooney
St Vincent's University Hospital, Dublin, Ireland

School of Medicine, University College Dublin, Dublin, Ireland

© The Author(s), under exclusive license to Springer Nature Switzerland AG 2023
T. M. Leucker, G. Gerstenblith (eds.), *Cardiovascular Disease in the Elderly*, Contemporary Cardiology, https://doi.org/10.1007/978-3-031-16594-8_1

guidelines frequently focus on recommendations for optimal management of a single CVD disease, rarely embracing the complexities imposed by multimorbidity (such as polypharmacy, therapeutic competition, and frailty) [5, 6]. These factors all create unique challenges for the clinician when considering the optimal preventive strategy for an older patient.

Moreover, physiological changes of aging mean that older patients are also at an increased risk for complications related to both pharmacological and non-pharmacological interventions. Therefore, a key priority in preventive care in older adults requires finding a balance between the risks of a given preventive intervention and the potential benefits. It should not be assumed that outcomes reported in trials of younger and healthier patients are automatically applicable to older adults. Compared to hard outcomes, such as death or myocardial infarction (MI) for example, outcomes important to older patients, such as maintaining independence, good quality of life, or reducing the burden of medication side effects, are infrequently reported in major clinical trials [7]. This adds complexity to meaningful discussions with older patients when reviewing the potential benefits of a preventive intervention.

In the subsequent two chapters we aim to provide a detailed but pragmatic discussion on some of the key priorities and unique challenges faced when considering primary and secondary prevention of atherosclerotic CVD (ASCVD) in older patients. We will use the ABCDE approach as a framework for the discussion, highlighting the relevant available evidence base as well as current guideline recommendations [8–10].

2 Assessment

> **Box 1**
>
>
>
> - The cornerstone of the preventive care of all older patients involves balancing the risk-benefit ratio of a given intervention.
> - While all guidelines recommend using risk scores to quantify a patient's overall risk of ASCVD, these should not be used in isolation.
> - Risk scores overestimate ASCVD risk in ethnically diverse populations, those with higher socioeconomic backgrounds, or those already receiving preventive care.
> - They can also underestimate ASCVD risk in those with lower socioeconomic status or those with chronic inflammatory conditions.

- Risk is a continuum and there is no exact point above which a given intervention is automatically indicated or below which an intervention should not be used.
- Therefore, final judgements on risk-benefit decisions should include a quantitative risk score assessment, combined with clinical judgement based on an individual patient's preferences, consideration of comorbidities and the potential for adverse effects, as well as the presence of additional risk modifiers.
- A shared clinician-patient decision model is key.

While the risks of developing incident CVD increase substantially with age, so too, in general, do the risks of adverse events from interventions. Therefore, the cornerstone of the preventive care of all older patients involves balancing the risk-benefit ratio of intervention, with each treatment decision tailored to an individual patient following a clinician-patient discussion. When considering the relative benefits of CVD prevention interventions, it is important to realise that older populations, particularly those over the age of 75 years, have been largely underrepresented in preventive trials. This can have important implications when considering an individual patient's potential net benefit from a given preventive strategy. In addition, when considering trial data, particular attention should be paid to the inclusion and exclusion criteria, with many trials excluding persons with multiple comorbidities or evidence of frailty, both of which are common in older adults. These points will be discussed in further detail under the relevant sections below with an overview provided in Box 1 and Fig. 1.

2.1   Risk Scores in Older Adults

In order to identify those at highest risk of developing incident CVD events, and hence those most likely to benefit from more intensive preventive measures, all major guidelines currently recommend quantifying a person's absolute risk of developing CVD events (typically over the next 10 years) using a validated scoring system [11–14] (Table 1). Using these estimates, patients are then grouped into various risk categories (e.g., low, moderate, or high) to guide the appropriate intensity of preventive treatments. While it is tempting to rely on these rigid risk-based cut-offs, this approach can be problematic, particularly in older patients who are almost always considered high risk based on age alone (noting that all CVD risk scores are heavily influenced by age). Furthermore, the accuracy of these scores has been questioned in contemporary populations. Overestimation of risk in ethnically diverse populations and underestimation of risk in those with lower socioeconomic backgrounds is a problem across all age groups [15]. Similarly, overestimation of risk is also more likely in those already receiving preventive care [16]. In contrast, risk may be underestimated in those with lower socioeconomic status or those with chronic inflammatory conditions. With that, it should be remembered

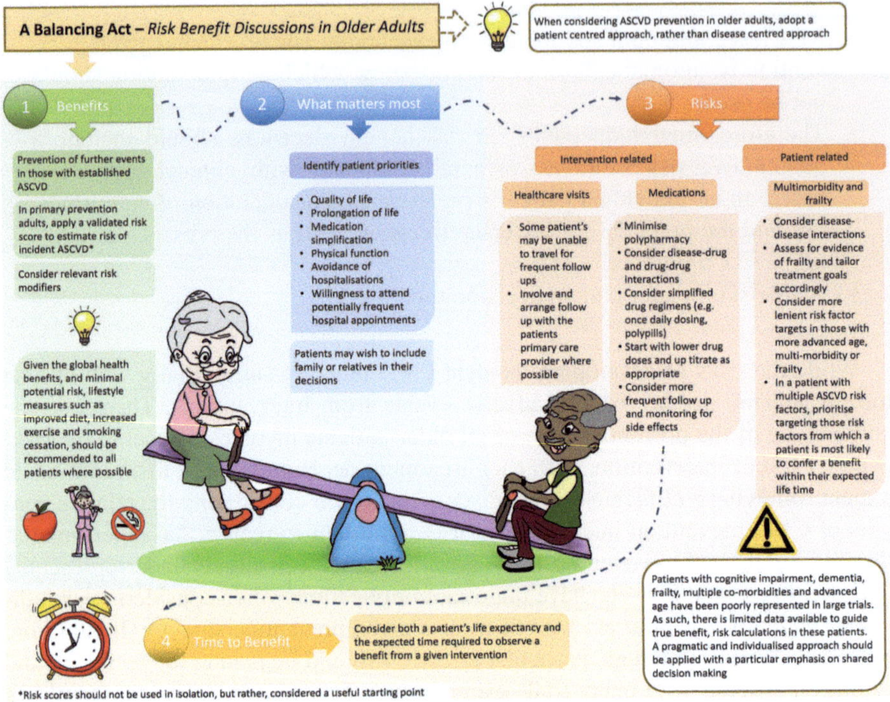

Fig. 1 A balancing act: risk-benefit discussions in older adults. *ASCVD* atherosclerotic cardiovascular disease

that risk is a continuum and there is no exact point above which a given intervention is automatically indicated or below which intervention should not be used. Considering this, there is now increased emphasis on clinician-patient shared decision making, particularly when applying intensive lifestyle measures or pharmacological therapies [16].

In addition to the above, there are a number of particularly important caveats to consider when applying risk scores to older adults. Most of the scoring systems estimate risk over 10 years, which may not be the most meaningful time frame for an older person, particularly among those with very advanced age. It is also worth noting the outcome measure for the score being used. For example, the Systematic COronary Risk Evaluation (SCORE) [17], which was previously recommended by the European Society of Cardiology (ESC) Guidelines, estimates the 10-year risk of CV mortality and therefore does not capture the risk of potential non-fatal events that could significantly impair quality of life (e.g., stroke). A later guideline, the Pooled Cohort Equation (PCE) [18], which is recommended by American guidelines, estimates a patient's 10-year risk of non-fatal MI or coronary heart disease (CHD) death or fatal or non-fatal stroke.

Most of the CVD risk estimators currently recommended by guidelines have performed poorly in older individuals [19, 20]. There are several potential reasons for this. As noted above, most risk scores place a large emphasis on age, meaning that patients over the age of 75 years would automatically be classified as either

Table 1 Comparison of risk estimators used by major Guidelines

Risk estimator	SCORE [17]	SCORE2-OP [24]	PCE [18]	Framingham risk score [27]	QRISK2 [28]	Mesa score [29]	WHO [30]
Components	Age Gender Total cholesterol or total cholesterol: high-density lipoprotein cholesterol ratio Systolic BP Smoking status	Age Gender Non-HDL cholesterol Systolic BP Smoking status	Age Gender Race Total cholesterol High-density lipoprotein cholesterol Systolic BP Diabetes mellitus Current smoking status	Age Sex Total cholesterol Systolic blood pressure Antihypertensive medication use Current smoking Diabetes mellitus	Ethnicity Age Sex Smoking status Systolic blood pressure BMI Family history Townsend deprivation score Treated hypertension RA Chronic renal disease Type 2 diabetes Atrial fibrillation	Age Gender Race/ethnicity Diabetes mellitus Current smoking Total and HDL cholesterol Use of lipid-lowering medication Systolic blood pressure Use of anti-hypertensive medication Any family history of a heart attack in a first-degree relative Coronary artery calcium score	Age Sex Blood pressure Diabetes Smoking status Cholesterol level
Outcome	10-year risk of CVD mortality	5- and 10-year risk of CVD events (non-fatal MI, non-fatal stroke, and cardiovascular mortality) Option of including hospitalisation for heart failure	10-year ASCVD (non-fatal MI or CHD death or fatal or non-fatal stroke)	10-year CVD risk (CHD death, MI, coronary insufficiency, angina, ischemic stroke, haemorrhagic stroke, TIA, intermittent claudication, and heart failure)	10-year risk of CVD event (CHD, stroke, or TIA)	10-year coronary heart disease risk	10-year risk of fatal or non-fatal CV event (myocardial infarction or stroke)

(continued)

Table 1 (continued)

Risk estimator	SCORE [17]	SCORE2-OP [24]	PCE [18]	Framingham risk score [27]	QRISK2 [28]	Mesa score [29]	WHO [30]
Validated age group	40–65 years	70–89 years	40–79 years	30–74 years	35–74 years	45–85 years	30–79 years
Age interactions	Not included	Age interactions included for all variables	Age interactions included for all variables	Not included	Age interactions included for all variables	Age interactions included for all variables	Not included
Recommended by	ESC	ESC	AHA	CCS	NICE	–	–

AHA American Heart Association, *ASCVD* atherosclerotic cardiovascular disease, *BP* blood pressure, *BMI* body mass index, *CCS* Canadian Cardiovascular Society, *CHD* coronary heart disease, *CV* cardiovascular, *CVD* cardiovascular disease, *ESC* European Society of Cardiology, *HDL* high-density lipoprotein, *MI* myocardial infarction, *NICE* National Institute for Health and Care Excellence, *SCORE* Systematic COronary Risk Evaluation, *PCE* pooled cohort equation, *TIA* transient ischemic attack

intermediate or high-risk of cardiovascular disease based on age alone [21]. Yet, neither SCORE, QRISK2, nor the PCE risk equations have been validated in those over 65, 75, and 79 years respectively. While traditional CVD risk factors are still very much relevant in older populations, the relative strengths of their effects change with increasing age [22, 23]. This, coupled with the competing risk of non-CVD mortality, leaves the potential for an overestimation of the possible benefits of CVD risk factor treatment in older populations when using risk scores validated in younger population cohorts [24]. Overestimation of risk, in turn, leads to the potential for overtreatment, which can have significant deleterious effects in older adults, subjecting patients to polypharmacy, increased risk of drug-drug interactions, adverse events, reduced quality of life, and increased costs. As a result, guidelines place a heavy emphasis on clinician-patient shared decision making in those over 75 years [11].

More recently, attempts have been made to create CVD risk sores specifically designed to estimate risk in older adults [24, 25]. For example, the SCORE2-OP model has recently been validated across four different risk regions in Europe in those over the age of 70 years and is recommended in the most recent ESC CVD Prevention guidelines [14, 24]. Significantly this score was developed to account for competing risk of non-CVD death and includes age interactions for all risk factors to account for differences in the relationship between risk factors and outcomes across different ages. It was also developed to estimate both a 5- and 10-year risk of incident CVD events. The shorter time frame of 5 years may be particularly relevant for those with more advanced age or increased frailty when balancing a time to benefit vs. life expectancy. Furthermore, SCORE2-OP includes a prediction of both fatal and non-fatal CV events (non-fatal MI, non-fatal stroke, and cardiovascular mortality). With increasing age and a limited life expectancy, non-fatal CVDs may be of particular clinical importance as they may severely impact a patient's quality of life. Finally, the 2021 ESC guideline also introduces, for the first time, different CVD risk thresholds for designation of high and very-high risk in younger vs. older adults, which is intended to reduce overtreatment in the elderly. Specifically, 10-year fatal and non-fatal CVD risk thresholds of >7.5% for persons <50 years, >10% for persons in the age group of 50–69 years, and >15% for persons >70 years are recommended for the designation of very-high risk by the ESC [14].

In conclusion, risk scores should not be used in isolation. Particularly among the elderly, they should be considered a useful starting point, rather than a final arbiter, for decision making in the primary prevention of CVD [16, 26]. Final judgements on risk-benefit decisions should include a quantitative risk score assessment, combined with clinical judgement based on an individual patient's preferences, consideration of comorbidities and the potential for adverse effects, as well as the presence of additional risk modifiers as discussed further below.

2.2　*Risk Modifiers for More Accurate Risk Assessment*

There is increasing recognition that the presence of certain phenotypes, which are not included in traditional risk scores, so-called "risk modifiers", can independently increase a patient's risk of CVD (Fig. 2) [9, 14, 26, 31]. Presence of such risk

Risk Modifiers	If measured in selected patients
Ethnicity (eg., South Asian populations, notably those from India and Pakistan)	hs-CRP ≥2mg/L
Family history of premature ASCVD	ApoB ≥130mg/dL (corresponds to an LDL-C of ≥160mg/dL). Consider measuring in those with triglyceride levels ≥200mg/dL
CKD (eGFR 15-59ml/min) with or without albuminuria	ABI <0.9
Chronic inflammatory conditions (e.g., HIV, AIDs, RA, psoriasis, SLE)	Elevated Lp(a) levels (>50mg/dL). Consider measuring in those with a family history of premature ASCVD
Conditions specific to women (e.g., preeclampsia, menopause before age 40)	Elevated coronary artery calcium (e.g., ≥100 Agatston units or ≥75% age-matched percentile)
Hypercholesterolemia (LDL-C ≥160mg/dL or non-HDLC>190 mg/dL)	Carotid artery plaque (focal wall thickening ≥50% greater than the surrounding vessel wall or a focal region with an intima-media thickness of ≥1.5mm) may be useful if CAC is not feasible
Metabolic syndrome (presence of 3 of the following; increased waist circumference, elevated BP, elevated glucose and low HDL-C)	
Persistently elevated triglycerides (≥175mg/ml) on 3 occasions	
Diabetes mellitus of long duration (≥ 10 years for type 2 diabetes or ≥20 years for type 1 diabetes) or DM with evidence of retinopathy, neuropathy or nephropahty	

Fig. 2 Risk modifiers in older adults. *ASCVD* atherosclerotic cardiovascular disease, *CKD* chronic kidney disease, *HIV* human immunodeficiency virus, *AIDS* acquired immunodeficiency syndromes, *RA* rheumatoid arthritis, *SLE* systemic lupus erythematosus, *LDL-C* low-density lipoprotein cholesterol, *HDL-C* high-density lipoprotein cholesterol, *BP* blood pressure, *hs-CRP* high sensitivity C-reactive protein, *ApoB* apolipoprotein B, *ABI* ankle-brachial index, *Lp(a)* lipoprotein (a), *DM* diabetes mellitus, *CAC* coronary artery calcium

modifiers should prompt consideration of more intensive treatment in selected patients. Chronic kidney disease and long-standing diabetes are two frequently encountered risk modifiers in older patients.

There is some evidence that increased levels of certain biomarkers are linked to increased CVD risk. Chronic inflammation, with an elevation of C reactive protein (CRP) is at least modestly associated with CVD risk [32, 33]. At the same time, emerging evidence suggests that treatment to reduce inflammation (using a humanised monoclonal antibody to interleukin 1β), reduces cardiovascular risk [34]. With this, there have been attempts to refine risk prediction of established scores in older patients by including these biomarkers. Authors from the Atherosclerosis Risk in Communities (ARIC) study compared the traditional PCE model to a "complete" model (PCE variables plus high sensitivity cardiac troponin T, high-sensitivity CRP, and pro-B-type natriuretic peptide to the PCE) [35]. They demonstrated improved prediction of short-term (follow-up of approximately 4 years) incident global CVD (incident CHD, stroke, HF hospitalisation) in older adults (mean age 75.4 years) [35]. Others have previously suggested that the presence of increased Interleukin-6 (IL-6) and or multiple carotid plaques could be useful predictors of mortality in older patients [36]. However, while these markers may be useful in selected patients, there is a risk that routinely adding such markers may complicate assessments and reduce the cost-effectiveness of risk estimation.

Coronary artery calcium scoring is also established as a particularly useful tool to help refine a patient's risk and is now provided a class 2 recommendation in American and European guidelines to help make therapeutic decisions in cases where a patient is considered at intermediate risk of CVD [14, 26]. Coronary artery calcium scoring is minimally invasive, low risk and can be performed with the same radiation exposure as a mammogram. In appropriately selected patients, a coronary artery calcium score of 0 equates to a low 10-year risk of CVD, even among the elderly, meaning that identification of such patients can avoid potentially harmful treatments [9, 37].

2.3 Frailty as Part of the Assessment

There is an increasing recognition that chronological age is only a rough proxy of a person's susceptibility to adverse health outcomes [38]. With that, the concept of frailty has now become a high-priority theme in the area of preventive cardiology [39]. Considered a biological syndrome, frailty reflects a state of "decreased physiological reserve and vulnerability to stressors" [39]. The association of frailty with worse health outcomes and as a predictor of CVD events is well established [39, 40]. Not only do frail patients have a higher prevalence of CV comorbidities but they are also less likely to be receiving guideline-based therapies [41, 42]. Frailer patients are also at higher risk of adverse outcomes following therapeutic interventions, and so recognition of this phenotype is particularly relevant when making risk benefits decisions. With upward of 20 frailty tools available, the lack of a practical road map on how to integrate frailty assessments into day-to-day decision-making remains a challenge [39]. Nonetheless, future validation of CVD risk estimation tools in older patients should consider concerns such as frailty, cognition, falls, and disability [43].

While those identified as frail do have higher risks of adverse events, it is equally important to avoid the common misconception that frailty should be used as a reason to withhold care. Instead, the identification of a frail patient should act as a prompt to restructure their preventive care towards a more personalised form. Furthermore, consideration must be given to interventions that might target and reduce the individual's frailty. One particularly important aspect of a personalized approach for CVD prevention among frail older adults is the concept of competing risk. A competing risk is an event whose occurrence precludes the occurrence of the primary event of interest. For example, in a study examining time to death attributable to CVD, death attributable to non-CVD causes is a competing risk. Therefore, a frail elderly adult with a preponderance of CVD risk factors (including importantly chronic kidney disease) is at particularly high CVD risk and may benefit most from CVD preventive care whereas a frail elderly adult with CVD risk factors but also other major non-CVD comorbidities (e.g., active cancer as an archetypal example) is at higher competing risk for non-CVD death and may be suitable for more lenient management of CVD risk factors. All frail adults may benefit from shorter follow-up periods to monitor for side effects of CVD prevention therapies.

2.4   *Life Expectancy, Competing Risk, and Time to Benefit*

Ultimately the goals of prevention are to prevent illness, morbidity, and mortality. However, preventive therapies have limited value if they are initiated for conditions that are unlikely to cause symptoms or problems during an individual's lifetime. In other words, if, in the setting of high competing risk, a person's life expectancy is less than the estimated time to benefit (TTB) for a CVD prevention intervention, the patient is unlikely to benefit from the intervention and is instead exposed to the risks of said intervention [44]. As most preventive measures will take years to accrue benefits (Table 2), consideration of a patient's life expectancy and estimated time to benefit should be included in patient-clinician discussions when initiating preventive strategies among older adults.

Table 2 Estimated time to benefit for main primary preventive strategies in older adults

Primary prevention	Time to benefit
Antiplatelets	Not currently recommended in those over the age of 70 years
Anti-hypertensives	1–2 years [44–46]
Diabetes	Intensive glycaemic control (HbA1c <7%) vs. more lenient control—between 5 and 10 years for intensive control, 2–5 years for GLP1 agonists, and <1 year for SGLT2i [47]. Summarised in Table 2 of chapter "Atherosclerotic Cardiovascular Disease Prevention in the Older Adult: Part 2"
Diet	DASH trail: Improved BP control observed within 8 weeks in a younger population cohort (although mean age 44 years) [48] TONE trial: Improved BP control and approximately 30% reduction in need for antihypertensive medication by reducing sodium intake about 40 mmol/day or by reducing average body weight by about 3.5 kg over a follow-up period ranging from 9 to 30 months (mean age 66.5 years) [49]

Table 2　(continued)

Primary prevention	Time to benefit
Statins	Meta-analysis by Gencer et al., including a combination of primary and secondary prevention for older adults over the age of 75 years (mean age 79 years) observed a 26% relative risk reduction in major vascular events for every 1 mmol/L reduction in LDL cholesterol (Rate ratio 0.74; 95% CI 0.61–0.89; $p = 0.0019$) over a median follow-up period of 2.2–6 years [50]. Similarly, relative risk reductions in cardiovascular death, myocardial infarction, stroke and coronary revascularisation were 15%, 20%, 27%, and 20%, respectively for each 1 mmol/L reduction in LDL
Smoking	Cessation at 60 years of age leads to an increase in life expectancy of 3 years compared to those who continue to smoke [51] Cessation at 65 years of age leads to an increase in life expectancy of 2 years in men and 3.7 years in women, compared to those who continue to smoke [52] Significant reduction in CV mortality within 5 years in those who quit, compared to those who continue to smoke [53]
Exercise	Reducing sedentary time by 1 h per day is associated with a 12% lower risk of CVD and 26% lower risk of heart disease in older women followed over 4.9 years [54]

CV cardiovascular, *CVD* cardiovascular disease, *GLP1* glucagon-like peptide-1, *SGLT2i* sodium-glucose cotransporter-2 inhibitors

3　Antiplatelets

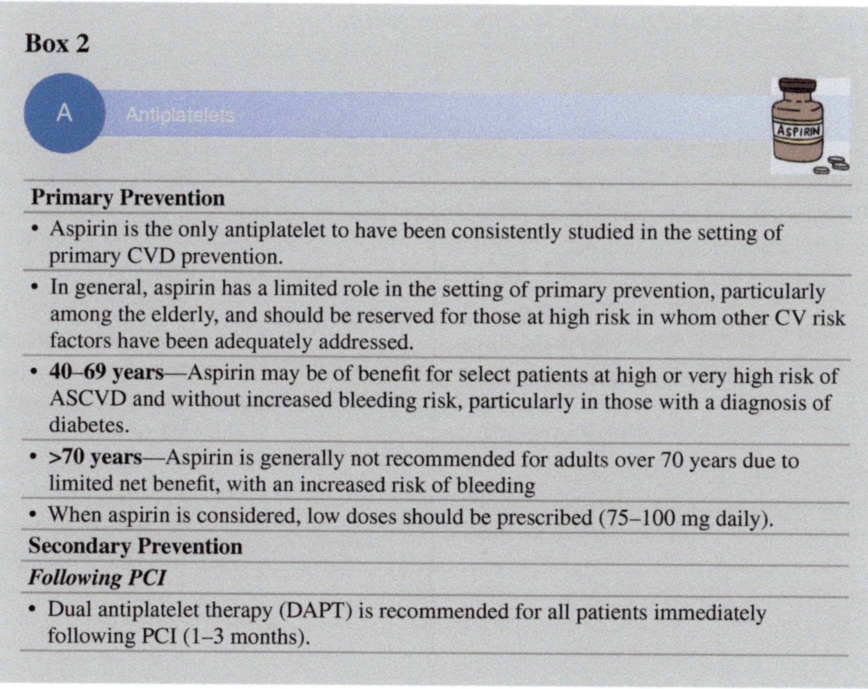

Box 2

Primary Prevention

- Aspirin is the only antiplatelet to have been consistently studied in the setting of primary CVD prevention.

- In general, aspirin has a limited role in the setting of primary prevention, particularly among the elderly, and should be reserved for those at high risk in whom other CV risk factors have been adequately addressed.

- **40–69 years**—Aspirin may be of benefit for select patients at high or very high risk of ASCVD and without increased bleeding risk, particularly in those with a diagnosis of diabetes.

- **>70 years**—Aspirin is generally not recommended for adults over 70 years due to limited net benefit, with an increased risk of bleeding

- When aspirin is considered, low doses should be prescribed (75–100 mg daily).

Secondary Prevention

Following PCI

- Dual antiplatelet therapy (DAPT) is recommended for all patients immediately following PCI (1–3 months).

- In patients with low bleeding risk, DAPT should be continued for 12 months.
- In patients with increased bleeding risks, early discontinuation of aspirin (1–3 months post-PCI), with a continuation of $P2Y_{12}$ inhibitor monotherapy for 6–12 months is one strategy to decrease bleeding risk.
- Of the $P2Y_{12}$ inhibitors, clopidogrel may have the best safety profile, particularly in those >70 years.
- In carefully selected, healthy older adults, with a long life expectancy, increased ischemic risk, and low bleeding risk, the addition of low dose rivaroxaban to aspirin beyond 12 months after the index event may reduce further ischemic events, with the trade-off of increased bleeding risk.

Post ischemic stroke/TIA

- Following a minor ischemic stroke (NIHSS ≤3) or high-risk TIA ($ABCD^2$ score of ≥4), DAPT, with aspirin and clopidogrel, is recommended for 21 days.
- Following the initial period of DAPT, single antiplatelet therapy (SAPT) should be continued long term.
- For patients with moderate to severe strokes, aspirin monotherapy is recommended.

Peripheral arterial disease

- Aspirin (75–325 mg daily) or clopidogrel (75 mg daily) is recommended for all patients with symptomatic peripheral arterial disease.
- Aspirin for all asymptomatic carotid stenosis.
- American guidelines consider aspirin reasonable in asymptomatic disease with an ABI ≤0.9.

3.1 Antiplatelets in Primary Prevention

3.1.1 The Aspirin Debate

Since it was first produced in 1897, aspirin remains one of the most commonly used medications worldwide, with recent data estimating that nearly half of those aged 70 years and older report taking primary prevention aspirin [55, 56]. Significantly, the self-reported use of aspirin for primary prevention increases with age (34.7% in those aged 60–69 years, compared to 46.2% in those ≥80 years) [55]. Notably, Jacobsen et al. have reported that over 80% of patients in the USA obtain aspirin over the counter [57]. While these figures come with the limitations of self-reported patient data, they highlight the widespread belief among the older population that regular aspirin use confers a benefit in reducing the incidence of ASCVD. However, despite its widespread use, aspirin's role in primary prevention has always been controversial [58]. Emerging data in a changing population context have led to an evolution in recommendations of how aspirin should be used in the setting of primary CVD prevention (Box 2) [59].

The use aspirin for primary prevention first gained traction after the Physicians Health Study (PHS) reported a 44% reduction in the risk of fatal and non-fatal MI (RR, 0.56; 95% CI 0.45–0.70; $p < 0.00001$) in a group of US Physicians who had received 325 mg aspirin every other day, compared to those assigned to a placebo group [60]. These results were deemed so significant at the time that the trial was terminated early, despite not having met its prespecified primary outcome, a reduction in CV mortality. Despite the apparent benefit of aspirin observed in the PHS, a similar trial published in the same year, the British Male Doctors study, failed to show a benefit of 500 mg aspirin daily in reducing MI, stroke, or death, compared to no aspirin in a group of British male doctors [61]. What both trials did agree on was an increased risk of bleeding in those who received aspirin. These divergent results of the first primary prevention trials involving aspirin set the scene for the subsequent debate surrounding its benefit.

Up until the 2000s, accruing trial evidence largely reported reductions in both MI and stroke in younger populations who had received primary prevention aspirin, with a consistent trade-off of an increased bleeding risk (Table 3). By 2002, both the AHA and United States Preventive Services Task Force (USPSTF) recommended aspirin for patients at high risk of CVD [62, 63]. By 2007 European guidelines adopted a similar recommendation [64]. However, aspirin trials in the later 2000s appeared to suggest a temporal reduction in aspirin's efficacy in the setting of modern primary prevention, inspiring further contemporary trials.

In 2018, three separate major trials were published that resulted in a pivotal shift in guideline recommendations. The first trial in this group, the Aspirin to Reduce Risk of Initial Vascular Events (ARRIVE) trial, found that treatment with 100 mg of enteric-coated aspirin did not result in a reduction in the primary end point (a composite outcome of time to first occurrence of confirmed MI, stroke, CV death, unstable angina, or TIA) in a group of 12,546 nondiabetic patients (mean age 63.9 years; 55% $\geq$65 years) at moderate risk of coronary heart disease (10–20% 10-year risk) compared to those who received a placebo (HR 0.96; 95% CI 0.81–1.13; $p = 0.6038$) [65]. While subsequent per protocol analyses did reveal a reduction in hazard ratios for combined fatal/non-fatal MI (HR 0.53; 95% CI 0.36–0.79; $p = 0.0014$) and non-fatal MI (HR 0.55; 95% CI 0.36–0.84; $p = 0.0056$) in those who received aspirin, these results are less causally valid. As with previous trials, gastrointestinal bleeding was significantly more common in those who had received aspirin (HR 2.11; 95% CI 1.36–3.28; $p = 0.0007$). Participants were not excluded from ARRIVE on the basis of older age.

The subsequent ASCEND (A Study of Cardiovascular Events in Diabetes) trial, recruited 15,480 diabetic patients (mean age 63 years; 23.5% $\geq$70 years) and observed a reduction in the primary outcome of a first vascular event (a composite of nonfatal MI, nonfatal stroke, TIA, or death from any vascular cause excluding intracranial haemorrhage) in those who were assigned to receive 100 mg enteric-coated aspirin (rate ratio 0.88; 95% CI 0.79–0.97; $p = 0.01$) [66]. Again, there was a significantly higher rate of bleeding in those who received aspirin (Rate ratio; 1.29; 95% CI 1.09–1.52; $p = 0.003$), almost half of which (41.3%) were due to gastrointestinal bleeding. Participants were not excluded from ASCEND on the basis of older age but were excluded if they had clinically significant conditions that might limit adherence to the trial regimen for at least 5 years.

Table 3 Randomised trials of aspirin in primary prevention

Study	BMD [61]	PHS [60, 72]	TPT [73, 74]	HOT [75, 76]	PPP [77]	WHS [78]	POPADAD [79]	JPAD [80]	AAA [81]	JPPP [82]	ARRIVE [65]	ASCEND [66]	ASPREE [67, 69]	TIPS-3 [71]
Year	1988	1989	1998	1998	2001	2005	2008	2008	2010	2014	2018	2018	2018	2020
No. participants	5139	22,071	5085	18,790	4495	39,876	1276	2539	3350	14,464	12,546	15,480	19,114	5713
Design	Randomised (computer), unblinded (2:1 randomisation in favour of the aspirin group)	Randomised double blind, placebo-controlled trial 2 × 2 factorial design	Randomised, double blind, placebo-controlled trial 2 × 3 factorial design	Prospective randomised double-blind placebo (aspirin arm), BP arm was open with end point evaluation was blinded 2 × 2 factorial design	Centrally randomised, open label trial 2 × 2 factorial design	Randomised double blinded placebo controlled 2 × 2 factorial design	Multicentre randomised, double bind, placebo-controlled trial 2 × 2 factorial design	Multicentre, randomised, open label trial (blinded end point assessment)	Double blind, randomised controlled trial	Multicentre, open label, randomised, parallel group trial	Double blinded multicentre, placebo controlled	Randomised, double blind Factorial design	Randomised, double blind, placebo-controlled trial	Double blind, randomised, placebo-controlled trial with a 2 × 2 × 2 factorial design
Aspirin dose	500 mg daily aspirin	325 mg every other day	75 mg controlled aspirin	75 mg aspirin daily	100 mg enteric coated aspirin	100 mg every other day	100 mg aspirin daily	81 mg or 100 mg of aspirin daily	100 mg aspirin daily	Enteric-coated aspirin 100 mg daily	100 mg enteric-coated aspirin	100 mg enteric-coated aspirin	100 mg enteric-coated aspirin	Enteric-coated aspirin 75 mg per day
Comparison	No aspirin	Placebo	Placebo	Placebo	No aspirin	Placebo	Placebo	No aspirin	Placebo	No aspirin	Placebo	Placebo	Placebo	Placebo
Population	Male doctors in the UK between 50 and 78 years	Male doctors in USA aged between 40 and 84 years	Men between aged 45 and 69 years at high risk	Men (9907) and women (8883) between the age of 50 and 80 years with a diastolic BP between 100 and 115 mmHg on two occasions	Men (1912) and women (2583) ≥50 with at least one of the major recognised cardiovascular risk factors	Healthy female health professionals ≥45 years	Men and women ≥40 years with diabetes and ABI ≤0.99	Men and women aged 30–85 years with diabetes	Men and women aged 50–75 years with ABI ≤0.95	Men and women aged 60–85 years with hypertension, hyperlipidaemia or diabetes	Men aged ≥55 years with 2–4 cardiovascular risk factors; women aged ≥60 years with ≥3 cardiovascular risk factors	Men and women aged ≥40 years with diabetes	Men and women aged ≥70 years	Men aged >50 years and women aged ≥55 years with an elevated INTERHEART score (intermediate or high risk)

Relevant exclusions	Already on aspirin, unable to take aspirin, history of PUD, stroke, or definite MI	History of MI, stroke or TIA, cancer, current liver or renal disease, PUD, or gout, contraindications to aspirin, current use of aspirin or NSAIDs, current use of vitamin A	Past or present history of PUD, hiatus hernia or oesophagitis, past history of bleeding tendency, known or suspected alcohol abuse, a past history of cerebrovascular disease, a range of other conditions including liver disease and malignant disease and other illnesses at the discretion of the GP	Malignant hypertension, secondary hypertension, DBP >115 mmHg, stroke or MI within 12 months prior to randomisation, decompensated heart failure, patients with a serious concomitant disease that would affect survival within 2–3 years, insulin treated diabetes, known contraindication to low dose aspirin, hypersensitivity to felodipine, patient who requires a BB, ACEI or diuretic for reasons other than hypertension	Treatment with antiplatelet drugs, chronic use of anti-inflammatories or anticoagulants, contraindications to aspirin, disease with predictable poor short-term prognosis, predictable psychological or logistical difficulties affecting compliance with the trial	History of coronary artery disease, cerebrovascular disease, cancer, or other major chronic illness, history of side effects to the study medications, taking NSAIDS more than once a week, on anticoagulants or corticosteroids	Symptomatic CVD, those on aspirin already, PUD, severe dyspepsia, a bleeding disorder, or intolerance to aspirin, those with suspected serious physical illness which might have been expected to curtail life expectancy, those with psychiatric illness, those with congenital disease, those unable to give informed consent	History of coronary heart disease, history of cerebrovascular disease, history of arteriosclerotic disease necessitating medical treatment, atrial fibrillation, use of antiplatelet or antithrombotic therapy, a history of severe gastric or duodenal ulcer, severe liver dysfunction, severe renal dysfunction, allergy to aspirin	History of MI, stroke, angina, PAD, currently used aspirin or another antiplatelet or an anticoagulant, had severe indigestion, had chronic liver or kidney disease, were receiving chemotherapy, had contraindications to aspirin	History of CAD or cerebrovascular disease, a fib, atherosclerotic disease requiring surgery or intervention, PUD or conditions associated with bleeding, serious blood abnormalities, patients with aspirin sensitive aspirin, those on anticoagulants or antiplatelets or long-term treatment with NSAIDs	History of a vascular event, relevant arrhythmias, congestive cardiac failure (CCF) or vascular intervention, requiring antiplatelet therapy, high risk of GI and other bleeding, requiring anticoagulation or frequent use of NSAIDS, history of diabetes	A clear indication for aspirin or a contraindication to aspirin, the presence of other co-morbidities that might limit adherence to the trial regimen for a least 5 years	Coronary heart disease, overt cerebrovascular disease, atrial fibrillation, dementia, clinically significant physical disability, high risk of bleeding, anaemia, regular use of anticoagulants or antiplatelets, SBP ≥ 180 or DBP ≥ 105, a condition that would result in death within 5 years, inability to take aspirin	Indication, contraindication, preference for or intolerance to statins, betablockers, ACEI, diuretics, aspirin or clopidogrel; PUD, dyspepsia or bleeding, long term use of anticoagulants, hypercalcemia or hyperparathyroidism, regular use of vitamin D, systolic BP <120 mmHg, known vascular disease, symptomatic hypotension, severe renal impairment, history of malignancy, other serious condition likely to interfere with study participation, inability to attend follow up for at least 5 years

Participant characteristics

Age	<60 = 47% 60–69 = 39% 70–79% = 14%	40–49 = 41% 50–59 = 34% 60–69 = 19% 70–84 = 7%	Mean 57.5 years	Mean 62 years	Mean 64 years	Mean 55 years	Mean 60 years	Mean 65 years	Mean 62 years	Mean 71 years	Mean 64 years	Mean 63 years	Median 74 years	Mean 63.9 years
Age breakdown (where available)			–	–	50–59 = 29% 60–69% = 45% 70–79 = 24% ≥80 = 3%	45– 54 = 60.2% 55– 64 = 29.5% ≥65 = 10.3%	–	<65 = 46% ≥65 = 54%	–	<70 = 44.9% ≥70 = 55.1%	<65 = 56% ≥65 = 44%	<60 = 36.1% 60 to <70 = 40.4% ≥70 = 23.5%	65–73 = 49.9% ≥74 = 50%	Aspirin vs. placebo: ≤61 = 40% 61–66 = 28% >66 = 31.5%
Men	100%	100%	100%	53%	42%	0%	44%	54%	28%	42%	70%	63%	44%	47%

Outcome data

Follow up (years)	Median 5.5	Median 5	Median 6.8	Mean 3.8	Mean 3.6	Mean 10.1	Median 6.7	Median 4.4	Mean 8.2	Median 5	Median 5	Median 7.4	Median 4.7	Mean 4.6

(continued)

Table 3 (continued)

Study	BMD [61]	PHS [60, 72]	TPT [73, 74]	HOT [75, 76]	PPP [77]	WHS [78]	POPADAD [79]	JPAD [80]	AAA [81]	JPPP [82]	ARRIVE [65]	ASCEND [66]	ASPREE [67, 69]	TIPS-3 [71]
Primary endpoint (aspirin vs. control)	Definite MI or stroke resulting in death (63.2 vs. 62.3 per 10,000 person-years; p = NS)	Cardiovascular mortality (81 vs. 83; RR 0.96; 95% CI 0.6–1.54)	IHD (154 vs. 190 events; p = 0.04) Excluding warfarin arm (p = NS)	Major cardiovascular events not including silent MI (315 vs. 368; RR 0.85; 95% CI 0.73–0.99; p = 0.03)	Major cardiovascular events (45 vs. 64; RR 0.71; 85% CI 0.48–1.04)	Major cardiovascular events (477 vs. 522; RR 0.91; 95% CI 0.80–1.03; p = 0.13)	Major cardiovascular (116 vs. 117; RR 0.98; 95% CI 0.76–1.26; p = 0.86); cardiovascular death (43 vs. 35; RR 1.23; 95% CI 0.79–1.93; p = 0.36)	Major cardiovascular events (68 vs. 86; HR 0.80; 95% CI 0.58–1.10; p = 0.16)	Major cardiovascular events (13.7 vs. 13.3 per 1000 person-years; HR 1.03; 95% CI 0.84–1.27)	Major cardiovascular events (193 vs. 207; HR 0.94; 95% CI 0.77–1.15; p = 0.54)	Major cardiovascular events (269 vs. 281; HR 0.96; 95% CI 0.81–1.13; p = 0.60)	Major cardiovascular events (658 vs. 743; rate ratio 0.88; 95% CI 0.79–0.97; p = 0.01)	Death, dementia or persistent disability (21.5 vs. 21.2 per 1000 person-years; HR 1.01; 95% CI 0.92–1.11; p = 0.79)	Death from CV causes, MI or stroke Aspirin vs. placebo; (116 vs. 134; HR 0.86; 95% CI 0.67–1.10)
Secondary endpoint (aspirin vs. control)	Non-fatal stroke (32.4 vs. 28.5 per 10,000 person years; p = NS) and non-fatal MI (42.4 vs. 43.3 per 10,000 person years; p = NS)	Myocardial infarction (139 vs. 239; RR 0.56; 95% CI 0.45–0.70; p < 0.0001); stroke (119 vs. 98; RR 1.22; 85% CI 0.93–1.60; p = 0.15)	Stroke (47 vs. 48; 2.9 vs. 3.0 per 1000 person years; p = NS)	Myocardial infarction (82 vs. 127; RR 0.64; 95% 0.49–0.85; p = 0.002); stroke (146 vs. 148; RR 0.98; 95% CI 0.78–1.24; p = 0.08); cardiovascular mortality (133 vs. 140; RR 0.95; 95% CI 0.75–1.20; p = 0.65)	Total cardiovascular events (141 vs. 187; RR 0.77; 95% CI 0.62–0.95); cardiovascular death (17 vs. 31; RR 0.56; 95% CI 0.31–0.99); all-cause mortality (62 vs. 68; RR 0.81; 95% CI 0.58–1.13)	Fatal MI (14 vs. 12; RR 1.16; 95% CI 0.54–2.51; p = 0.70); fatal stroke (23 vs. 22; RR 1.04; 95% 0.58–1.86; p = 0.90); cardiovascular death (120 vs. 126; RR 0.95; 95% CI 0.74–1.22; p = 0.68)	All-cause mortality; non-fatal MI; other vascular events—no significant difference between groups	Cardiovascular mortality (1 vs. 10); HR 0.10; 95% CI 0.01–0.79; p = 0.0037); coronary heart disease events (28 vs. 35; HR 0.81; 95% CI 0.49–1.33; p = 0.40)	Composite of primary endpoint or angina, claudication, or TIA (22.8 vs. 22.9 per 1000 person-years; HR 1.00; 95% CI 0.85–1.17) and all-cause mortality	Composite of primary endpoint or atherosclerosis (280 vs. 319; HR 0.89; 95% CI 0.75–1.04; p = 0.14); cardiovascular death (58 vs. 57; HR 1.03; 95% CI 0.71–1.48; p = 0.89)	Composite and individual outcomes of the time to cardiovascular death, MI, or stroke; time to UA, time to TIA; and time to death (p = NS for all endpoints)	Any major vascular vent (833 vs. 936; rate ratio 0.88; 95% CI 0.80–0.97); GI cancer (157 vs. 158; rate ratio 0.99; p = NS)	Major cardiovascular events (10.7 vs. 11.3 per 1000 person years; HR 0.95; 95% CI 0.83–1.08)	Death from cardiovascular causes, MI or stroke or cancer (153 vs. 177; HR 0.86; 95% CI 0.69–1.07)
Safety endpoint	Extracranial bleeding (10.6 vs. 7.4 per 10,000 person-years; p = NS)	Bleeding requiring transfusion (48 vs. 28; RR 1.71; 95% CI 1.09–2.69; p = 0.02)	Major bleeding event (8 vs. 4; p = NS); intermediate bleeding event (48 vs. 33; p = NS)	Fatal bleeds (7 vs. 8); non-fatal major bleeds (129 vs. 70; RR 1.8; p < 0.001)	Severe bleeding (24 vs. 6; p < 0.0008)	GI bleeding requiring transfusion (127 vs. 91; RR 1.40; 95% 1.07–1.83; p = 0.02)	GI bleeding (28 vs. 31; RR 0.90; 95% CI 0.53–1.52; p = 0.69)	Haemorrhagic stroke or severe GI bleeding (10 vs. 7; p = NS)	Major haemorrhage requiring hospitalisation (34 vs. 20; HR 1.71; 95% CI 0.99–2.97)		GI bleeding events (61 vs. 29; HR 2.11; 95% CI 1.36–3.28; p = 0.0007)	Major bleeding event (314 vs. 245; rate ratio 1.29; 95% CI 1.09–1.52; p = 0.003)	Major haemorrhage (8.6 vs. 6.2 per 1000 person years; HR 1.38; 95% CI 1.18–1.62; p < 0.0001)	

Baseline characteristics represent an average of the complete trial population (i.e., both control and treatment arms)

BMD British Male Doctors, *PHS* Physicians Health Study, *TPT* Thrombosis Prevention Trial, *HOT* Hypertension Optimal Treatment, *PPP* Primary Prevention Project, WHS Women's Health Study, *POPADAD* Progression of arterial disease and diabetes, *JPAD* Japanese primary prevention of atherosclerosis with aspirin for diabetes, *AAA* aspirin for asymptomatic atherosclerosis, *JPPP* Japanese primary prevention project, *ARRVIE* aspirin to reduce risk of initial vascular events, *ASCEND* a study of cardiovascular events in diabetes, *ASPREE* aspirin in reducing events in the elderly, *TIPS-3* the international polycap study-3, *ACEI* angiotensin converting enzyme inhibitor, *BB* betablocker, *BP* blood pressure, *CAD* coronary artery disease, *CI* confidence interval, *DBP* diastolic blood pressure, *GI* gastrointestinal, *IHD* ischemic heart disease, *LDL-c* low density lipoprotein cholesterol, *MI* myocardial infarction, *NS* non-significant, *NSAIDs* non-steroidal anti-inflammatory drugs, *PPI* proton pump inhibitor, *PUD* peptic ulcer disease, *SBP* systolic blood pressure, *TIA* transient ischemic attack, *UA* unstable angina, *UK* United Kingdom

Finally, the Aspirin in Reducing Events in the Elderly (ASPREE) trial, became the first landmark randomised double-blinded placebo controlled trial to compare aspirin to placebo in a group of primary prevention adults over the age of 70 years ($\geq$65 years of age among blacks and Hispanics) [67–69]. As it stands, the ASPREE trial provides the largest body of trial evidence on aspirin use in the primary prevention of CVD among older adults. Enrolling 19,114 patients, with a median age of 74 years, the trial was stopped prematurely due to futility after it failed to show a benefit of 100 mg of enteric-coated aspirin in reducing CVD events (HR 0.95; 95% CI 0.83–1.08). Notably, there was a significantly higher rate of major haemorrhagic events in the aspirin group (hazard ratio, 1.38; 95% CI, 1.18–1.62; $p < 0.001$) with an unexpected trend towards increased mortality (HR 1.14; 95% CI 1.01–1.29), primarily attributed to cancer-related deaths. Low dose aspirin did not prolong disability-free survival over the study period of 5 years (HR 1.01; 95% CI 0.92–1.11; $p = 0.79$), which may represent a more meaningful outcome in older patients [69, 70]. Significantly, the trial excluded older patients with life-limiting chronic illnesses, dementia, or physical disability, meaning that these results cannot reliably be extrapolated to more frail older individuals.

Since the three trials of 2018, there has been one further large trial, the TIPS-3 study (The International Polycap Study 3) [71]. Here patients were randomised to receive aspirin plus placebo, polypill (simvastatin, atenolol, hydrochlorothiazide, and ramipril) plus placebo, double placebo, or double active treatment. The investigators did report a decrease in the occurrence of the primary outcome in those assigned to polypill plus aspirin compared to placebo. However, they observed no benefit when comparing aspirin alone to placebo, suggesting that the benefit observed in the double treatment group was largely driven by the polypill component. Notably, they also observed no increased rate of bleeding in the aspirin groups, which would be completely at odds with all previous trials, and thus raises questions with regards to the trial methodology (i.e., was the randomised allocation complied with and how well were bleeding events captured?) [59].

3.1.2   Putting It All Together: Meta-analyses

There have been several meta-analyses concluding that primary prevention aspirin may confer a benefit in lowering the risk of non-fatal MI, TIA, and ischemic stroke in younger patients at higher CVD risk (mean age of included participants <65 years) [83–85]. By contrast, the ASPREE trial, which is the only trial to target an older population (median age of 74 years), failed to demonstrate a beneficial effect of primary prevention aspirin on MI [67, 68]. One potential explanation for this difference is that older patients may be inherently different from younger patients with respect to their response to drug therapy [86]. Concurrently, any modest benefits observed with aspirin use have consistently been balanced by an increased risk of major bleeding, intracranial haemorrhage, and major gastrointestinal bleeding, which is particularly salient for older adults. Also worth noting when considering aspirin for elderly patients is that aspirin's benefit on the reduction in TIA and ischemic stroke is offset by the increased rate of haemorrhagic stroke, resulting in a similar rate of all strokes in those who receive aspirin compared to those who do not [83].

3.1.3   Additional Considerations

Minimising the Bleeding Risk

While aspirin's efficacy in primary prevention has always been an area of debate, its association with increased bleeding, particularly upper gastrointestinal bleeding, has been consistent. This risk of bleeding is dose-dependent. Among older patients, the odds ratio of bleeding with daily doses of aspirin of 75 mg, 150 mg, and 300 mg are 2.3, 3.2, and 3.9, respectively and so, when aspirin is used in primary prevention, low doses (75–100mg daily) are recommended [11, 87].

Proton pump inhibitors have been shown to decrease bleeding risk in those assigned to aspirin therapy in other settings and are recommended prophylactically in those considered at increased bleeding risk (history of gastroduodenal ulcers or GI bleeding, age over 60 years, corticosteroid use, dyspepsia or GERD symptoms, concomitant anticoagulant therapy, dual antiplatelet therapy) [88]. To date, the major aspirin primary prevention trials have infrequently reported on the use of PPIs and how these may influence bleeding outcomes in this setting. For example, while the ASPREE trial did not prevent the use of PPIs, (25% of patients were taking a PPI at trial entry), because of the double-blinded nature of the trial patients assigned to the (blinded) aspirin arm were not able to be considered for prophylactic PPI use. As such, the trial may not truly reflect the risk of GI haemorrhage in older patients in an everyday clinical setting, given that many of these patients would typically be offered prophylactic PPIs in this context [86]. Therefore, while aspirin should not be routinely recommended in older patients, co-prescription with proton pump inhibitors in those deemed at very high CV risk and with an otherwise good quality of life, may reduce the bleeding risk, therefore shifting the risk-benefit ratio in these select group of patients.

Drug Interactions

Co-administration of aspirin with other NSAIDs can lead to a drug interaction where the aspirin is prevented from irreversibly binding to COX-1, leading to rapid elimination of aspirin, and thus, decreased clinical benefit despite the increased bleeding risk. As it is estimated that approximately 14% of older adults are taking NSAIDS, this is an important point to consider when using aspirin in this population [86].

Areas of Uncertainty

While contemporary trials have favoured enteric-coated aspirin, definitive evidence for a reduction in bleeding risk with such formulations is lacking [89, 90]. Simultaneously, evidence is emerging that such formulations may reduce oral bio-availability and thus rendering aspirin's antithrombotic effects less pronounced. This effect seems to be particularly marked in patients with diabetes mellitus, with as many as half of such patients being non-responders to enteric-coated aspirin [91]. Patients with diabetes have an increased platelet turnover and so it has been suggested that twice daily dosing may be more effective.

There may also be an interaction between body weight and treatment response to aspirin. A recent post-hoc meta-analysis suggested that low doses of aspirin (75–100 mg) were only effective in preventing vascular events in patients weighing less than 70 kg [92]. However, other studies have not indicated a body weight interaction [93].

3.1.4 Guideline Recommendations for Aspirin in Primary Prevention

As it stands, most guidelines currently agree that aspirin should not be routinely prescribed for most patients without established ASCVD, particularly in those over the age of 70 years [11] (Table 4). Instead, intensive management of co-morbidities and other ASCVD risk factors will likely yield greater individual benefits. Low dose aspirin may provide a benefit in selected younger patients at high or very high risk of CVD, following an individualised patient-clinician discussion [14]. While there is broad international agreement that aspirin should not be commenced routinely for primary prevention in older adults, no trial or guideline has clearly addressed the question as to whether healthy older adults who are already taking aspirin should continue its use or should stop (and, if the latter, at what age should they stop).

3.2 Antiplatelets in Secondary Prevention

While antiplatelet therapies continue to play a pivotal role in the setting of secondary prevention of ASCVD, the advent of newer, more potent, antiplatelet drugs, such as the $P2Y_{12}$ inhibitors, mean that the options for antiplatelet therapies have expanded dramatically in recent years.

Table 4 Current guidelines on the use of aspirin in the setting of primary prevention of ASCVD in older adults

Guideline	Year	Recommendation
Australian [94]	2013	Aspirin and other antiplatelet agents are no longer routinely recommended for use in the primary prevention of CVD, including for people with diabetes or high absolute CVD risk
ACC/AHA [11]	2019	Low dose aspirin (75–100 mg daily) might be considered for the primary prevention of ASCVD among select adults 40–70 years of age who are at higher ASCVD risk but not at increased bleeding risk (Class IIb) Low dose aspirin (75–100 mg) should not be administered on a routine basis for the primary prevention of ASCVD among adults >70 years of age (Class III: Harm) Low dose aspirin (75–100 mg) should not be administered for primary prevention in adults at any age who are at increased risk of bleeding (Class III: Harm)
NICE [95]	2020	Do not routinely prescribe antiplatelet treatment for the primary prevention of CVD Consider aspirin in people with a high risk of stroke or MI. There is limited evidence of benefit even in people with multiple risk factors and there is a risk of harm. If aspirin is being considered, discuss the likely benefits and risks with the person
Canadian Stroke Best Practice [96]	2020	The use of aspirin is not recommended for primary prevention of a first vascular event (evidence level A) This recommendation pertains to individuals with vascular risk factors who have not had a vascular event (evidence level A) and to healthy older individuals without vascular risk factors (evidence level B) The net benefit of aspirin in individuals with asymptomatic atherosclerosis is uncertain (evidence level B)
ESC/EAPC [14]	2021	In patients with DM at high or very high CVD risk, low-dose aspirin may be considered for primary prevention in the absence of clear contraindications (Class IIb) Antiplatelet therapy is not recommended in individuals with low/moderate CV risk due to the increased risk of major bleeding
ADA [97]	2021	Aspirin therapy (75–162 mg/day) may be considered as a primary prevention strategy in those with diabetes who are at increased cardiovascular risk, after a comprehensive discussion with the patient on the benefits versus the comparable increased risk of bleeding (A)
USPSTF [98]	2021	The decision to initiate low-dose aspirin use for primary prevention in adults aged 40–59 years who have a 10% or greater 10-year CVD risk should be an individual one. Evidence indicates that the net benefit of aspirin use in this group is small. Persons who are not at increased risk for bleeding and are willing to take low-dose aspirin daily are more likely to benefit Recommend against low-dose aspirin use for primary prevention of CVD in those ≥60 years old

3.2.1 Antiplatelets in Patients with Recent Percutaneous Coronary Intervention (PCI)

Duration of Therapy

Dual antiplatelet therapy (DAPT) with aspirin and an oral $P2Y_{12}$ inhibitor continues to be the mainstay of antithrombotic treatment following PCI. Aspirin is recommended for all patients in the immediate period (1–3 months) following PCI, with the recent ADAPTABLE trial confirming that lower doses of aspirin (81 mg) appear to be as effective as higher doses (325 mg) in preventing subsequent ischemic events [99, 100]. However, more recently, the traditional approach of DAPT for a minimum of 6–12 months following PCI for a chronic coronary syndrome (CCS) or acute coronary syndrome (ACS) respectively, followed by the ubiquitous requirement for life-long aspirin has come into question [101]. Contemporary trials have begun to evaluate early discontinuation of DAPT, as well as continuing a maintenance $P2Y_{12}$ monotherapy in place of aspirin [59, 101, 102]. There have been two recent meta-analyses, including 32,145 patients across five trials (mean age 64.7 years) who underwent PCI in the setting of either CCS or ACS, both of which concluded that discontinuation of aspirin within 1–3 months post-PCI, while continuing $P2Y_{12}$ inhibitor monotherapy (most frequently clopidogrel), was associated with a significant reduction in major bleeding by almost 40%, without increasing the ischemic risk or a patient's mortality [103, 104]. The mean age across the five included trials was only 65 years meaning that there is limited data available for those over 70 years. However, this approach to abbreviated DAPT could be especially important for older patients at higher bleeding risks. While statistically inconclusive, the meta-analyses do suggest that 3 months of DAPT may be superior to 1 month in terms of balancing bleeding and ischemic risks in these post-PCI patients [103]. There are currently several ongoing trials further evaluating DAPT combinations and durations post PCI [102]. As it stands, most guidelines continue to recommend 12 months of DAPT as the standard, but with the option to either shorten or extend the duration depending on the balance of ischemic and bleeding risks. How future iterations of guidelines will change based on recent trials of 1–3 months DAPT remains to be determined.

As there is increasing emphasis on individualising the duration of antiplatelet therapy to a given patient's risk, tools such as PRECISE DAPT have been developed in an attempt to aid the identification of those at high risk of bleeding (PRECISE DAPT $\geq$25) who may benefit from shortened durations of DAPT [105]. Whether single antiplatelet therapy (SAPT) with a $P2Y_{12}$ inhibitor is preferable to SAPT with aspirin, following the initial period of DAPT, requires further study, however, a recent meta-analysis suggested that the risk of all-cause mortality, vascular death, and stroke does not differ between patients receiving a $P2Y_{12}$ inhibitor monotherapy vs. aspirin monotherapy [106]. The authors did; however, report a borderline trend towards a reduction for the risk of MI in those who received a $P2Y_{12}$ inhibitor compared to aspirin (Odds radio 0.81; 95% CI 0.66–0.99), with no difference in major bleeding events (odds radio 0.90; 95% CI 0.74–1.10), albeit these results are from a younger population.

Choice of Antiplatelet Agent

Both ticagrelor and prasugrel have been favoured as first-line $P2Y_{12}$ inhibitors, particularly in European guidelines, following PCI in the setting of acute coronary syndromes [107–109]. However, while they are considered more potent, have a more rapid onset, and have been shown to be superior in reducing cardiovascular death, MI, and stroke compared to clopidogrel in certain groups, both ticagrelor and prasugrel have also been associated with an elevated bleeding risk [110, 111]. Bleeding post-PCI is not a benign phenomenon, and it is now well established that there is a consistent association between bleeding and death in this setting [112]. A subgroup analysis of the TRITON-TIMI 38 trial (Trial to Assess Improvement in Therapeutic Outcomes by Optimising Platelet Inhibition with Prasugrel-Thrombolysis in Myocardial Infarction 38), failed to show a net benefit of prasugrel in a subgroup of patients 75 years and older due to elevated bleeding rates [111]. As a result, prasugrel should be used with caution in this age group, with dose reductions recommended [107, 113, 114]. Prasugrel should also be avoided in those with low body weight ($\leq$60 kg) or a history of TIA or stroke due to increased bleeding risks [109, 111]. The recent POPular AGE study, suggests that clopidogrel may be the preferred $P2Y_{12}$ inhibitor in those over 70 years (mean age 77 years) presenting with NSTE-ACS, as it was found to lead to fewer bleeding events (HR 0.71; 95% CI 0.54–0.94; $p = 0.02$ for superiority), without increasing a combined endpoint of all-cause death, myocardial infarction, stroke, or bleeding, when compared to ticagrelor (28% vs. 32%; absolute risk difference -4%; 95% CI -10 to 1.4; $p = 0.03$ for noninferiority) [115]. It should be noted that the trial was not powered to find statistical differences in all-cause mortality between groups, however. The previous TOPIC trial also demonstrated that switching from a more potent $P2Y_{12}$ inhibitor to clopidogrel 1 month following PCI in the setting of an ACS did not confer an elevated risk in major ischemic outcomes, but did result in a marked reduction in bleeding risk, and so this may also be an option for older patients who have both a high ischemic and bleeding risk [116].

More recently, European guidelines have introduced recommendations to consider the use of very low dose rivaroxaban (2.5 mg twice daily), in addition to aspirin, beyond 12 months posttreatment for ACS in those at increased ischemic risk (e.g., those with diabetes or polyvascular disease) [107]. This recommendation is largely based on results of the COMPASS trial (mean age 68 years), which found that a very low dose rivaroxaban (2.5 mg twice daily) plus aspirin 100 mg daily reduced the risk of the combined ischemic endpoint of CV death, stroke or MI (HR 0.76; 95% CI 0.66–0.86; $p < 0.001$), all-cause mortality (HR 0.82; 95% CI 0.71–0.96; $p = 0.01$), and CV mortality (HR 0.78; 95% CI 0.64–0.96; $p = 0.02$) in patients with known CAD or PAD or both [117]. There was an increased risk of bleeding however in the combination group (HR 1.70; 95% CI 1.40–2.05; $p < 0.001$) compared to aspirin alone. A similar trial evaluated the addition of low-dose rivaroxaban to clopidogrel in the setting of recent ACS (with participants enrolled within 7 days after admission) and again noted a reduction in ischemic events with a trade-off of major bleeding [118]. While reductions in ischemic events are always attractive, it should be remembered that bleeding risks increase with more advanced age and so may modify the risk benefits gained in older adults, particularly in those with a more limited life expectancy. A summary of current recommendations is provided in Box 2.

Triple Therapy: When Less Is More

A commonly encountered clinical scenario is one in which patients undergoing PCI have a coexisting underlying indication for oral anticoagulation (OAC). This simultaneous requirement for DAPT and an OAC, commonly referred to as "triple therapy", is most frequently encountered in the setting of a patient with underlying atrial fibrillation who has a requirement for PCI. It is estimated that between 17% and 46% of patients with atrial fibrillation have coronary artery disease and between 5% and 15% of those patients will eventually require PCI at some point during their lives and, with an increasing prevalence of atrial fibrillation and an aging population, this number is likely to increase [119]. While OAC is superior to DAPT in preventing thromboembolic disease in the setting of atrial fibrillation, DAPT is considered superior to OAC in preventing stent thrombosis around the time of PCI. However, triple therapy significantly increases a patient's bleeding risk, particularly in those >90 years of age, with CHA_2DS_2-VASc scores of 7–9 or those with a history of major bleeding [120, 121]. Therefore, patients who have an indication for both DAPT and oral anticoagulation pose a real practical dilemma for clinicians when balancing thrombotic risk against bleeding risk, particularly in older patients in the immediate period following PCI. Guidelines now recommend shortened durations of triple therapy (as short as 1 month depending on the balance of ischemic and bleeding risks), followed by a combination of single antiplatelet therapy (best data is available on the $P2Y_{12}$ inhibitor, clopidogrel) and OAC for up to a year [122, 123]. Following that, the previously recommendation for long-term aspirin is no longer considered necessary for secondary prevention of adults with a lifelong indication for monotherapy with OAC. PPIs are recommended for all older patients on dual or triple therapy [122].

3.2.2 Antiplatelets in Secondary Prevention of TIA/Stroke

Following a non-cardioembolic ischemic stroke or TIA, all patients should receive either aspirin, clopidogrel, or a combination of aspirin and extended-release dipyridamole [124, 125]. More recently, investigators have begun to evaluate the role of DAPT poststroke. Two recent landmark trials, CHANCE (Clopidogrel in High-Risk Patients with Acute Nondisabling Cerebrovascular Events) and POINT (Platelet-Orientated Inhibition in New TIA and Minor Ischemic Stroke), have resulted in major guideline changes [126, 127]. The earlier CHANCE trial suggested that adding clopidogrel (at an initial dose of 300 mg, followed by 75 mg daily) to aspirin for 90 days could lead to reductions in new stroke events (HR 0.68; 95% CI 0.57–0.81;

$p < 0.001$), without significantly increasing bleeding risk (any bleeding event: HR 1.41; 95% CI 0.95–2.10; $p = 0.09$) in patients who had suffered a minor ischemic stroke (defined as an NIHSS $\leq$3) or high-risk TIA within the previous 24 h (ABCD^2 score of $\geq$4) [126]. More recently, data from the POINT trial confirmed similar findings, suggesting that a combination of aspirin and clopidogrel (600 mg on day 1, followed by 75 mg daily) in a similar setting resulted in a lower risk of major ischemic events (HR 0.75; 95% CI 0.59–0.95; $p = 0.02$) compared to those who received aspirin alone, albeit with a higher risk of major haemorrhage at 90 days (HR 2.32; 95% CI 1.10–4.87; $p = 0.02$) [127]. The median ages of both trials were 63.5 and 65 years, respectively. The THALES (Acute or Transient Ischemic Attack Treated with Ticagrelor and ASA for Prevention of Stroke and Death) study evaluated the benefit of DAPT with ticagrelor and aspirin (mean age 65 years), and while they also observed a reduction in the composite outcome of stroke or death at 30 days (5.5% vs. 6.6%; HR 0.83; 95% CI 0.71–0.96; $p = 0.02$), there was a significant increase in severe bleeding (HR 3.99; 95% CI 1.74–9.14; $p = 0.001$) without improvements in disability (defined as a score >1 on the modified Rankin scale; odds ratio 0.98; 95% CI 0.89–1.07; $p = 0.61$) [128]. The CHANCE-2 trial is currently underway and aims to compare DAPT with ticagrelor and aspirin to DAPT with clopidogrel and aspirin (NCT04078737) [129]. While no trial to date has exclusively recruited older patients, a recent meta-analysis of available data suggested that DAPT is superior to aspirin therapy alone but may be equivalent to clopidogrel monotherapy in those aged 65 years or older with a recent stroke or TIA [130]. This highlights the need for further large RCTs in this area and population group.

Largely on the basis of the CHANCE and POINT trials, guidelines now recommend DAPT with clopidogrel and aspirin, following a non-cardioembolic minor ischemic stroke or high-risk TIA, ideally to be commended within 12–24 h post symptom onset and to be continued for 21 days [124, 131]. The current European Stroke Organisation (ESO) guidelines are largely modelled around the CHANCE trial, recommending a loading dose of 300 mg of clopidogrel (followed by 75 mg maintenance) and 50–325 mg of aspirin (dose of aspirin at physician discretion) [131]. Other than references to the POINT and CHANCE trial, the AHA guidelines do not provide a specific loading dose recommendation, but do agree that 50–325 mg of aspirin daily, in combination with 75 mg clopidogrel daily should be used as maintenance therapy in the context of a non-cardioembolic minor ischemic stroke [124]. While the AHA guidelines include the option of a duration of DAPT for up to 90 days in this setting, a pooled analysis of data from CHANCE and POINT found that the benefit of DAPT appeared to be confined to the first 21 days, and so this duration may be more sensible for older adults at increased bleeding risk [132]. Following the initial period of DAPT, patients should be continued on single antiplatelet therapy. Long-term DAPT is not recommended due to increased bleeding risks [124, 133, 134]. For patients with moderate to severe strokes, aspirin monotherapy, without a second antiplatelet, is recommended [124].

3.2.3   Antiplatelets in Peripheral Arterial Disease

Antiplatelet therapy also remains the mainstay of treatment in symptomatic peripheral arterial disease, with both American and European guidelines recommending either aspirin (75–325 mg) or clopidogrel (75 mg daily) as first-line agents [135, 136]. While the AHA guidelines consider aspirin reasonable in asymptomatic individuals with an ABI $\leq$0.9 and may even be considered in those with an ABI of 0.91–0.99, European guidelines recommend against its use in this setting [135, 136]. European guidelines recommend aspirin for all asymptomatic carotid stenosis [135]. A recent meta-analysis suggested that DAPT may be superior to aspirin monotherapy in those with lower extremity peripheral arterial disease, although this has not been adopted by guidelines to date [137]. As discussed previously, the COMPASS trial demonstrated that very low dose rivaroxaban in addition to aspirin may improve ischemic outcomes in patients with PAD [117].

4   Blood Pressure

The prevalence of hypertension increases dramatically with age. Data from the NHANES survey (National Health and Nutrition Examination Survey) in the USA have estimated the prevalence of hypertension (defined as a blood pressure $\geq$130 and/or $\geq$80) to be over 70% in those $\geq$65 years of age (77% between 2015 and 2018) [42]. Similarly, the Framingham Heart Study has estimated that more than 90% of patients with normal blood pressure at 55 years of age will eventually develop hypertension [138]. Our understanding of preventive medicine in the area of hypertension among older adults has evolved dramatically over the last 60 years. As late as the 1960s, high blood pressure was considered an unavoidable and, indeed "essential", component of ageing [139]. A prominent opinion piece summarised that "a benign course was the rule, not the exception" in hypertensive patients [140]. These opinions contributed to an underappreciation of the importance of treating hypertension in older patients. Thankfully, there is now unquestionable evidence that, similar to younger patients, hypertension is a strong but treatable risk factor for incident heart failure, myocardial infarction, stroke, peripheral arterial disease, and all-cause mortality in older adults [141].

While there are many similarities in the assessment and management of blood pressure in older adults compared to their younger counterparts, there are some notable differences and challenges, particularly when it comes to deciding on an appropriate target [142].

4.1 Measuring Blood Pressure in Older Adults

Accurately measuring blood pressure is the first step to initiating an appropriate management plan in any hypertensive patient. Masked hypertension has been shown to be present in up to 12% of older patients and is associated with significantly higher cardiovascular risk, and so undertreatment of these patients can have significant negative consequences [143]. Conversely, overzealous treatment in those with white coat hypertension may lead to deleterious effects of treatments such as orthostatic hypotension and injurious falls, which can have serious consequences in older patients. Therefore, the gold standard to confirm the diagnosis of hypertension remains the use of a 24-h ambulatory blood pressure monitor (ABPM). However, ABPM may be problematic for some older patients, where travel to and from clinics may be difficult, so home blood pressure monitoring (HBPM) has been shown to be a useful alternative to office measurements in such patients and is supported by most guidelines [144].

4.2 Benefits of Treating Hypertension in Older Adults

Lewington et al. reported a meta-analysis of observational studies, which indicated that the risks for both stroke and ischemic heart disease start to increase progressively from as low as 115 mmHg, even among those >80 years [145]. The benefits of treating hypertension in patients over the age of 60 years have been recently summarised in an updated Cochrane systematic review by Musini et al., which combined data from 26,795 healthy ambulatory adults $\geq$60 years across 16 randomised trials that compared antihypertensive treatment to no treatment or placebo [146]. The average age of participants within the review was 73.8 years with a mean baseline blood pressure of 182/95 mmHg. Treatment of hypertension resulted in a reduction in all-cause mortality (risk ratio 0.91, 95% CI 0.85–0.97; participants 25,932; $I^2 = 8\%$; $p = 0.01$), primarily due to a significant reduction in fatal stroke and fatal myocardial infarction. On subgroup analysis, this benefit was mainly seen in those aged 60–79 years (risk ratio, 0.86; 95% CI 0.79–0.95; $I^2 = 48\%$), with a non-significant effect in those over the age of 80 years (risk ratio, 0.97; 95% CI 0.87–1.10; $I^2 = 52\%$). Cardiovascular morbidity and mortality were also significantly reduced (risk ratio, 0.72; 95% CI 0.68–0.77; $I^2 = 64.98\%$; $p < 0.0001$), representing an absolute reduction from 136 events (in the no treatment/placebo group) to 98 events per 1000 participants (in those treated) over a mean duration of treatment of 3.7 years. Relevantly, on subgroup analysis, this benefit extended to those $\geq$80 years (risk ratio, 0.75; 95% CI 0.65–0.87; $I^2 = 0\%$), with no significant subgroup effect between those aged 60–79 years and those $\geq$80 years. This would suggest that age does not modify the effect of antihypertensive treatment in comparison to placebo or no treatment. Treatment of hypertension not only impacts CV disease prevention but has also been shown to lower the risks of dementia and cognitive impairment [147].

4.3   Target BP: The Debate

4.3.1   The J-Shaped Curve and Potential Risks with Treatment

While there is no doubt that treatment of hypertension is of benefit in most older adults, a significantly controversial area remains the decision surrounding an appropriate blood pressure target [148, 149]. A particularly apt example of the disagreements on this issue comes from the Eight Joint National Committee (JNC 8) in 2014, which provided a recommendation to raise the SBP goal to <150 mmHg for patients aged 60 years or older [150]. This decision was viewed as so controversial at the time, that some members of the committee refused to endorse this recommendation and published a minority report to advocate for a target of SBP of less than 140 mmHg in persons 60 years or older [149]. Two of the authors of this minority report would ultimately go on to author the landmark trial SPRINT [45].

The question becomes, is lower simply better? Or is there a middle ground that we should be aiming for? The idea that there is a nadir point at which further lowering of a patient's blood pressure becomes associated with an increased cardiovascular risk has become known as the J-shaped or U-shaped curve [151]. Observational data have previously suggested that there may be an increased risk with lowering SBP below 110–120 mmHg or DBP below 60–70 mmHg [152]. However, this may be in part due to confounding or reverse causation; for example, where those with a higher number of co-morbidities may have a lower BP and are hence less likely to survive. In support of this theory, a large community-based study including adults ≥85 years in the Netherlands reported an inverse relationship between blood pressure and mortality, in that 5-year mortality was higher among those who had a DBP <65 mmHg (compared to those with higher DBP) and among those with a systolic BP <125 mmHg (compared to those with higher SBP) [153]. Significantly, however, this inverse relationship between blood pressure and all-cause mortality disappeared after adjustment for health status and frailty [153]. The existence of the J-shaped curve has recently been further challenged by the landmark trial SPRINT, which did not find increased adverse outcomes in those treated to a mean BP of 121.5 mmHg. Indeed, SPRINT demonstrated a benefit on the primary CVD endpoint that was consistent across baseline quintiles of diastolic BP [45].

Significant fear of lowering blood pressure excessively in older adults is the increased risk of adverse events. The use of anti-hypertensive medications has been associated with an increased risk of falls, orthostatic hypotension, fractures, strokes, cognitive problems, depression, and reduced survival [154–159]. However, the risk of serious fall injuries seems to be highest within the first 14 days, with a recent meta-analysis suggesting no overall long-term risk once this period has passed [160–162].

4.3.2 Targets in Those Aged 60–79 Years

A summary of trials recruiting those over the age of 60 years with systolic/diastolic hypertension and isolated systolic hypertension is summarised in Table 5.

One of the first major hypertension trials to target an exclusively older population was the European Working Party High Blood pressure in the Elderly (EWHPE) trial, which recruited participants $\geq$60 years old with an SBP between 160 and 239 mmHg and a DBP in the range 90–119 mmHg and compared treatment with hydrochlorothiazide to placebo [163]. The trial was terminated early after a 27% reduction in all cardiovascular mortality was seen ($p = 0.037$), achieving a mean BP of 150/85 in the treatment group at the 5-year follow-up. A year later, Coope and Warrender published the results of a small randomised controlled trial comparing treatment with antihypertensive therapy (this time starting with beta blocker therapy) to usual care in those 60–79 years (mean age 68.75) with an SBP 170–280 mmHg or DBP 105–120 mmHg [164]. They achieved a consistent difference of approx. 18/11 mmHg between groups, and noted a significant reduction in stroke (rate ratio 0.58; 95% CI 0.35–0.96; $p < 0.03$), but no reduction in fatal coronary events, left ventricular failure, cardiovascular or all-cause mortality. Meanwhile, the SHEP (Systolic Hypertension in the Elderly Program) trial was underway. This was the first trial to target patients with isolated systolic hypertension (>160 mmHg at the time) [169]. This double-blind, placebo-controlled trial randomised 4736 patients $\geq$60 years (mean age 71.6 years) with isolated systolic hypertension to placebo or treatment (46% received chlorthalidone, and 23% atenolol, 21% other, 9% no medication), targeting a blood pressure of $\leq$159 mmHg (or a reduction in BP of at least 20 mmHg for those with a baseline BP between 160 and 170 mmHg). After an average follow-up of 4.5 years, the treatment group had achieved a mean BP of 143/68 mmHg with a notable 36% reduction in the incidence of stroke (relative risk of 0.64; 95% CI, 0.5–0.82; $p = 0.003$). In contrast to the previous trials, the incidence of nonfatal MI and coronary death was 27% lower in the active treatment group, when compared to those assigned to the placebo group. All-cause mortality was 13% lower in the treatment group, although this did not reach statistical significance. There was a higher rate of some adverse events in the treatment group, for example, the prevalence of falls was 12.8% in the treatment group vs. 10.4% in the placebo group.

STOP hypertension recruited a slightly older cohort (mean age 75.65), and showed that reducing a blood pressure to 167/87 mmHg, using either a beta blocker or beta blocker thiazide combination, reduced stroke from 31.3 events per 1000 patient years in those receiving placebo, to 16.8 events per 1000 patient years in those receiving treatment (relative risk 0.53; 95% CI 0.33–0.86; $p = 0.0081$) [172]. The investigators also observed a significant reduction in all-cause mortality (relative risk 0.57 (95% CI 0.37–0.78); $p = 0.0079$). The Syst Eur and Sys China trials both recruited patients over the age of 60 and compared antihypertensive treatment with nitrendipine to placebo [176, 178]. Syst-Eur was stopped early following a 42% reduction in occurrence of fatal and nonfatal strokes ($p = 0.003$), reaching a mean end of treatment BP of 150.8/78.5 mmHg in the nitrendipine group. All-cause

Table 5 Summary of major hypertension trials recruiting patients ≥60 with systolic/diastolic or isolated systolic hypertension (excludes trials focusing on isolated diastolic hypertension)

	EWHPE [163]	Coope et al. [164]	SHEP pilot [165–168]	SHEP [169–171]	STOP hypertnesion [172, 173]	MRC trial [174]	STONE [175]	Syst-Eur [176, 177]	Syst-China [178]	HYVET pilot [157, 179, 180]	HYVET [181–183]	JATOS [184, 185]	VALISH [186, 187]	Wei et al., [188]	SPRINT SENIOR [189]
Year published	1985	1986	1989	1991	1991	1992	1996	1997	1998	2003	2008	2008	2010	2013	2016
Trial design	Double-blind, randomised, placebo-controlled trial	Open-label, multicentre, randomised, controlled trial	Randomised, double-blind, placebo-controlled trial	Double-blind, randomised, placebo-controlled, multicentre trial	Prospective, randomised, double-blinded, multicentre, trial	Participant blinded, placebo controlled trial	Single-blind controlled trial	Double-blind placebo-controlled, multicentre trial	Placebo-controlled, multicentre trial	Randomised, multicentre, open, pilot study	Randomised, double blind, placebo controlled trail	Prospective, randomised, open label trial with blinded assessment of endpoints	Multicentre, parallel-group, prospective, randomised, open label, blinded end point	Prospective, randomised, open-label, blinded endpoint assessment study	Randomised, controlled, open label, multicentre trial. Outcome adjudicator blinded
Country	Multiple centres across Europe (? I think 5 couldn't access the whole protocol)	13 General Practices in England and Wales	USA	16 centres across the US	116 centres throughout Sweden	226 general practices in the UK	China	197 centres, in 23 countries in Europe	31 centres in China	10 European countries	195 centres in 13 countries including Europe, China, Australasia and North Africa	Japan	Japan	China	102 clinical sites in the US
Inclusion	≥60 years Sitting BP 160–239, DBP 90–119	60–79 years SBP 170–280 mmHg DBP 105–120	≥60 years Isolated systolic hypertension: SBP ≥160 and diastolic BP <90	≥60 years Isolated systolic hypertension (SBP ≥160 with diastolic BP <90 mmHg)	70–84 years BP >180/90 or a diastolic BP >105 irrespective of the systolic pressure	65–74 years SBP 160–209 mmHg DBP <115 mmHg	60–79 years of age BP ≥160 and/or ≥96 mmHg	≥60 years BP Systolic BP ≥160 and ≤219 mmHg Diastolic <95 mmHg Standing BP had to be at least 140 mmHg	≥60 years BP Systolic BP ≥160 and ≤219 mmHg	≥80 years Persistent hypertension Systolic blood pressure: 160–219 mmHg Diastolic BP 95–109 mmHg Standing BP must be ≥140 mmHg	≥80 years Persistent hypertension Systolic blood pressure: 160–199 mmHg Diastolic BP 90–109 mmHg Standing BP must be ≥140 mmHg	65-85 years old BP consistently ≥160 mmHg while receiving no antihypertensive drugs or receiving the same antihypertensive drugs for at least 4 weeks	≥70 and <85 ISH: BP >160 and diastolic BP <90 Drug used: valsartan and others as required	>70 years BP ≥150 and/or ≥90 or were diagnosed with hypertension and currently receiving antihypertensive treatment	Age ≥75 years Systolic blood pressure 130–180 mmHg

(continued)

Table 5 (continued)

	EWHPE [163]	Coope et al. [164]	SHEP pilot [165–168]	SHEP [169–171]	STOP hypertension [172, 173]	MRC trial [174]	STONE [175]	Syst-Eur [176, 177]	Syst-China [178]	HYVET pilot [157, 179, 180]	HYVET [181–183]	JATOS [184, 185]	VALISH [186, 187]	Wei et al., [188]	SPRINT SENIOR [189]
Exclusion	Curable causes of hypertension, certain complications of hypertension (grade III or IV retinopathy, CCF, history of cerebral or subarachnoid haemorrhage), concurrent illnesses such as hepatitis or cirrhosis, malignancy, diabetes requiring insulin	Atrial fibrillation, AV heart block, ventricular failure, bronchial asthma, diabetes mellitus requiring pharmacological treatment, or any serious concomitant disease limiting the prospect of fruitful living, untreated hypertension with levels persistently above 280 mmHg systolic or 120 mmHg diastolic, or patients already being treated for hypertension within 3 months	CABG within 2 years, heart attack within 6 months, stroke with residua, current treatment with antihypertensive drugs and physician judges not able to discontinue, insulin or anticoagulants; allergy to study meds, specified arrhythmias or a pacemaker, uncontrolled CCF, serum creatinine ≥2 mg/dL; alcohol abuse, cancer or other life threatening disease, COPD, PVD with tissue injury, senile dementia, residence in a nursing home, carotid bruit with history of TIA, history of malignant hypertension	Atrial fibrillation or flutter, AV block, multifocal VPB, bradycardia <50 bpm or permanent pacemaker, recent MI, recent stroke with residua, carotid artery disease, history of TIA with a bruit matched with TIA localisation, 2 or more TIAs and signs or symptoms in a single neurological distribution, coronary bypass surgery during the previous 6 months, insulin-dependent diabetes, dementia, history of renal insufficiency, or alcohol abuse	SBP >230 mmHg and/or 120 mmHg diastolic, isolated SBP (≥180 mmHg with a diastolic <90 mmHg), orthostatic hypotension, contraindications to any of the drugs, MI, or stroke during the previous 12 months, angina pectoris requiring treatment with drugs other than GTN, other severe or incapacitating illnesses	Suspected secondary hypertension, were taking antihypertensive drugs, had a cardiac failure or any other accepted indication for antihypertensive treatment, were receiving treatment for angina pectoris, had a history of MI or stroke within the preceding 3 months, had impaired renal function, were diabetic, had asthma, had any serious intercurrent disease, including malignancy known to be present at the time of examination or had a serum potassium concentration of <3.4 or >5 mmol/L.	SBP ≥220 mmHg DBP ≥125 mmHg, secondary hypertension, severe arrhythmia (frequent ventricular premature beats, >10/min) or multifocal premature beats, atrial fibrillation, second degree AV block, strokes, CCF, angina pectoris, MI, azotemia, and the presence of other diseases, including asthma, emphysema, cirrhosis, cancer, and diabetes mellitus	Secondary hypertension that required specific medical or surgical treatment; retinal haemorrhage or papilledema, CCF, dissecting aortic aneurysm, creatinine ≥180 µmol/L, history of severe nose bleeds, stroke, or MI in the year before, dementia, substance abuse; and any disorder prohibiting a sitting or standing position; and any severe concomitant cardiovascular or non-cardiovascular disease	Serum creatinine ≥180 µmol/L or patients with severe concomitant cardiovascular or non-cardiovascular disorders	Serum creatinine >150 µmol/L, accelerated hypertension, CCF requiring treatment, need for blood pressure decreasing treatment because of angina, etc., inability to stand, a cerebral or subarachnoid haemorrhage in the past 6 months, the presence of gout, renal artery stenosis, demented, and a condition expected to limit survival severely	Contraindications to trial medications Accelerated hypertension Secondary hypertension Haemorrhagic stroke in the previous 6 months Heart failure requiring treatment with anti-hypertensive medications Serum creatinine >150 µmol Serum potassium <3.5 mmol/L or >5.5 mmol/L Gout A diagnosis of dementia Requirement of nursing home Inability to stand up or walk	Diastolic BP ≥120 nmHg, secondary hypertension, recent stroke (<6 months previously) or signs and symptoms of stroke, a recent MI or coronary angioplasty (<6 months previously), angina pectoris requiring hospitalisation, HF with an NHYA class II or higher, persistent arrhythmia such as atrial fibrillation, dissecting aneurysm of the aorta or occlusive arterial disease, hypertensive retinopathy, serum AST more than double the upper limits of normal, poorly controlled diabetes, serum creatinine ≥1.5 mg/dL, malignant disease or collagen disease. Patients considered unsuitable as subjects were also excluded	Secondary hypertension or malignant hypertension; patients with a seated systolic blood pressure of ≥220 mmHg or diastolic ≥90 mmHg, patients with a history of cerebrovascular disorder or MI within 6 months prior to enrolment, patients who underwent coronary arterioplasty within 6 months prior to enrolment, patients NYHA ≥3 heart failure, patients with severe AS or valvular disease, patients with atrial fibrillation, atrial flutter or serious arrhythmia, patients with a serum creatinine ≥2 mg/dL, patients with serious liver dysfunction, other patients who are judged to be inappropriate for the study by the investigator or subinvestigator, patients with a history of hypersensitivity to valsartan	Secondary hypertension, valvular heart disease, CKD (serum creatinine ≥3 mg/dL), previous MI or stroke within the past 6 months, NYHA class III or higher CCF, LVEF <40%, hepatic dysfunction, autoimmune disorders, malignant tumour, Alzheimer's disease and other non-cardiovascular diseases potentially causing death before the end of the study	Nonadherence to a blood pressure medication that the patient had an indication for Known secondary cause of hypertension that posed concern regarding safety of the protocol 1 min standing BP <110 mmHg Significant proteinuria Arm circumference too large or small to allow accurate blood pressure measurement Diabetes mellitus History of stroke Polycystic kidney disease GFR <20 mL/min/1.73m² Glomerulonephritis treated with/likely to be treated with immunosuppressive therapy Symptomatic heart failure in the past 6 months or LV EF <35% A medical condition likely to limit survival to less than 3 months, or cancer diagnosed and treated within the last 2 years that would compromise a participants ability to comply with the protocol and complete the trial Any factors judged by the clinic team to be likely to limit adherence to interventions including; a history of poor compliance with medications or attendance at clinics, residence in a nursing home, clinical diagnosis of dementia Lack of informed consent Currently participating in another clinical trail Organ transplant Unintentional weight loss >10% in last 6 months Pregnant

Intervention group	Active treatment: 25 mg hydrochlorothiazide and 50 mg triamterene Methyldopa if required	Step 1: atenolol 100 mg daily Step 2: bendroflumethiazide 5 mg daily Step 3: methyldopa 500 mg daily Step 4: any recognised therapy In the last 2 years of the trial, nifedipine was also used	Step 1: Chlorthalidone 25 mg or 50 mg Step 2: additional antihypertensives Goal: <159 systolic or a 20 mmHg drop, whichever was lower	Chlorthalidone, betablockers, reserpine Target: for those with a baseline SBP >179, the goal was to reduce to ≤159 mmHg; for those with a baseline of 160–179, the goal was reduction by at least 20 mmHg	Treatment: atenolol 50 mg daily, hydrochlorothiazide 25 mg plus amiloride 2.5 mg, metoprolol 100 mg or pinodolol 5 mg (choice of regimen left up to the centre)	If run in BP was <180 mmHg then target was ≤150 If run in BP was ≥180 mmHg the target was ≤160 mmHg Potassium sparing diuretic regimen (amiloride, hydrochlorothiazide) or atenolol	Blood pressure target 140–159 mmHg and ≤90 mmHg diastolic Treatment: nifedipine	Reduce the systolic BP by at least 20–<150 mmHg Drug used: nitrendipine as first line. If necessary, this was combined or replaced by enalapril, hydrochlorothiazide or both	Reduce the systolic BP by at least 20–<150 mmHg Drug used: nitrendipine as first line. If necessary, this was combined or replaced by captopril, hydrochlorothiazide or both	Target BP <150/80 mmHg Treatment: diuretic group ACEI group	Indapamide (sustained release 1.5 mg) ± perindopril (2 mg or 4 mg) to a target BP of <150 mmHg systolic and 80 mmHg diastolic	Strict treatment target BP <140 mmHg Drug used: efonidipine and others as required	Strict control: <140 Drug used: valsartan and others as required	Intensive treatment target BP <140/90 mmHg Drugs used: ACEI, BB, CCB, diuretic; added in stepwise fashion	Blood pressure target <120 mmHg (intensive treatment) Most common medications used: ACEI or ARBs, diuretics, calcium channel blockers, beta blockers, alpha 1 blockers
Control	Placebo	Usual care (control)	Placebo	Placebo	Placebo	Placebo	Placebo	Placebo	Placebo	No treatment	Placebo	Mild treatment target BP: 140–160 mmHg Drug used: efonidipine and others as required	Lenient control: ≥140 and <150 Drug used: valsartan and others as required	Standard treatment target BP <150/90 mmHg Drugs used: ACEI, BB, CCB, diuretic; added in stepwise fashion	Blood pressure target 130–140 mmHg (standard treatment)
Method of BP measurement	Sitting blood pressure	Seated BP using Hawksely random zero sphygmomanometer	Sitting after 5 min of rest. Average of 4 readings taken with a random-zero sphygmomanometer	Seated BP, taken by certified technicians using the Hawksley random-zero manometer (manual BP)	Measured by the same observer for each patient throughout the study. Measured after 5 min of rest in supine position and after 1 min of standing using a mercury sphygmomanometer	Hawksley random zero sphygmomanometer	NR in primary paper	Manual BP measurement Twice after 2-min rest in supine, twice after 5-min rest sitting, twice after 3 min standing, repeated at 3 separate visits (6 measurements each)	Sitting blood pressure. Method not specified in primary paper	Sitting BP after rest for 5 min using sphygmomanometer	Observed blood pressure taken after the patient had been sitting for 5 min. BP was recorded using either a mercury sphygmomanometer or a validated automated device	Seated BP taken by sphygmomanometer with patients seated for at least 5 min	Seated BP but method otherwise not specified	Auscultatory method using a sphygmomanometer with patients in the seated position for 5–10 min	Unobserved automated Omron BP measurement, average of 3 readings each taken 1 min apart
Followup	Mean 4.6 years	Mean 4.4 years	Mean 34 months	Mean 4.5 years	25 months	Mean 5.8 years	Mean 30 months	Median 2 years	Median 3 years	Mean 13 months	Median duration of followup = 1.8 years (mean 2.1 years, range 0–6.5)	2 years	2.85 years (mean) 3.07 years (median)	4 years	3.14 years for primary outcome
Participants															
Number of participants	840	884	551	4736	1627	4396	1632	4695	2394	1283	3845	4418	3079	724	2636
Sex (female)	69.75%	69.5%	63.5%	56.8%	63%	58.23%	53%	66.85%	35.7%	63.4%	60.5%	61.2%	62.4%	33.7%	38%

(continued)

Table 5 (continued)

	EWHPE [163]	Coope et al. [164]	SHEP pilot [165–168]	SHEP [169–171]	STOP hypertnesion [172, 173]	MRC trial [174]	STONE [175]	Syst-Eur [176, 177]	Syst-China [178]	HYVET pilot [157, 179, 180]	HYVET [181–183]	JATOS [184, 185]	VALISH [186, 187]	Wei et al., [188]	SPRINT SENIOR [189]
Age, years (mean)	72	68.75	72.1 ≥70 = 62.5%	71.6 60–69 = 41.5% 70–79 = 44.8% ≥80 = 15.9%	75.65 70–74 = 44% 75–70 = 40% ≥80 = 16.5%	70.32	66.43 ≥70 = 28.4%	70.25	66.55	83.8	83.6	73.6 65–74 = 57.7% 75–85 = 42.3%	76.1	76.6	79.9
Blood pressure (sitting)	SBP 182.5 DBP 101	196.4 systolic 98.85 diastolic	Sitting 172/75	170.3 mmHg systolic 76.6 mmHg diastolic	Supine: 195/102	SBP 184.5 DBP 90.83 mmHg	169/98 mmHg SBP >180 = 25% SBP > 200 = 5%	Seated systolic 173.9 Seated diastolic: 85.5	Seated systolic 170.45 Seated diastolic: 86 mmHg	181.5 ± 11.3 mmHg 99.6 ± 3.4 mmHg	Seated 173 mmHg systolic 90.8 mmHg diastolic	Systolic 171.55 mmHg 89.1 mmHg diastolic	Systolic 169.55 mmHg Diastolic: 81.45 mmHg	Systolic 159.55 Diastolic 84.25	Seated 141.6 mmHg systolic 71.2 mmHg diastolic
History of cardio-vascular disease	35.5%	–	Angina: 3.3% Prior MI (>6 months ago); 4.4% Controlled CCF: 0.5% TIA within the past year 1.1%	MI: 4.9% Stroke: 1.4% Carotid bruits: 7.1%	Previous MI = 2.05% Previous stroke = 4.25%	% with ischemic ECG changes = 16.5% (1, 4, 5 on the Minnesota code)	–	Cardiovascular complications: 29.85%	Cardiovascular complications: 11.25% 224 (9.36%) had symptoms or signs suggestive of coronary heart disease or MI 1.42% had a history of stroke	MI: 3% Stroke: 4.5%	11.8% Stroke: 6.8% MI: 3.15% HF: 2.9%	Cerebrovascular disease = 4.4% Cardiac and vascular disease = 3%	Stroke (6.6%) IHD (4.95%)	History of stroke: 6.65% History of atrial fibrillation: 18% in the intensive treatment group CAD: 7.5% in the intensive treatment group	24.6%
Diabetes mellitus	–	Fasting blood glucose: 4.71 mmol/L	–	10.1%	7.9%	–	Blood glucose: 85.35 mg/dL (mean)	–	–	–	6.9%	11.8%	13%	23.35%	Excluded
Antihy-perten-sive treatment	–	–	Prior treatment for hypertension: 47%	33.3% on treatment at initial contact	52.5% previously treated	Excluded if previously on antihypertensive medications	–	Previous antihypertensive medication: 46.55%	Previous antihyperten-sive medication: 69.55%	Previously treated: 47.9%	64.65% on treatment at randomisation	56% on prior anti-hypertensive treatment	49.95% on antihypertensives at trial beginning	Mean number of years of hypertension diagnosis: 13 years	Mean number of antihypertensive agents taken at baseline visit = 1.9 (standard deviation 1)
Smoking	–	24.5%	11%	12.7% (current smokers)	8%	18.17%	<10 per day = 13.68% >10 per day = 8.25%	7.3%	Current smokers: 30.9%	4.2%	6.5%	13.5% (current smokers)	19.2%	24.85%	–
Frailty status	–	–	Activity limitation = 7%	No limitations of ADLs = 94.6% Post hoc analysis: PAL: 258 in treated group vs. 287 in placebo group	–	–	–	–	–	–	Post hoc calculation; 2656 participant data Frailty index (IQR) 0.17	–	–	–	Frailty status: Frailty index: 0.18 (median) Fit (frailty index ≤0.10) 13.25% Less fit (frailty index >0.10 to ≤0.21) 55.25% Frail (frailty index >0.21) 30.9%

Outcomes

Primary outcome	? Not specified	No primary outcome stated	Given this was a pilot study, no primary outcome was.specified	**Fatal or nonfatal stroke:** 103 (4.36%) vs. 159 (6.7%); relative risk of 0.64; 95% CI, 0.5–0.82; $p = 0.003$ **Nonfatal stroke:** 96 (4.06%) vs. 149 (6.28%); relative risk 0.63 (95% CI 0.49–0.82) **Fatal stroke:** 10 (0.42%) vs. 14 (0.59%); relative risk 0.71 (95% CI 0.31–1.59)	Stroke, myocardial infarction and other cardiovascular death—see below	**Fatal and nonfatal stroke** 101 (4.6%) vs. 134 (6.1%): % difference (active group minus placebo group); 25%; 95% CI 3–42; $p = 0.04$ **Fatal stroke:** 37 (1.69%) vs. 42 (1.89%): % difference (active group minus placebo group); 12%; 95% CI −37 to 44	No primary outcome specified	**Fata and non fatal stroke:** 47 vs. 77; % rate (active minus placebo): −42%; 95% CI −60 to −17; $p = 0.003$ **Fatal stroke:** 16 (0.67%); vs. 21 (0.91%); % rate (active minus placebo): −27%; 95% CI −62 to 39; $p = 0.33$ **Nonfatal stroke:** 34 (1.42%) vs. 57 (2.48%); % rate (active minus placebo): −44%; 95% CI −63 to −14; $p = 0.007$	**Fatal stroke:** 10 (0.8%) vs. 20 (1.75%); % rate (active drug minus placebo): 58% (95% CI 14–80); $p = 0.02$ **Nonfatal stroke:** 35 (2.79%) vs. 41 (3.59%); % rate (active drug minus placebo): 30% (95% CI −10 to 58); $p = 0.12$	**Main endpoints:** Stroke events, total mortality and cardiovascular, cardiac and stroke mortality	**Fatal or nonfatal stroke:** 51 (0.03%) vs. 69 (3.6%) events (unadjusted HR 0.7; 95% CI 0.49–1.01; $p = 0.06$) **Fatal stroke:** 27 (1.4%) vs. 42 (2.2%); unadjusted HR 0.61; 95% CI 0.38–0.99; $p = 0.046$)	Composite of cerebrovascular disease (cerebral haemorrhage, cerebral infarction, TIA and subarachnoid), cardiac and vascular disease (MI, angina pectoris requiring hospitalisation, heart failure, sudden death, dissecting aneurysms of the aorta and occlusive arterial disease) and renal failure (acute or chronic) **Nonfatal:** 86 (3.89%) vs. 86 (3.9%), $p = 0.99$ 22.6 per 1000 patient years (95% CI 18.1–27.9) vs. 22.7 (95% CI 18.2–28.1) $p = 0.98$ **Fatal:** 9 (0.41%) vs. 8 (0.36%); $p = 0.81$ 2.4 per 1000 patient years (95% CI 1.1– 4.5) vs. 2.1 per 1000 patient years (0.9–4.2); $p = 0.82$	Composite of cardiovascular events (sudden death, fatal or nonfatal stroke, fatal or nonfatal MI, death because of heart failure, other cardiovascular death, unplanned hospitalisation for CV disease and renal dysfunction) 47 (3.04%) vs. 52 (3.39%); HR 0.89; 95% CI 0.60–1.31; $p = 0.383$	Composite incidence of fatal/nonfatal stroke, acute MI and other cardiovascular deaths (sudden death and heart failure death) 40 (11%) vs. 67 (18.6%); $p = 0.004$	Composite of nonfatal myocardial infarction, acute coronary syndrome not resulting in a myocardial infarction, nonfatal stroke, nonfatal acute decompensated heart failure and death from cardiovascular causes 2.59% per year vs. 3.85% per year (HR 0.66; 95% CI, 0.51–0.85; $p = 0.001$)
End of treatment BP	**After 1 year:** Active 151/88 (300 participants) Placebo: 172/23 (287 participants) **3 years:** Active 149/85 (187 participants) Placebo: 172/94 (171 participants) **5 years:** Active: 150/85 (108 participants) Placebo 171/95 (93 participants)	Consistent difference of approximately 18/11 mmHg between treatment group and no treatment	142/68 in treatment group 157/71 in placebo group Systolic BP <160 at year 3: Treatment group: 60% Placebo: 33%	Treatment group: 143 systolic 68 diastolic Placebo: 155.1 systolic 72 diastolic	Supine BP 167/87 in the active treatment group 186/96 in the placebo group	Numbers not reported—only graphical reported	Nifedipine group: Decline SBP 21.65 ± 17.96 and DBP 13.14 ± 9.84 Placebo: Decline SBP 13.21 ± 16.56 mmHg and DBP 7.59 ± 10.08	Active group: 150.8/78.5 Placebo group: 160.9 mmHg/83.5 mmHg	After 2 years Treatment group: 150.7/81.1 mmHg Placebo: 159.3/84 mmHg	Diuretic based group: 152/84 ACEI based group: 151/84 No treatment group: 174/95	Treatment group: Systolic 143.5 mmHg Diastolic 77.9 mmHg Placebo: 158.5 84	Strict treatment group: 135.9 ± 11.7 78.1 ± 8.9 Mild treatment group: 145.6 ± 11.1 78.1 ± 8.9	Strict treatment group: 136.6 systolic 74.8 diastolic Mild treatment group: 142/76.5	Intensive treatment group: 135.7 + −9 76.2 + −6.1 Standard treatment group 149.7 + −11 82.1 + −7.5	Intensive treatment: 123.4 systolic 62.0 diastolic Standard treatment: 134.8 mmHg systolic 67.2 mmHg diastolic

(continued)

Table 5 (continued)

	EWHPE [163]	Coope et al. [164]	SHEP pilot [165–168]	SHEP [169–171]	STOP hypertnesion [172, 173]	MRC trial [174]	STONE [175]	Syst-Eur [176, 177]	Syst-China [178]	HYVET pilot [157, 179, 180]	HYVET [181–183]	JATOS [184, 185]	VALISH [186, 187]	Wei et al., [188]	SPRINT SENIOR [189]
MI	**Fatal:** 7 vs. 16; % change: −60% (95%CI −84 to −4; $p = 0$: 0.43)	**Fatal coronary artery deaths** (sudden death and MI combined) 13.6 per 1000 patient years vs. 13.6 per 1000 patient years (ratio ratio 1.00; 95% CI 0.58–1.71; $p =$ NS)	**MI:** 6.3 per 1000 person years vs. 6.5 per 1000 person years (NS) **Fatal MI:** 1.6 per 1000 person years vs. 3.3 per 1000 person years (NS)	**Nonfatal:** 50 (2.11%) vs. 74 (3.12%); relative risk 0.67; 95% CI 0.47–0.96 **Fatal:** 15 (0.63%) vs. 26 (1.1%); relative risk 0.57; 95% CI 0.3–1.08	**All MI:** 14.4 per 1000 patient years vs. 16.5 per 1000 patient years (relative risk 0.87; 95% CI 0.49–1.56) **Fatal MI:** 3.4 per 1000 patient years vs. 4.5 per 1000 patient years (relative risk 0.75; 95% CI 0.21–2.47)	**Coronary events (fatal and nonfatal MI as well as sudden death thought to be due to a coronary cause):** 128 (5.86%) vs. 159 (7.18%); % difference: 19% (95% CI −2 to 36); $p = 0.08$ **Fatal coronary event:** 85 (3.89%) vs. 110 (4.97%); % difference: 22% (95% CI −4 to 41)	**All MI's** Relative risk 0.94; 95% CI 0.13–6.66	**Nonfatal MI:** 26 (1.08%) vs. 31 (1.35%); % rate: (active minus placebo): −20%; 95% CI −53 to 34; $p = 0.40$ **Fatal MI:** 7 (0.29%) vs. 15 (0.65%); % rate: (active minus placebo); −56%; 95% CI −82 to 9; $p = 0.08$	**Nonfatal MI:** 4 (0.32%) vs. 4 (0.35%); % rate (active drug minus placebo): 18 (95% CI −231 to 80); $p = 0.78$ **Fatal MI:** 5 (0.4%) vs. 3 (0.26%); % rate (active drug minus placebo): −36% (95% CI −449 to 66); $p = 0.66$	–	**Fatal or nonfatal:** 9 (0.47%) vs. 12 (0.63%); unadjusted HR 0.72; 95% CI 0.3–1.70; $p = 0.45$	**Nonfatal MI:** 6 (0.27%) vs. 6 (0.25%), $p =$ NR **Fatal MI:** 1 (0.05%) vs. 0 (0%), $p =$ NR	**Fatal and non-nonfatal MI:** 5 (0.32%) vs. 4 (0.26%); HR 1.23; 95%CI 0.33–4.56; $p = 0.761$	**Acute MI:** 9 (2.5%) vs. 9 (2.5%); $p = 0.991$ **Fatal MI:** 8 (2.2%) vs. 7 (1.9%); $p = 0.803$	**Nonfatal MI:** 0.92% per year vs. 1.34% per year (HR 0.69; 95% CI 0.45–1.05; $p = 0.09$)
Stroke	**Fatal cerebrovascu-lar events:** Per protocol: 12 vs. 19; % change: −43; (95% CI −72 to +18); $p = 0.15$ **Non-termi-nating[a] cerebrovascu-lar events (ischemic stroke, or TIA):** Per protocol: 13 vs. 24; % change: −52% (95% CI −76 to −7); $p = 0.026$	**All strokes:** 12.5 per 1000 patient years vs. 21.4 per 1000 patient years (rate ratio 0.58; 95% CI 0.35–0.96; $p < 0.03$) **Fatal stroke:** 22 per 1000 patient years vs. 73 per 1000 patient years (Rate ratio 0.30; 95% CI 0.11–0.84; $p < 0.025$) **Major stroke:** 27 per 100 patient years vs. 29 per 1000 patient years (rate ratio 0.70; 95% CI 0.23–2.12; $p =$ NS)	**Stroke:** 14.3 per 1000 person years vs. 32.5 per 1000 person years (NS) **Fatal stroke:** 1.6 per 1000 person years vs. 6.5 per 1000 person years (NS)	See primary outcome	**All stroke:** 16.8 per 1000 patient years vs. 31.3 per 1000 patient years (relative risk 0.53; 95% CI 0.33–0.86); $p = 0.0081$ **Fatal stroke:** 2.3 per 1000 patient years vs. 8.4 per 1000 patient years (relative risk 0.27; 95% CI 0.06–0.84)	See primary outcome	All strokes: 16 vs. 36 (Relative risk 0.43; 95% CI 0.24–0.77)	See primary outcome	See primary outcome	**Combined treatment groups for fatal plus nonfatal strokes:** Relative hazard ratio 0.46; 95% CI 0.24–0.91; $p = 0.02$ **Fatal stroke:** Diuretic group: relative hazard ratio, 0.52 (95% CI 0.19–1.42) ACEI group: relative hazard ratio, 0.60 (95% CI 0.23–1.55)	See primary outcome	**Nonfatal cerebral infarction:** 36 (1.63%) vs. 30 (1.36%), $p =$ NR **Nonfatal cerebral haemorrhage:** 7 (0.32%) vs. 8 (0.36%), $p =$ NR **Fatal cerebral infarction:** 2 (0.09%) vs. 0 (0%) **Fatal cerebral haemorrhage:** 0 (0%) vs. 1 (0.05%), $p =$ NR	**Fatal and nonfatal stroke:** 16 (1.04%) vs. 23 (1.50%); HR 0.68; 95% CI 0.36–1.29; $p = 0.237$	**Fatal/nonfatal stroke:** 21 (5.8%) vs. 36 (10%); $p = 0.036$ **Fatal stroke:** 7 (1.9%) vs. 21 (5.8%); $p = 0.007$	**Fatal and nonfatal stroke:** 0.67% per year vs. 0.85% per year (HR 0.72; 95% CI 0.43–1.21; $p = 0.22$) **Nonfatal stroke:** 0.62% per year vs. 0.83% per year (HR 0.68; 95% CI 0.40–0.1.15; $p = 0.15$)

Heart failure	**Terminating[a] nonfatal severe CCF; not controlled by digitalis alone** 7 vs. 17; % change: −63% (95% CI −85 to −10); p = 0.014 **Non-terminating[a] moderate CCF** 12 vs. 6; % change: not calculated	**Fatal ventricular failure:** 22 per 1000 patient years vs. 19 per 1000 patient years (rate ratio 0.28–4.45; p = NS) **Nonfatal ventricular failure:** 9.8 per 1000 patient years vs. 15.6 per 1000 patient years (rate ratio 0.35–1.11; p = NS)	**Left ventricular failure:** 4.8 per 1000 person years vs. 6.5 per 1000 person years (NS) **Fatal LV failure:** 2.4 per 1000 person years vs. 0 (NS)	**Nonfatal LV failure:** 48 (2.03%) vs. 102 (4.30%); relative risk 0.46; (95% CI 0.33–0.65) **Fatal LV failure:** 8 (0.34%) vs. 7 (0.3%)	19 events vs. 39 events	–		**Nonfatal HF:** 29 (1.21%) = vs. 43 (1.87%); % rate (active minus placebo); −36%; 95% CI −60 to 2; p = 0.06 **Fatal HF:** 8 (0.33%) = vs. 10 (0.44%); % rate (active minus placebo); −24%; 95% CI −70 to 93; p = 0.57	**Fatal HF:** 3 (0.24%) vs. 4 (0.35%); % rate (active drug minus placebo): 38% (95% CI −173 to 86); p = 0.52	–	**Fatal HF:** 6 (0.31) vs. 12 (0.63%); unadjusted HR 0.48; 95% CI 0.18–1.28; p = 0.14 **Fatal or nonfatal HF:** 22 (1.14%) vs. 57 (2.98%); unadjusted HR 0.36; 95% CI 0.22–0.58; p < 0.001	**Nonfatal HF:** 8 (0.36%) vs. 7 (0.32%), p = NR **Fatal HF:** 4 (0.18%) vs. 1 (0.05%), p = NR	–	**Fatal HF:** 6 (1.7%) vs. 16 (4.4%); p = 0.029	0.86% per year to 1.41% per year (HR 0.62; 95% CI 0.40–0.95; p = 0.03) **Nonfatal heart failure:** 0.86% per year vs. 1.39% per year (HR 0.63; 95% CI 0.40–0.96; p = 0.03)
Cardio-vascular mortality	**Cardiovascular mortality (intention to treat analysis)** 67 (16.11%) vs. 93 (21.93%); % change: −27% (95% CI −46 to −1); p = 0.037 **On randomised treatment:** 42 vs. 61; % change for active treatment; −38; 95% CI −58 to −8; p = 0.023	**Cardiovascular deaths** (excluding PE) 19 per 1000 patient years vs. 24.3 per 1000 patient years (rate ratio 0.78; 95% CI 0.51–1.20; p = NS)	**Sudden death** 5.5 per 1000 patient years vs. 6.5 per 1000 patient years; p = NS	**Cardiovascular deaths:** 90 (3.8%) vs. 112 (4.72%); relative risk 0.80; 95% CI 0.57–1.13	**Other CV death** (excluding stroke, MI) 2.3 per 1000 patient years vs. 7.7 per 1000 patient years (relative risk 0.30; 95% CI 0.43–0.85)	**All cardiovascular deaths:** 161 (7.38%) vs. 180 (8.13%); % difference: 9%; 95% CI −12 to 27	**Cardiovascular deaths:** 11 vs. 14 (Relative risk 0.74; 95% CI 0.34–1.62)	**Cardiac mortality:** 32 (1.33%) vs. 42 (1.93%); % rate (active minus placebo); −27% (−51 to 11); p = 0.14	**All cardiovascular:** 33 (2.63%) vs. 44 (3.86%); % rate (active drug minus placebo); 39% (95% CI 4–61); p = 0.03	**Cardiovascular mortality Treatment groups combined:** RHR 1.13 (95% CI 0.66–1.94) **Diuretic group:** RHR 1.17 (0.63–2.14) **ACEI group:** RHR 1.09 (95% CI 0.58–2.03)	**Cardiovascular mortality:** 99 (5.12%) vs. 121 (6.33%); unadjusted HR 0.77; 95% CI 0.60–1.01; p = 0.06				
All cause mortality	**Intention to treat analysis:** 135 (32.45%) vs. 149 (35.14%); % change: −9% (95% CI −28 to +15); p = 0.41 **On treatment analysis:** 73 (17.54%) vs. 89 (20.99%); % change for active treatment: −26%; 95% CI −45 to 1; p = 0.077	32.5 per 1000 patient years vs. 33.6 per 1000 patient years (rate ratio 0.97; 95% CI 0.70–1.42; p = NS)	25.4 per 1000 person years vs. 22.7 per 1000 person years (OR 1.12; 95% CI 0.48–2.62) (NS)	213 (9%) vs. 242 (10.2%); relative risk 0.87; (95% CI 0.73–1.05)	20.2 per 100 patient years vs. 35.4 per 1000 patient years; relative risk 0.57 (95% CI 0.37–0.78); p = 0.0079	301 (13.78%) vs. 315 (14.23%); % difference (active group minus placebo group); 3%; 95% CI −14 to 18		123 (5.13%) vs. 137 (5.96%); % rate (active minus placebo); −14% (−33 to 9); p = 0.22	61 (4.87%) vs. 82 (7.19%); % rate (active drug minus placebo); 39% (95% CI 16–56); p = 0.003	**Treatment groups combined:** RHR 1.23 (95% CI 0.75–2.01) **Diuretic group:** Relative hazard ratio 1.31 (95% CI 0.75–2.27) **ACEI group:** Relative hazard ratio 1.14 (95% CI 0.65–2.02)	196 (10.14%) vs. 235 (12.29%); unadjusted HR 0.79; 95% CI 0.65–0.95; p = 0.02	54 (2.44%) patients vs. 42 (1.90%) patients (p = 0.22)	24 (1.55%) vs. 30 (1.96%); HR 0.78; 95% CI 0.46–1.33; p = 0.362	51 (14%) vs. 87 (24.1%), p = 0.001	1.78% per year vs. 2.63% per year (HR 0.67; 95% CI 0.49–0.91; p = 0.009)

(continued)

Table 5 (continued)

	EWHPE [163]	Coope et al. [164]	SHEP pilot [165–168]	SHEP [169–171]	STOP hypertnesion [172, 173]	MRC trial [174]	STONE [175]	Syst-Eur [176, 177]	Syst-China [178]	HYVET pilot [157, 179, 180]	HYVET [181–183]	JATOS [184, 185]	VALISH [186, 187]	Wei et al., [188]	SPRINT SENIOR [189]
Adverse events															
Serious adverse events	–	Approx 25% were unable to tolerate atenolol due to side effects; most commonly include: general fatigue, muscular weakness and breathlessness on exertion Severe dizziness: 5 (1.4%) vs. 4 (1.1%) Moderate dizziness: 29 (8.33%) vs. 26 (6.9%)	None	Faintness on standing 12.8% vs. 10.6%; feelings of unsteadiness or imbalance, 33.7% vs. 32.9% Falls, 12.8% vs. 10.4%	58 patients on active treatment and 47 patients on placebo discontinued randomised treatment because of subjective side effects not classified as any specific clinical event (difference not significant)	Higher rates of adverse events in both the beta blocker and diuretic groups compared to placebo. Overall the beta blocker group had more frequent side effects (333—30.2%) when compared to the diuretic group (160—14.8%) or control (82—3.7%)	–	Safety endpoint: **Bleeding** (excluding cerebral and retinal haemorrhage) 20 vs. 19; % rate (active minus placebo) −10% (95% CI −52 to 69); $p = 0.74$ **Fatal and nonfatal cancer** 73 (3.04%) vs. 82 (3.57%); % rate (active minus placebo) −15% (95% CI −38 to 16); $p = 0.29$	–	No patient was withdrawn because of renal problems; otherwise adverse events not reported	Serious adverse events: 358 (18.52% vs. 448 (23.43%); $p = 0.001$ 5 of these events were classified by the local investigator as possibly having been due to trial medications	Treatment discontinued because of adverse events in 36 (1.63%) patients in the strict treatment group and 36 (1.63%) patients in the mild treatment group ($p = 0.99$)	5.6% vs. 5.2%; $p = 0.61$	–	48.4% vs. 48.3% (HR 0.99; 95% CI 0.89–1.11; $p = 0.895$)

*Definition of terminating events: Terminating events were those that resulted in death or any cerebral haemorrhage or SAH, development of hypertensive retinopathy grade III or IV, dissecting aneurysm, congestive cardiac failure not controllable without diuretics or antihypertensive drugs, hypertensive encephalopathy, severe increase in left ventricular hypertrophy, and a rise in blood pressure exceeding the defined limits

mortality was not significantly different between the two groups and while there was a 27% reduction in deaths from cardiovascular causes, this did not reach statistical significance ($p = 0.07$). Syst China also showed a 39% reduction in cardiovascular mortality and a 58% reduction in stroke mortality, reaching a BP of 150.7/81.1 mmHg in the treatment group. In contrast to Sys-Eur, all-cause mortality was reduced by 39% in the active treatment group ($p = 0.003$).

Between 2008 and 2013, three trials, JATOS, VALISH and Wei et al. compared more intense BP control (SBP <140/90 mmHg) to more lenient control (SBP <150 or <160 mmHg) in older Asian adults (mean age 75 years across the three trials) [184, 186, 188]. Notably, Wei et al. observed a significant reduction in all-cause mortality, CV mortality, fatal/nonfatal stroke and heart failure on lowering a blood pressure to 135.6/76.2 mmHg. A meta-analysis combining the three trials deemed the evidence insufficient to determine which treatment arm was superior, however, there was significant heterogeneity between the studies [190]. This is likely due to the fact that both JATOS and VALISH noted no difference in cardiovascular events between treatment arms.

Following the publication of the landmark trial, SPRINT (Systolic Blood Pressure Intervention Trial), 2015 became a pivotal year for hypertension management with subsequent major reforms across guidelines [45]. This randomised, controlled, open label trial recruited 9361 patients ≥50 years with a systolic blood pressure of ≥130 mmHg and an increased cardiovascular risk, across 102 clinical sites in the US and Puerto Rico and assigned participants to an intensive treatment arm (with a target blood pressure of <120 mmHg systolic) or a standard treatment arm (BP target of <140 mmHg systolic). The mean age of recruited participants was 67.9 years. SPRINT immediately attracted widespread attention after the trial was stopped early by the data and safety monitoring board, after a median follow-up of 3.26 years, following an observed 25% lower relative risk of major cardiovascular events in the intensive treatment arm compared to the standard group (1.65% per year vs. 2.19% per year; HR 0.75; 95% CI 0.64–0.89; $p < 0.001$). There was also a significant reduction in all-cause mortality (HR 0.73; 95% CI 0.60–0.90; $p = 0.003$). SPRINT challenged the status quo of aiming for a blood pressure <140/90 mmHg, demonstrating that achieving a mean systolic blood pressure of 121.5 mmHg (measured using automated devices mostly while the participant was left in a room unattended) was associated with improved outcomes [191]. Significantly, a pre-specified subgroup analysis of 2636 participants ≥75 years (mean age 79.9) with a baseline BP of 141.6 mmHg/71.2 mmHg showed similar results [189]. There was a statistically significant reduction in the primary outcome between groups (HR 0.66; 95% CI, 0.51–0.85; $p = 0.001$), with a 33% reduction in incident cardiovascular disease and a reduction in all-cause mortality of 32% between the treatment groups. There was also a significant reduction in heart failure (HR 0.62; 95% CI 0.40–0.95; $p = 0.03$), nonfatal heart failure (HR 0.63; 95% CI 0.40–0.96; $p = 0.03$) and all-cause mortality (HR 0.67; 95% CI 0.49–0.91; $p = 0.009$). Interestingly, though the point estimates were in the direction of benefit, there was no statistically significant difference in the occurrence of stroke (HR 0.72; 95% CI 0.43–1.21; $p = 0.22$), and nonfatal stroke (HR 0.68; 95% CI 0.40–1.15; $p = 0.15$), which was a contrast to previous trials [169, 176, 178]. Notably, frailty did not impact these results ($p = 0.84$ for interaction) and the rate of overall serious adverse events between groups was similar, with 637 (48.4%) participants experiencing an SAE in the intensive treatment group, compared with 637 (48.3%) participants experiencing a SAE in the standard treatment group.

While the results of SPRINT have already changed major guidelines, a critical question remains: are these results applicable to the general population, particularly comorbid and older patients [192, 193]? The debate surrounding the applicability of hypertensive trial data to the general population isn't new [194]. Even prior to SPRINT, Messerli et al. made the point that many of the large hypertension trials exclusion criteria mean that trial results may not be appliable to a general non-trial elderly population cohort [195]. They applied the exclusion criteria of 13 large hypertension trials to a cohort of elderly patients with hypertension in general practices in Poland. 71.3% would have met at least one of the exclusion criteria of these trials. SPRINT notably excluded patients with adherence issues, a 1-min standing BP <110 mmHg, diabetics, those with a history of stroke, symptomatic heart failure or those with an ejection fraction of <35%, a limited life expectancy, a diagnosis of dementia or residence in a nursing home. The exclusion of these common comorbidities have led to the external validity of these results being challenged [196]. Bress et al. estimated that only 7.6% of US adults, 16.7% of those with treated hypertension, and 5% without treated hypertension, met the SPRINT eligibility criteria [197].

Adding to the debate, the findings of SPRINT are contrasted to the similar ACCORD trial, which included a younger cohort (mean age 62.2 years). In contrast to SPRINT, ACCORD recruited patients with type 2 diabetes. Similar to SPRINT, trial participants were randomised to either an intensive treatment arm (with a target blood pressure of <120 mmHg systolic) or a standard treatment arm. There was no observed significant difference in the primary outcome between intensive and standard treatment groups (HR 0.88; 95% CI, 0.73–1.06; $p = 0.20$), though there was a significant reduction in stroke [198]. This may be due to a slightly different definition in primary outcome, with ACCORD including a composite outcome of nonfatal MI, nonfatal stroke or death from cardiovascular causes. SPRINT's primary outcome was more expansive, including ACS not resulting in MI and nonfatal episodes of HF. Analyses combining the results of both trials have reported a reduction in outcomes in the intensive treatment arm [199]. Given that ACCORD excluded those over 80 years, the SPRINT criteria have not been tested in diabetic patients ≥80 years.

One of the major concerns of lowering BP excessively is the increased risk of orthostatic hypotension and falls. Notably, the SPRINT authors reported no difference in the occurrence of serious adverse events in those ≥75 comparing those assigned to the intensive treatment group vs. standard treatment (HR 0.99; 95% CI 0.89–1.11; $p = 0.895$). Significantly, the risk of hypotension or injurious falls was the same across both groups. However, the composite outcome of hypotension leading to a SAE or ER visit was increased in the intensive arm (3.3% vs. 2%; HR 1.66; 95% CI 1.03–2.73; $p = 0.039$). These results are in keeping with findings in the ACCORD trial, albeit the latter was a much younger cohort [200].

The method of BP measurement used in SPRINT has also generated significant controversy [201]. In an attempt to avoid the effects of white coat hypertension, BP in SPRINT was recorded using an average of three automated office BP measurements following 5 min of quiet rest with participants mostly left unattended (i.e., the health care provider left the room for the measurement) [189]. This is in contrast to all other major hypertension trials (Table 5), and most everyday clinical practices, where attended (or observed) measurements are the common practice. Blood pressures taken in an observed fashion in routine clinical practice have been shown in some studies to vary significantly from those taken in a research setting, or by ambulatory methods [202]. It has been argued that BP measured in this unobserved fashion could result in blood pressure readings up to 5–10 mmHg lower than when measured manually, or in an observed setting [201, 203].

Unlike many other trials, SPRINT also pre-specified that participants in the standard treatment arm should not achieve a BP of <130 mmHg on any occasion or <135 mmHg on two consecutive occasions [204]. In fact, 87% of patients in the standard treatment group required at least one reduction in their medications to maintain systolic blood pressure in the range of 135–139 mmHg [205]. While these reductions were required to test the hypothesis of SPRINT, it would not be standard of care to withdraw treatment in an asymptomatic hypertensive patient with these blood pressure readings, and this nuance; therefore, is worth noting when interpreting the SPRINT results [206].

A meta-analysis including SPRINT, combined data on 65,890 patients $\geq$50 years (mean age of 69.4 years) demonstrated that treating to a mean blood pressure of 140.7/79.1 compared to 150.1/83.5, results in a significant reduction in major cardiovascular events (risk ratio 0.74, 95% CI 0.64–0.86; $p = 0.000$; $I^2 = 79.71\%$), stroke (risk ratio 0.72; 95% CI 0.64–0.82; $p = 0.000$; $I^2 = 32.45\%$), heart failure (Risk ratio 0.53; 95% CI 0.43–0.66; $p = 0.000$; $I^2 = 1.23\%$), CV mortality (risk ratio 0.76; 95% CI 0.66–0.89; $p = 0.000$; $I^2 = 39.74\%$) and all-cause mortality (risk ratio 0.83; 95% CI 0.73–0.93; $p = 0.001$; $I^2 = 53.09\%$) [207].

4.3.3 Targets in Those Over 80 Years

A large observational study carried out among primary care practices in the UK aimed to assess the associations between systolic blood pressure (SBP) and all-cause mortality, cardiovascular events and fragility fractures in those over 80 years [208]. They included 79,376 patients over the age of 80 years diagnosed with hypertension, prescribed at least one class of antihypertensive and who were free of dementia, recent cancer, stroke, heart failure, coronary heart disease and end stage renal disease. Patients with these conditions were excluded in an effort to minimise confounding on the outcomes. After a mean (±SD) follow-up of 4.4 years (±2.9), the results demonstrated that the lowest mortality was in those with an on-treatment SBP of 135–154 mmHg. A systolic blood pressure of <135 mmHg being associated with a greater morality (HR 1.25; 95% CI 1.19–1.31), suggesting a J-shaped association between SBP and outcomes in this observational cohort [208]. The risk of incident stroke increased once the SBP was about 145–154 mmHg. Incident heart failure increased at both lower pressures (SPB <125 mmHg; HR 1.2; 95% CI 1.02–1.4) and rose progressively at higher blood pressures (SBP above 145–154mmHg). By contrast, the authors noted that the risk of incident MI increased in an approximately linear fashion with increasing BP. As an example, those with an SBP <125 mmHg had an HR of 0.6 (95% CI 0.43–0.84) compared to an HR of 0.85 (95% CI 0.76–0.94) for those with an SBP of 135–144 or an HR of 1.12 (95% CI 1.01–1.24) for those with an SBP of 155–164 mmHg for example. The observational nature of the study has its limitations, including the possibility of confounding or reverse causation explaining the J-shaped associations reported.

By 1999 no trial had exclusively recruited patients over the age of 80 [209]. Gueyffier et al. therefore combined the data on those $\geq$80 from available trials, demonstrating a 34% reduction in stroke in those receiving antihypertensive therapy, as well as significant reductions in heart failure and overall cardiovascular events [209]. However, when including only double blinded trials, they observed a 14% ($p = 0.05$) increase in total mortality.

Since then, the first and only trial to exclusively recruit patients over the age of 80 is the HYVET trial [182, 210]. A double blind, placebo-controlled trial, the investigators recruited 3845 patients with a mean age of 83.86 years, a baseline systolic blood pressure of 160–199 mmHg and diastolic BP 90–109 mmHg. Participants were randomised to either receive 1.5 mg sustained release indapamide (aiming for a target BP <150/80 mmHg), or a placebo. The trial was terminated early due to a significant reduction in both the primary outcome (fatal or nonfatal stroke), as well as an unexpected reduction in all-cause mortality. Over a median follow up of 1.8 years, there was a 30% reduction in the primary outcome of fatal or nonfatal stroke (unadjusted HR 0.70; 95% CI 0.49–1.01; $p = 0.06$). There was a significant reduction in all-cause mortality of 21% in the active treatment group (unadjusted HR 0.79; 95% C9 0.65–0.95; $p = 0.02$) as well as fatal or non-fatal heart failure events (unadjusted HR 0.36; 95% CI 0.22–0.58, $p < 0.001$). Death from cardiovascular causes was also reduced ($p = 0.06$). Notably, they reported fewer serious adverse events in the treatment group (358 vs. 448; $p = 0.001$). With a mean end of trial blood pressure of 143.5/77.9 mmHg in those who received treatment (compared to 173/90.8 mmHg at baseline), results of the HYVET trial suggest that lowering a SPB <150 mmHg/80 in those over 80 is both safe and associated with significant benefits. Relevantly, the observed benefits began to appear within the first year of the trial. There remain a number of caveats when interpreting these results. Similar to previous hypertension trials, the HYVET trial included a relatively healthy trial population, excluding co-morbid patients such as those with heart failure requiring treatment with antihypertensives, a creatinine >150 μmol/L, dementia and those requiring nursing care. Because the trial was ended prematurely, the follow up time was also short (median of 1.8 years). While HYVET provides some data on those over 80 years old, the mean age of participants was only 83.86 years, meaning that we have little information about those in their late 80s or nonagenarians [211].

In 2010, a meta-analysis by Bejan-Angoulvant et al., combined all available data on hypertensive patients ≥80 from eight major hypertension trials or pilots at the time that had compared active treatment to no treatment or placebo in this patient cohort [212]. This included data from SHEP, SHPP, SYST-EUR, EWPHE, STOP, HYVET Pilot, Coope and Warrender and HYVET. Cumulatively, these trials included over 6701 patients over the age of 80 years. A weakness of this meta-analysis was the use of aggregate and not participant-level data. Contrary to the findings of HYVET, there was no significant reduction in relative mortality (relative risk 1.06; 95% CI 0.89–1.25; $p = 0.54$; $I^2 = 45.7\%$). Antihypertensive therapy was; however, associated with a 35% reduction in stroke (relative risk 0.65; 95% CI 0.52–0.83; $p < 0.001$; $I^2 = 0\%$), 27% reduction in cardiovascular events (relative risk 0.73; 95% CI 0.62–0.86; $p < 0.001$; $I^2 = 0\%$) and 50% reduction in heart failure (relative risk 0.50; 95% CI 0.33–0.76; $p = 0.001$; $I^2 = 21\%$).

Despite the results of HYVET, and the above meta-analysis, there continues to be a debate in relation to treatment targets and benefits in this age group [213]. The recently published OPTIMISE trial included 569 patients ≥80 years of age recruited through primary care centres, who had a SBP <150 mmHg and were receiving two or more antihypertensive medications [214]. The aim of the trial was to assess if reducing the intensity of a patient's anti-hypertensive regime would significantly impact the number of patients meeting a target BP of <150 mmHg after 12 weeks. Participants were deemed eligible if they were felt to potentially benefit from medication reduction due to either polypharmacy, co-morbidities, non-adherence, dislike of the medications or frailty by their general practitioner. Participants were then randomised to either a medication reduction arm or usual care. The mean systolic BP at baseline was 129.4 mmHg in the medication reduction group, compared to 130.5 mmHg in the usual care group. After 12 weeks of follow-up the mean SBP was 133.7 mmHg in the medication reduction group and 130.8 in the usual care group. 86.4% of patients in the medication reduction group had a BP SBP <150 mmHg compared to 87.7% in the usual care group (adjusted relative risk; 0.98; 95% CI 0.92 to infinity). Participants in the medication reduction group were taking 0.6 fewer antihypertensive medications than the usual care group at 12-week follow-up, indicating that some older adults might be able to de-intensify anti-hypertensive drug treatment without major increases in SBP. Unfortunately, the follow up period of 12 weeks was extremely short and there were no reports on long-term clinical outcomes.

With increasing numbers of co-morbidities and an increased prevalence of frailty with age, it seems probable that those over 80 are more likely to be a heterogenous group. A personalised stepwise approach, aiming for a target of <140/90 as long as treatment is well tolerated, with the goal of going lower or higher in some older adults depending on patient preferences, side effects, and individual comorbidities, would seem a practical approach [215].

The Impact of Frailty on Setting a Blood Pressure Target

The use of chronological age to classify patients into CVD risk categories (and in so doing to influence hypertensive treatment targets) may not be the optimum approach in producing meaningful outcomes [171]. The likelihood of encountering frailty or an impaired level of functioning in the context of managing hypertension is high, with observational data suggesting that 72% of frail individuals have hypertension, while 14% of those with hypertension may be considered frail [216]. A lower BP in these patients may in fact be a marker of declining health, with higher BP a marker of good health [203]. With this comes the concept that lowering blood pressure in frailer patients may have less therapeutic benefit compared to healthier adults, and may in fact be associated with increased harm [217–219]. Using data from 2340 patients from the NHANES study, Odden et al. demonstrated that in slower walkers (gait speed <0.8 m/s), a blood pressure ≥140/90, was not associated with increased mortality [220]. Bromfield et al. examined the relationship between six frailty markers (low body mass index, cognitive impairment, depressive symptoms, exhaustion, limited mobility and a history of falls), blood pressure level, antihypertensives and falls [219]. They included 5236 Medicare patients with a mean age of 73 and a mean BP 133/76 mmHg, of which 55.7% had no indicators of frailty, 26.6%, 11.8% and 5.9% had 1, 2 or ≥3 indicators of frailty, respectively. Following multivariable adjustment, they found that having ≥2 indicators of frailty was associated with a significantly increased risk of falls. In contrast, taking antihypertensive medications at baseline, SBP, DBP and the number of antihypertensive medications prescribed, were not associated with an increased risk of serious injurious falls after multivariant adjustment. This adds important context when considering blood pressure targets, as well as anti-hypertensive medications in older adults. Frailty may be a more powerful indicator of adverse outcomes in older adults being treated for hypertension compared to the blood pressure value or chronological age itself. This finding suggests that interventions to prevent or reverse frailty may be a better approach to reducing falls than de-intensification of BP therapy in hypertensive older patients.

Almost three decades after the initial trial results were published, the SHEP study group published a post hoc analysis of the trial data, which suggested that the presence of self-reported physical ability limitations (PAL) modified the observed benefits of the antihypertensive therapy [171]. The analysis found that those in the treatment group who reported no PAL, had a lower rate of death (8.3% vs. 8.8%; HR 0.82; 95% CI 0.66–1.00), CV death (3.7% vs. 8.4%; HR 0.71; 95% CI 0.51–0.98), and MI (3.3% vs. 4%; HR 0.57; 95% CI 0.40–0.81) compared to those who received placebo [171]. In adjusted Cox proportional hazard models, treatment was protective against cardiovascular death in those with no PAL (HR 0.71; 95% CI 0.51–0.98), but not for those with a PAL (HR 1.27; 95% CI 0.71–2.28) Similar patterns were seen for MI. In contrast, treatment remained protective for stroke, regardless of self-reported PAL status. The investigators observed a higher rate of falls in those on treatment with a PAL, although this failed to reach statistical significance. HYVET also did a similar post hoc analysis on their trial data using a frailty index, which suggested that both frailer and fitter older adults with hypertension appear to benefit equally from treatment when targeting a blood pressure of <150/80 mmHg [183].

Because both of these reports are post-hoc analyses their results should be interpreted with some caution. There are several potential explanations for the discrepant results between SHEP and HYVET. Whereas SHEP analyzed functional status using a self-reported questionnaire, HYVET employed a frailty index derived from a mix of 60 self-reported and objectively measured variables. Secondly, the HYVET population had a lower prevalence of comorbid health conditions compared to a general community dwelling population, making it a healthier population. Finally, while both SHEP and HYVET used diuretics as the primary medication class, the secondary drug was a beta blocker in SHEP and an ACEI in HYVET.

The SPRINT group carried out an exploratory subgroup analysis that demonstrated higher events rates in those with increasing frailty (assessed using a frailty index), but ultimately absolute events rates were lower in the intensive treatment group (mean on-treatment SBP 121.5 mmHg) compared to standard treatment (mean SBP 134.6 mmHg) [45, 189]. These analyses need to be interpreted with caution, as they were exploratory in nature and were not prespecified in the trial protocol [221].

Carrying out a frailty assessment prior to starting or intensifying antihypertensive therapy in older adults might be considered to identify patients at high risk of adverse outcomes. From a practical perspective, easy-to-use tools to aid with the identification of frailer adults that can be used by non-geriatricians need to be agreed upon so that they can be incorporated into busy clinical practices for those making decisions in relation to blood pressure management in older adults [222]. One approach suggested by Mühlbauer et al. is to target an SBP of 150 mmHg for those with a gait speed <0.8 m/s, with a target of 130–139 mmHg for those with a gait speed >0.8 m/s [223]. However, as it stands, there is insufficient evidence to provide a definitive BP target for frailer adults and the preponderance of data suggests that, while frailty is a high-risk state and one that is accompanied by significant competing risks for non-CVD death, frail adults appear to benefit just as much from good BP control as non-frail adults. It is also worth remembering that, though in some patients the best achievable BP without medication side effects may be higher than a recommended target, any amount of BP lowering is likely to be of benefit, particularly in preventing incident stroke and heart failure.

Blood Pressure Targets in Nursing Home Residents and Those with Dementia

The primary reason for considering these cohorts in a separate paragraph is that most of the hypertension trials to date, including SPRINT, have excluded nursing home residents or those with dementia. Therefore, trial data for hypertension targets in these patients are lacking. Observational data suggests that intensive approaches to antihypertensive therapies may not be of benefit in long-term nursing home residents [224]. Evidence is also emerging that de-intensifying of antihypertensive treatment in these patients does not result in increased adverse outcomes [225]. Those who are not expected to live beyond 2 years are unlikely to live long enough to experience the benefits of intensive BP control and therefore more lenient blood pressure targets seem pragmatic in this patient cohort [222]. In 2014, a consensus statement from the CRIME project (CRIteria to assess appropriate Medication use among Elderly complex patients), specifically recommended against targeting a blood pressure below 140/90 in those with dementia, cognitive impairment, limited function status or those with a limited life expectancy [226]. It should be noted; however, that not all nursing home residents are frail or have dementia, and so, as always, an individualised patient approach should be adopted, avoiding age or place of residence as a singular deciding factor in setting an appropriate BP target.

4.4 Choice of Antihypertensive Therapy: Practical Considerations

Anti-hypertensive choices remain the same in older patients as they are in younger patients, but with some special considerations. ACEI, ARBs, calcium channel blockers and thiazide diuretics are all generally suitable options [227]. The European guidelines also include beta blockers as a therapeutic option, however their use in older patients to exclusively treat hypertension, remains controversial [211]. Unless there is a concurrent indication, loop diuretics and alpha blockers should be avoided given their association with falls. Many patients will have co-morbidities or target organ damage to which the first drug should be tailored [228]. Given that the HYVET trial used thiazide diuretics and ACEI, these may be an appropriate first choice in those over 80 years [182]. Where the use of polypills is advocated in younger patients, consideration for starting with low dose monotherapy in those ≥80 or with increased frailty, may be more appropriate [229]. If considering a more intense treatment goal, the likelihood of polypharmacy increases. For example, in SPRINT-SENIOR, the majority of patients in the intensive treatment group were on either 2 or 3 medications (30.4% and 31.1% respectively), compared to 2 medications in the standard treatment group (30.9%) [189]. In that context, it becomes important to consider drug-drug interactions.

One of the main fears of starting antihypertensive therapy in older patients is the perceived increased risk of falls. This risk seems to be higher following initiation of treatment, and so closer follow-up should be considered during this period in older patients [158, 160, 161]. There are also suggestions that gaps in medication adherence can increase the risk of self-reported injurious falls by up to 18%, and so addressing adherence issues may be an important consideration in the oldest old or frailer patients [155].

4.5 Current Guideline Recommendations

The debate surrounding blood pressure targets highlighted above is reflected in the lack of unity seen across global hypertension guidelines Table 6. Encouragingly, older patients are now recognised in most guidelines although definitions remain

Table 6 Current guideline recommendations for diagnosis and management of hypertension

	JNC-8 [150]	NFA Australia [235]	ACC/AHA Guidelines [230]	American College of Physicians/ American Association of Family Physicians [236]	ESC/ESH Guidelines for the management of arterial hypertension [229]	NICE (UK) [231]	Hypertension Canada [233]	International Society of Hypertension Global Hypertension Practice Guidelines [232]
Year	2014	2016	2017	2017	2018	2019	2020	2020
Recognition of age in the guideline	≥60 years old	≥75 years old	≥65 years old	≥60 years old	Older ≥65 years[a] Very old ≥80 years[a]	≥80 years old	≥75 years old with SBP 130–180 mmHg are considered high risk	Reference "elderly" but no definition of the term given
Definitions								
Office measurements	–	Optimal <120 and <80 Normal 120–129 and/or 80–84 High normal 130–139 and/or 85–89 Grade 1: 140–159 and/or 90–99 Grade 2: 160–179 and/or 100–109 Grade 3: ≥180 and/or ≥110 Isolated systolic hypertension >140 and <90	Normal: <120 and <80 mmHg Elevated: 120–129 mmHg and <80 mmHg Stage 1: 130–139 mmHg or 80–89 mmHg Stage 2: >140 mmHg or ≥90 mmHg	–	Optimal <120 and <80 Normal: 120–129 and/or 80–84 High normal: 130–139 and/or 85–89 Grade 1 hypertension: 140–159 and/or 90–99 Grade 2 hypertension: 160–179 and/or 100–109 Grade 3 hypertension: ≥180 and/or ≥110 Isolated systolic hypertension ≥140 and <90	≥140/90 followed by either ABPM or HBPM to confirm diagnosis Stage 1: office BP 140/90 to 159/99 with subsequent ABPM daytime average or HBPM average of 135/85 to 149/94 mmHg Stage 2: Office BP of ≥160/100 mg but ≤180/120 mmHg with subsequent ABPM daytime average or HBPM average of ≥159/95 mmHg Stage 3: office of ≥180/120	Automated officed: SBP ≥135 and/or DBP ≥85 Observed office: SBP ≥140 and/or DBP ≥90 OR in diabetics SBP ≥130 and/or DBP ≥80	Normal <130 and <85 High normal 130–139 and/or 85–89 Grade 1 hypertension 140–159 and/or 90–99 Grade 2 hypertension ≥160 and/or ≥100

(continued)

Table 6 (continued)

	JNC-8 [150]	NFA Australia [235]	ACC/AHA Guidelines [230]	American College of Physicians/ American Association of Family Physicians [236]	ESC/ESH Guidelines for the management of arterial hypertension [229]	NICE (UK) [231]	Hypertension Canada [233]	International Society of Hypertension Global Hypertension Practice Guidelines [232]
Ambulatory	–	Daytime awake ≥135 and/or ≥85 Daytime over 24 h ≥130 and/or ≥80 ABPM night time ≥120 and/or ≥70	24-h mean >125/75 Daytime: 130/80 Nightime: 110/65	–	24-h mean ≥130 mmHg and/or ≥80 mmHg Daytime (or awake) mean: ≥135 mmHg and/or ≥85 mmHg Night-time (or asleep) mean: ≥120 mmHg and/or ≥70 mmHg	Daytime average ≥135/85 mmHg	Mean 24-h SBP ≥130 and/or DBP ≥80 Or mean daytime SBP ≥135 and/or DBP ≥85	24-h mean: ≥130 and or ≥80 mmHg Daytime (or awake) mean: ≥135 mmHg and/or ≥85 mmHg Night-time (or asleep) mean: ≥120 mmHg and/or ≥70 mmHg
Home BP	–	≥135 and/or ≥85	>130/80	–	≥135 mmHg and/or ≥85 mmHg	≥135/85 mmHg	SBP ≥135 or DBP ≥85	≥135 mmHg and/or ≥85 mmHg
Measurement	–	If clinic BP is ≥140/90 or hypertension is suspected, ambulatory and/or home monitoring should be offered to confirmed	Repeated office BP measurements OR Out of office BP measurement with ABPM and/or HBPM	–	Repeated office BP measurements OR Out of office BP measurement with ABPM and/or HBPM	Repeated office BP measurements and then using ABPM or home monitoring to confirm the diagnosis	Electronic upper arm devices preferred for office measurements in an automated fashion OR observed, ABPM or HBPM	Repeated office BP measurements Out of office BP measurement with ABPM and/or HBPM

When to start drug treatment (in addition to lifestyle interventions)							
In patients ≥60, start pharmaco-logical treatment at a SBP ≥150 or diastolic BP ≥90 If CKD or DM start treatment at ≥140/90	Low absolute cardiovascular risk (5-year risk, <10%) with a persistent BP ≥160/100 (grade: strong; level: I) Moderate absolute CV risk (5-year risk, 10–15%) with a persistent BP ≥140 and ≥90 (grade: strong; level: I)	Secondary prevention: patients with CVD and a BP ≥130 mmHg and/or ≥80 mmHg (Class I) Primary prevention in patients with an estimated 10-year ASCVD risk of ≥10% and a BP >130 mmHg and/or ≥80 mmHg (class I) Primary prevention in adults with an estimated 10-year risk of ASCVD of <10% and a BP ≥140 and/or ≥90 mmHg (Class I)	SBP persistently ≥150 Consider initiating or intensifying treatment in adults ≥60 with a history of stroke or TIA to achieve a target of <140 mmHg Initiate or intensifying treatment in some adults ≥60 years at high cardiovascular risk to achieve a target of <140	Drug treatment and lifestyle interventions in all patients with Grade 2 or 3 hypertension at any level of CV risk (class I) Grade 1 hypertension: Drug treatment and lifestyle interventions in high or very high-risk patients with CVD, renal disease or hyperten-sion-mediated organ damage (HMOD)—class I High normal: Consider drug treatment in very high-risk patients with CVD, especially CAD (class IIb). Lifestyle interventions recommended for all (class I) Specifies that fit older adults (even those >80 years) should be treated if SBP >160 mmHg—class 1 Do not recommend drugs for those over 80 with an isolated systolic BP 140–159 mmHg. Antihypertensive treatment may also be considered in frail older patients if tolerated (Class IIb) Withdrawal of BP lowering treatment on the basis of age, even when patients attain an age of ≥80 years, is not recommended, provided that treatment is well tolerated (Class III)	Stage 2 hypertension Discuss starting drug treatment for adults <80 years with persistent stage 1 hypertension who have 1 or more of the following: target organ damage, established cardiovascular disease, renal disease, diabetes, an estimated 10-year risk of CVD of ≥10% Consider drug treatment for adults <60 years with stage 1 hypertension and an estimated 10 year risk <10% Consider drug treatment for people >80 years with stage 1 hypertension if their clinic BP is >150/90 mmHg	High risk patients: ≥75 years with SBP 130–180 OR ≥50 years AND SBP 130–180 AND one of the following: CVD, CKD, 10-year CV risk ≥15%	Immediate drug treatment in those with grade 2 hypertension (≥160/100) Grade 1: immediate drug treatment in high-risk patients or those with CVD, CKD, DM or HMOD

(continued)

Table 6 (continued)

	JNC-8 [150]	NFA Australia [235]	ACC/AHA Guidelines [230]	American College of Physicians/ American Association of Family Physicians [236]	ESC/ESH Guidelines for the management of arterial hypertension [229]	NICE (UK) [231]	Hypertension Canada [233]	International Society of Hypertension Global Hypertension Practice Guidelines [232]
Targets in older adults	≥60, target SBP <150 and DBP <90 (Strong recommendation—Grade A) If pharmacological treatment for high BP results in a lower SBP (e.g., <140 mmHg) and treatment is well tolerated and without adverse effects on health or QoL then treatment doesn't need to be adjusted ≤140/90 if CKD or DM	<140/90 mmHg or lower if tolerated (grade: strong; level: I) In selected high CV risk populations a BP <120 can improve CV outcomes For patients >74 years of age, aiming for a SBP <120 mmHg has shown benefit where tolerated, unless there is concomitant diabetes	Known CVD or a 10-year ASCVD event risk of ≥10%: target of <130/80 mmHg (Class I) Hypertension without additional markers of increased CVD risk, a target of <130/80 may be reasonable	≥60 years, SBP <150 OR SBP <140 if patient has a history of stroke or TIA Consider SBP target <140 if the patient is ≥60 years and at high cardiovascular risk Insufficient evidence to recommend targeting treatment according to DBP	<140/90 in all patients and to 130/80 if possible ≥65 years • Systolic BP 130–139 mmHg • Close monitoring of adverse events Diastolic BP <80 mmHg for all patients (Class IIa)	Office BP <140/90 for anyone <80 years or ≤135/85 if ABPM or HBPM is used Office BP <150/90mmHg for those ≥80 years old or <145/85 if ABPM or HBPM used	High risk patients: SBP <120 (automated office reading)—which includes anyone over 75 with a SBP 130–180 DM: <130/80 Others: <140/90	Ideally to <140/90 mmHg Optimal: <65 years: target BP <130/80 mmHg if tolerated (but >120/70 mmHg) ≥65 years: BP target <140/90 mmHg if tolerated but consider an individualised BP target in the context of frailty, independence and likely tolerability of treatment

Special considerations for older patients		Start with the lowest dose and titrate slowly (grade: strong; level: –) If treatment being targeted to <120, close follow up is recommended (grade: strong; level: II) Clinical judgement should be used to assess benefit of treatment against risk of adverse effects in all older patients with lower grades of hypertension (grade: strong; level: –)	Treatment of hypertension with a SBP treatment goal of <130 mmHg is recommended for non-institution-alised ambulatory community dwelling adults (≥65 years of ago)—Class I For older adults (≥65) and a high burden of comorbidity and limited life expectancy, clinical judgement, patient preference, and a team-based approach to assess risk/benefit is reasonable for decisions regarding intensity of BP lowering and choice of antihypertensive drugs (Class IIa)	Individual assessment of benefits and harms is particularly important in adults ≥60 years	In those ≥80, it may be appropriate to start with monotherapy Start at the lowest available dose Monitor closely for postural BP Avoid loop diuretics or alpha blockers (unless required for other conditions) as there are associations with falls	Use clinical judgement for people of any age with frailty or multimorbidity Measure standing BP in those ≥80 years. In those with a significant drop on standing, treat to a blood pressure target based on standing BP	No specific guidance	In those ≥65 consider an individualised BP target in the context of frailty, independence and likely tolerability of treatment Assess for postural hypotension at time of diagnosis in elderly patients

ABPM ambulatory blood pressure monitoring, *ASCVD* atherosclerotic cardiovascular disease, *BP* blood pressure, *CKD* chronic kidney disease, *CV* cardiovascular, *CVD* cardiovascular disease, *HMOD* hypertension mediated organ damage, *HBPM* home blood pressure monitoring, *SBP* systolic blood pressure, *TIA* transient ischemic attack

[a] Acknowledgement that the definition of 'older' is complex

based on chronological ages and vary from ≥ 60 years to ≥ 80 years. While the European Society of Cardiology Guidelines (ESC), recommend a blood pressure target of <140/90, with consideration to aiming for 130/80 if tolerated, the American Heart Association (AHA) Guidelines recommend a target of <130/80, reflecting an emphasis on the results of the 2015 SPRINT trial [45, 229, 230]. NICE and the International Society of Hypertension Global Hypertension Practice Guidelines are in keeping with the ESC Guidelines, recommending a BP target of <140/90 [231, 232]. In contrast, guidelines from the American College of Physicians and the American Association of Family Practitioners, published in the same year as the AHA Guidelines, recommend a systolic blood pressure of <150 mmHg, 20 mmHg higher than most other societies, as does the JNC-8 (albeit published prior to SPRINT). Meanwhile, Hypertension Canada recommend an SBP target of <120 mmHg for those over 75 with an SBP between 130 and 180 mmHg [233]. These kind of discrepancies represent a real challenge for the physician treating hypertension in older patients, leaving ultimate choices to physicians [142, 234].

4.6 Practical Tips and Take-Home Points

While the guidelines may not be harmonised on what defines an older patient or on a recommended treatment target for this patient group, there is one thing that remains in consistent agreement. An individualised approach should be used for the older patient cohort making decisions based not on age alone, but on the overall medical, physical, social and mental characteristics of the patient [142]. While we do need to be mindful of potential adverse outcomes, it is a dangerous misconception to assume that increased age alone excludes a patient from a more intensive BP treatment plan. A summary of the above discussion points is provided in Box 3.

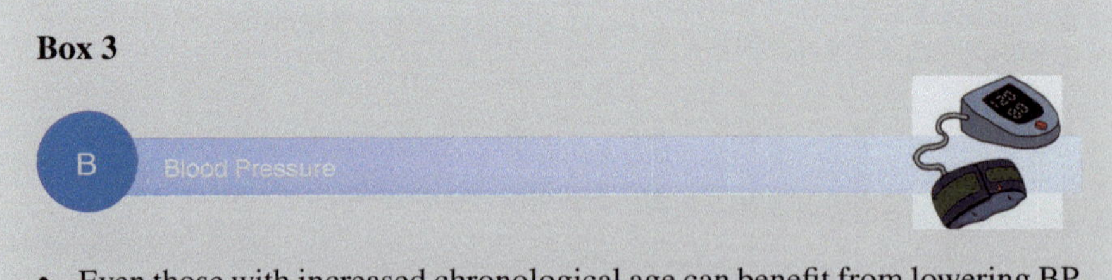

Box 3

- Even those with increased chronological age can benefit from lowering BP.
- While various guidelines may not currently be harmonised on targets, all guidelines currently agree that an individualised approach should be used for the older patient cohort making decisions based not on age alone, but on the overall medical, physical, social, and mental characteristics of the patient (including frailty assessment).

- In general, a target blood pressure of <140/90 is suitable for most older adults.
- More lenient control should be considered in those with multiple comorbidities (resulting in high competing risk for non-cardiovascular death) or those with evidence of severe frailty that is likely to limit lifespan.
- In contrast, a more intensive target of 130/80 can be considered in fitter older adults who do not experience side effects from anti-hypertensive therapy.
- We have no reliable data on patients in nursing homes or with dementia.
- We also have little data to guide decisions on targets and benefits in those >85 years.
- The highest risk of falls is around the time of initiation and intensification of medications—consider closer follow up in frail patients after changes are made to their antihypertensives.

Disclosures and Other Relevant Conflicts of Interest None Reported.

References

1. Virani SS, Alonso A, Aparicio HJ, et al. Heart disease and stroke statistics—2021 update. Circulation. 2021;143(8):e254–743. https://doi.org/10.1161/CIR.0000000000000950.
2. Yazdanyar A, Newman AB. The burden of cardiovascular disease in the elderly: morbidity, mortality, and costs. Clin Geriatr Med. 2009;25(4):563–77, vii. https://doi.org/10.1016/j.cger.2009.07.007.
3. Roth GA, Mensah GA, Johnson CO, et al. Global burden of cardiovascular diseases and risk factors, 1990–2019: update from the GBD 2019 Study. J Am Coll Cardiol. 2020;76(25):2982–3021. https://doi.org/10.1016/j.jacc.2020.11.010.
4. Rich MW, Chyun DA, Skolnick AH, et al. Knowledge gaps in cardiovascular care of the older adult population: a scientific statement from the American Heart Association, American College of Cardiology, and American Geriatrics Society. J Am Coll Cardiol. 2016;67(20):2419–40. https://doi.org/10.1016/j.jacc.2016.03.004.
5. Forman DE, Maurer MS, Boyd C, et al. Multimorbidity in older adults with cardiovascular disease. J Am Coll Cardiol. 2018;71(19):2149–61. https://doi.org/10.1016/j.jacc.2018.03.022.
6. Forman DE, Rich MW, Alexander KP, et al. Cardiac care for older adults. Time for a new paradigm. J Am Coll Cardiol. 2011;57(18):1801–10. https://doi.org/10.1016/j.jacc.2011.02.014.
7. O'Neill D, Forman DE. The importance of physical function as a clinical outcome: assessment and enhancement. Clin Cardiol. 2020;43(2):108–17. https://doi.org/10.1002/clc.23311.
8. Braunstein JB, Cheng A, Fakhry C, Nass CM, Vigilance C, Blumenthal RS. ABCs of cardiovascular disease risk management. Cardiol Rev. 2001;9(2):96–105. https://doi.org/10.1097/00045415-200103000-00008.
9. Arps K, Pallazola VA, Cardoso R, et al. Clinician's guide to the updated ABCs of cardiovascular disease prevention: a review Part 1. Am J Med. 2019;132(6):e569–80. https://doi.org/10.1016/j.amjmed.2019.01.016.

10. Arps K, Pallazola VA, Cardoso R, et al. Clinician's guide to the updated ABCs of cardio-vascular disease prevention: a review Part 2. Am J Med. 2019;132(7):e599–609. https://doi.org/10.1016/j.amjmed.2019.01.031.

11. Arnett DK, Blumenthal RS, Albert MA, et al. 2019 ACC/AHA guideline on the primary prevention of cardiovascular disease: a report of the American College of Cardiology/American Heart Association Task Force on Clinical Practice Guidelines. Circulation. 2019;140(11):e596–646. https://doi.org/10.1161/CIR.0000000000000678.

12. Pearson GJ, Thanassoulis G, Anderson TJ, et al. Canadian Cardiovascular Society guidelines for the management of dyslipidemia for the prevention of cardiovascular disease in the adult. Can J Cardiol. 2021; https://doi.org/10.1016/j.cjca.2021.03.016.

13. Cardiovascular disease: risk assessment and reduction, including lipid modification; 2014 (updated 2016).

14. Visseren FLJ, Mach F, Smulders YM, et al. 2021 ESC Guidelines on cardiovascular disease prevention in clinical practice: developed by the Task Force for cardiovascular disease prevention in clinical practice with representatives of the European Society of Cardiology and 12 medical societies With the special contribution of the European Association of Preventive Cardiology (EAPC). Eur Heart J. 2021;42(34):3227–337. https://doi.org/10.1093/eurheartj/ehab484.

15. DeFilippis AP, Young R, McEvoy JW, et al. Risk score overestimation: the impact of individual cardiovascular risk factors and preventive therapies on the performance of the American Heart Association-American College of Cardiology-Atherosclerotic Cardiovascular Disease risk score in a modern multi-ethnic cohort. Eur Heart J. 2017;38(8):598–608. https://doi.org/10.1093/eurheartj/ehw301.

16. Lloyd-Jones DM, Braun LT, Ndumele CE, et al. Use of risk assessment tools to guide decision-making in the primary prevention of atherosclerotic cardiovascular disease: a special report from the American Heart Association and American College of Cardiology. J Am Coll Cardiol. 2019;73(24):3153–67. https://doi.org/10.1016/j.jacc.2018.11.005.

17. Conroy RM, Pyörälä K, Fitzgerald AP, et al. Estimation of ten-year risk of fatal cardiovascular disease in Europe: the SCORE project. Eur Heart J. 2003;24(11):987–1003. https://doi.org/10.1016/s0195-668x(03)00114-3.

18. Goff DC, Lloyd-Jones DM, Bennett G, et al. 2013 ACC/AHA guideline on the assessment of cardiovascular risk. Circulation. 2014;129(25_Suppl_2):S49–73. https://doi.org/10.1161/01.cir.0000437741.48606.98.

19. Nanna MG, Peterson ED, Wojdyla D, Navar AM. The accuracy of cardiovascular pooled cohort risk estimates in U.S. older adults. J Gen Intern Med. 2020;35(6):1701–8. https://doi.org/10.1007/s11606-019-05361-4.

20. Koller MT, Steyerberg EW, Wolbers M, et al. Validity of the Framingham point scores in the elderly: results from the Rotterdam study. Am Heart J. 2007;154(1):87–93. https://doi.org/10.1016/j.ahj.2007.03.022.

21. Barry AR, O'Neill DE, Graham MM. Primary prevention of cardiovascular disease in older adults. Can J Cardiol. 2016;32(9):1074–81. https://doi.org/10.1016/j.cjca.2016.01.032.

22. Cooney MT, Selmer R, Lindman A, et al. Cardiovascular risk estimation in older persons: SCORE O.P. Eur J Prev Cardiol. 2016;23(10):1093–103. https://doi.org/10.1177/2047487315588390.

23. Ahmadi SF, Streja E, Zahmatkesh G, et al. Reverse epidemiology of traditional cardiovascular risk factors in the geriatric population. J Am Med Dir Assoc. 2015;16(11):933–9. https://doi.org/10.1016/j.jamda.2015.07.014.

24. SCORE2-OP working group and ESC Cardiovascular risk collaboration. SCORE2-OP risk prediction algorithms: estimating incident cardiovascular event risk in older persons in four geographical risk regions. Eur Heart J. 2021;42(25):2455–67. https://doi.org/10.1093/eurheartj/ehab312.

25. van Bussel EF, Richard E, Busschers WB, et al. A cardiovascular risk prediction model for older people: development and validation in a primary care population. J Clin Hypertens. 2019;21(8):1145–52. https://doi.org/10.1111/jch.13617.
26. Grundy Scott M, Stone Neil J, Bailey Alison L, et al. 2018 AHA/ACC/AACVPR/AAPA/ABC/ACPM/ADA/AGS/APhA/ASPC/NLA/PCNA guideline on the management of blood cholesterol: a report of the American College of Cardiology/American Heart Association Task Force on clinical practice guidelines. Circulation. 2019;139(25):e1082–143. https://doi.org/10.1161/CIR.0000000000000625.
27. D'Agostino RB, Vasan RS, Pencina MJ, et al. General cardiovascular risk profile for use in primary care. Circulation. 2008;117(6):743–53. https://doi.org/10.1161/CIRCULATIONAHA.107.699579.
28. Hippisley-Cox J, Coupland C, Vinogradova Y, et al. Predicting cardiovascular risk in England and Wales: prospective derivation and validation of QRISK2. BMJ. 2008;336(7659):1475–82. https://doi.org/10.1136/bmj.39609.449676.25.
29. McClelland RL, Jorgensen NW, Budoff M, et al. 10-Year coronary heart disease risk prediction using coronary artery calcium and traditional risk factors: derivation in the MESA (Multi-Ethnic Study of Atherosclerosis) with validation in the HNR (Heinz Nixdorf Recall) study and the DHS (Dallas Heart Study). J Am Coll Cardiol. 2015;66(15):1643–53. https://doi.org/10.1016/j.jacc.2015.08.035.
30. World Health Organization. Prevention of cardiovascular disease: guidelines for assessment and management of cardiovascular risk. World Health Organization; 2007.
31. Vega GL, Wang J, Grundy SM. Utility of metabolic syndrome as a risk enhancing factor in decision of statin use. J Clin Lipidol. 2021;15(2):255–65. https://doi.org/10.1016/j.jacl.2021.01.012.
32. Golia E, Limongelli G, Natale F, et al. Inflammation and cardiovascular disease: from pathogenesis to therapeutic target. Curr Atheroscler Rep. 2014;16(9):435. https://doi.org/10.1007/s11883-014-0435-z.
33. Cainzos-Achirica M, Miedema MD, McEvoy JW, et al. The prognostic value of high sensitivity C-reactive protein in a multi-ethnic population after >10 years of follow-up: The Multi-Ethnic Study of Atherosclerosis (MESA). Int J Cardiol. 2018;264:158–64. https://doi.org/10.1016/j.ijcard.2018.02.027.
34. Ridker PM, Everett BM, Thuren T, et al. Antiinflammatory therapy with canakinumab for atherosclerotic disease. N Engl J Med. 2017;377(12):1119–31. https://doi.org/10.1056/NEJMoa1707914.
35. Saeed A, Nambi V, Sun W, et al. Short-term global cardiovascular disease risk prediction in older adults. J Am Coll Cardiol. 2018;71(22):2527–36. https://doi.org/10.1016/j.jacc.2018.02.050.
36. Störk S, Feelders RA, van den Beld AW, et al. Prediction of mortality risk in the elderly. Am J Med. 2006;119(6):519–25. https://doi.org/10.1016/j.amjmed.2005.10.062.
37. Tota-Maharaj R, Blaha MJ, McEvoy JW, et al. Coronary artery calcium for the prediction of mortality in young adults <45 years old and elderly adults >75 years old. Eur Heart J. 2012;33(23):2955–62. https://doi.org/10.1093/eurheartj/ehs230.
38. Bergman H, Ferrucci L, Guralnik J, et al. Frailty: an emerging research and clinical paradigm—issues and controversies. J Gerontol A. 2007;62(7):731–7. https://doi.org/10.1093/gerona/62.7.731.
39. Afilalo J, Alexander KP, Mack MJ, et al. Frailty assessment in the cardiovascular care of older adults. J Am Coll Cardiol. 2014;63(8):747–62. https://doi.org/10.1016/j.jacc.2013.09.070.
40. Clegg A, Young J, Iliffe S, Rikkert MO, Rockwood K. Frailty in elderly people. Lancet. 2013;381(9868):752–62. https://doi.org/10.1016/s0140-6736(12)62167-9.
41. Newman AB, Gottdiener JS, McBurnie MA, et al. Associations of subclinical cardiovascular disease with frailty. J Gerontol A Biol Sci Med Sci. 2001;56(3):M158–66. https://doi.org/10.1093/gerona/56.3.m158.

42. Virani Salim S, Alonso A, Aparicio Hugo J, et al. Heart disease and stroke statistics—2021 update. Circulation. 2021;143(8):e254–743. https://doi.org/10.1161/CIR.0000000000000950.

43. Hawley CE, Roefaro J, Forman DE, Orkaby AR. Statins for primary prevention in those aged 70 years and older: a critical review of recent cholesterol guidelines. Drugs Aging. 2019;36(8):687–99. https://doi.org/10.1007/s40266-019-00673-w.

44. Lee SJ, Kim CM. Individualizing prevention for older adults. J Am Geriatr Soc. 2018;66(2):229–34. https://doi.org/10.1111/jgs.15216.

45. The Sprint Research Group. A randomized trial of intensive versus standard blood-pressure control. N Engl J Med. 2015;373(22):2103–16. https://doi.org/10.1056/NEJMoa1511939.

46. Beckett N, Peters R, Tuomilehto J, et al. Immediate and late benefits of treating very elderly people with hypertension: results from active treatment extension to Hypertension in the Very Elderly randomised controlled trial. BMJ. 2012;344:d7541. https://doi.org/10.1136/bmj.d7541.

47. Rodriguez-Gutierrez R, Gonzalez-Gonzalez JG, Zuñiga-Hernandez JA, McCoy RG. Benefits and harms of intensive glycemic control in patients with type 2 diabetes. BMJ. 2019;367:l5887. https://doi.org/10.1136/bmj.l5887.

48. Appel LJ, Moore TJ, Obarzanek E, et al. A clinical trial of the effects of dietary patterns on blood pressure. N Engl J Med. 1997;336(16):1117–24. https://doi.org/10.1056/NEJM199704173361601.

49. Whelton PK, Appel LJ, Espeland MA, et al. Sodium reduction and weight loss in the treatment of hypertension in older persons: a randomized controlled Trial of Nonpharmacologic Interventions in the Elderly (TONE). JAMA. 1998;279(11):839–46. https://doi.org/10.1001/jama.279.11.839.

50. Gencer B, Marston NA, Im K, et al. Efficacy and safety of lowering LDL cholesterol in older patients: a systematic review and meta-analysis of randomised controlled trials. Lancet. 2020;396(10263):1637–43. https://doi.org/10.1016/s0140-6736(20)32332-1.

51. Doll R, Peto R, Boreham J, Sutherland I. Mortality in relation to smoking: 50 years' observations on male British doctors. BMJ. 2004;328(7455):1519. https://doi.org/10.1136/bmj.38142.554479.AE.

52. Taylor DH Jr, Hasselblad V, Henley SJ, Thun MJ, Sloan FA. Benefits of smoking cessation for longevity. Am J Public Health. 2002;92(6):990–6. https://doi.org/10.2105/ajph.92.6.990.

53. Mons U, Müezzinler A, Gellert C, et al. Impact of smoking and smoking cessation on cardiovascular events and mortality among older adults: meta-analysis of individual participant data from prospective cohort studies of the CHANCES consortium. BMJ. 2015;350:h1551. https://doi.org/10.1136/bmj.h1551.

54. Bellettiere J, LaMonte MJ, Evenson KR, et al. Sedentary behavior and cardiovascular disease in older women. Circulation. 2019;139(8):1036–46. https://doi.org/10.1161/CIRCULATIONAHA.118.035312.

55. O'Brien CW, Juraschek SP, Wee CC. Prevalence of aspirin use for primary prevention of cardiovascular disease in the United States: results from the 2017 National Health Interview Survey. Ann Intern Med. 2019;171(8):596–8. https://doi.org/10.7326/M19-0953.

56. Boakye E, Uddin SMI, Obisesan OH, et al. Aspirin for cardiovascular disease prevention among adults in the United States: trends, prevalence, and participant characteristics associated with use. Am J Prev Cardiol. 2021;8:100256. https://doi.org/10.1016/j.ajpc.2021.100256.

57. Jacobsen Alan P, Lim Zi L, Chang B, et al. A transatlantic comparison of patient-reported access to and use of aspirin in contemporary preventive cardiology. J Am Coll Cardiol. 2021;78(11):1193–5. https://doi.org/10.1016/j.jacc.2021.07.015.

58. Raber I, McCarthy CP, Vaduganathan M, et al. The rise and fall of aspirin in the primary prevention of cardiovascular disease. Lancet. 2019;393(10186):2155–67. https://doi.org/10.1016/S0140-6736(19)30541-0.

59. Murphy E, Curneen J, McEvoy JW. Aspirin in the modern era of cardiovascular disease prevention. Methodist Debakey Cardiovasc J. 2021;17(4):36–47. https://doi.org/10.14797/mdcvj.293.
60. Steering Committee of the Physicians' Health Study Research Group. Final report on the aspirin component of the ongoing Physicians' Health Study. N Engl J Med. 1989;321(3):129–35. https://doi.org/10.1056/nejm198907203210301.
61. Peto R, Gray R, Collins R, et al. Randomised trial of prophylactic daily aspirin in British male doctors. Br Med J (Clin Res Ed). 1988;296(6618):313–6. https://doi.org/10.1136/bmj.296.6618.313.
62. Pearson Thomas A, Blair Steven N, Daniels Stephen R, et al. AHA guidelines for primary prevention of cardiovascular disease and stroke: 2002 update. Circulation. 2002;106(3):388–91. https://doi.org/10.1161/01.CIR.0000020190.45892.75.
63. Hayden M, Pignone M, Phillips C, Mulrow C. Aspirin for the primary prevention of cardiovascular events: a summary of the evidence for the U.S. Preventive Services Task Force. Ann Intern Med. 2002;136(2):161–72. https://doi.org/10.7326/0003-4819-136-2-200201150-00016.
64. Graham I, Atar D, Borch-Johnsen K, et al. †European guidelines on cardiovascular disease prevention in clinical practice: executive summary: Fourth Joint Task Force of the European Society of Cardiology and Other Societies on Cardiovascular Disease Prevention in Clinical Practice (Constituted by representatives of nine societies and by invited experts). Eur Heart J. 2007;28(19):2375–414. https://doi.org/10.1093/eurheartj/ehm316.
65. Gaziano JM, Brotons C, Coppolecchia R, et al. Use of aspirin to reduce risk of initial vascular events in patients at moderate risk of cardiovascular disease (ARRIVE): a randomised, double-blind, placebo-controlled trial. Lancet. 2018;392(10152):1036–46. https://doi.org/10.1016/s0140-6736(18)31924-x.
66. Bowman L, Mafham M, Wallendszus K, et al. Effects of aspirin for primary prevention in persons with diabetes mellitus. N Engl J Med. 2018;379(16):1529–39. https://doi.org/10.1056/NEJMoa1804988.
67. McNeil JJ, Wolfe R, Woods RL, et al. Effect of aspirin on cardiovascular events and bleeding in the healthy elderly. N Engl J Med. 2018;379(16):1509–18. https://doi.org/10.1056/NEJMoa1805819.
68. McNeil JJ, Nelson MR, Woods RL, et al. Effect of aspirin on all-cause mortality in the healthy elderly. N Engl J Med. 2018;379(16):1519–28. https://doi.org/10.1056/NEJMoa1803955.
69. McNeil JJ, Woods RL, Nelson MR, et al. Effect of aspirin on disability-free survival in the healthy elderly. N Engl J Med. 2018;379(16):1499–508. https://doi.org/10.1056/NEJMoa1800722.
70. Woods RL, Espinoza S, Thao LTP, et al. Effect of aspirin on activities of daily living disability in community-dwelling older adults. J Gerontol A. 2020; https://doi.org/10.1093/gerona/glaa316.
71. Yusuf S, Joseph P, Dans A, et al. Polypill with or without aspirin in persons without cardiovascular disease. N Engl J Med. 2021;384(3):216–28. https://doi.org/10.1056/NEJMoa2028220.
72. Steering Committee of the Physicians' Health Study Research Group. Preliminary report: Findings from the aspirin component of the ongoing Physicians' Health Study. N Engl J Med. 1988;318(4):262–4. https://doi.org/10.1056/nejm198801283180431.
73. Meade TW, Wilkes HC, Stirling Y, Brennan PJ, Kelleher C, Browne W. Randomized controlled trial of low dose warfarin in the primary prevention of ischaemic heart disease in men at high risk: design and pilot study. Eur Heart J. 1988;9(8):836–43. https://doi.org/10.1093/oxfordjournals.eurheartj.a062576.
74. The Medical Research Council's General Practice Research Framework. Thrombosis prevention trial: randomised trial of low-intensity oral anticoagulation with warfarin and low-dose aspirin in the primary prevention of ischaemic heart disease in men at increased risk. Lancet. 1998;351(9098):233–41. https://doi.org/10.1016/S0140-6736(97)11475-1.

75. The HOT Study Group. The hypertension optimal treatment study (the HOT Study). Blood Press. 1993;2(1):62–8. https://doi.org/10.3109/08037059309077529.

76. Hansson L, Zanchetti A, Carruthers SG, et al. Effects of intensive blood-pressure lowering and low-dose aspirin in patients with hypertension: principal results of the Hypertension Optimal Treatment (HOT) randomised trial. HOT Study Group. Lancet. 1998;351(9118):1755–62. https://doi.org/10.1016/s0140-6736(98)04311-6.

77. de Gaetano G, Collaborative Group of the Primary Prevention Project. Low-dose aspirin and vitamin E in people at cardiovascular risk: a randomised trial in general practice. Collaborative Group of the Primary Prevention Project. Lancet. 2001;357(9250):89–95. https://doi.org/10.1016/s0140-6736(00)03539-x.

78. Ridker PM, Cook NR, Lee IM, et al. A randomized trial of low-dose aspirin in the primary prevention of cardiovascular disease in women. N Engl J Med. 2005;352(13):1293–304. https://doi.org/10.1056/NEJMoa050613.

79. Belch J, MacCuish A, Campbell I, et al. The prevention of progression of arterial disease and diabetes (POPADAD) trial: factorial randomised placebo controlled trial of aspirin and antioxidants in patients with diabetes and asymptomatic peripheral arterial disease. BMJ. 2008;337:a1840. https://doi.org/10.1136/bmj.a1840.

80. Ogawa H, Nakayama M, Morimoto T, et al. Low-dose aspirin for primary prevention of atherosclerotic events in patients with type 2 diabetes: a randomized controlled trial. JAMA. 2008;300(18):2134–41. https://doi.org/10.1001/jama.2008.623.

81. Fowkes FGR, Price JF, Stewart MCW, et al. Aspirin for prevention of cardiovascular events in a general population screened for a low ankle brachial index: a randomized controlled trial. JAMA. 2010;303(9):841–8. https://doi.org/10.1001/jama.2010.221.

82. Ikeda Y, Shimada K, Teramoto T, et al. Low-dose aspirin for primary prevention of cardiovascular events in Japanese patients 60 years or older with atherosclerotic risk factors: a randomized clinical trial. JAMA. 2014;312(23):2510–20. https://doi.org/10.1001/jama.2014.15690.

83. Abdelaziz HK, Saad M, Pothineni NVK, et al. Aspirin for primary prevention of cardiovascular events. J Am Coll Cardiol. 2019;73(23):2915–29. https://doi.org/10.1016/j.jacc.2019.03.501.

84. Zheng SL, Roddick AJ. Association of aspirin use for primary prevention with cardiovascular events and bleeding events: a systematic review and meta-analysis. JAMA. 2019;321(3):277–87. https://doi.org/10.1001/jama.2018.20578.

85. Mahmoud AN, Gad MM, Elgendy AY, Elgendy IY, Bavry AA. Efficacy and safety of aspirin for primary prevention of cardiovascular events: a meta-analysis and trial sequential analysis of randomized controlled trials. Eur Heart J. 2019;40(7):607–17. https://doi.org/10.1093/eurheartj/ehy813.

86. McEvoy J, Keane M, Ng J. Primary prevention aspirin among the elderly: challenges in translating trial evidence to the clinic. Br J Cardiol. 2020;2020:31–3. https://doi.org/10.5837/bjc.2020.007.

87. Weil J, Colin-Jones D, Langman M, et al. Prophylactic aspirin and risk of peptic ulcer bleeding. BMJ. 1995;310(6983):827–30. https://doi.org/10.1136/bmj.310.6983.827.

88. Bhatt DL, Scheiman J, Abraham NS, et al. ACCF/ACG/AHA 2008 expert consensus document on reducing the gastrointestinal risks of antiplatelet therapy and NSAID use. Circulation. 2008;118(18):1894–909. https://doi.org/10.1161/CIRCULATIONAHA.108.191087.

89. Marquis-Gravel G, Roe MT, Harrington RA, Muñoz D, Hernandez AF, Jones WS. Revisiting the role of aspirin for the primary prevention of cardiovascular disease. Circulation. 2019;140(13):1115–24. https://doi.org/10.1161/CIRCULATIONAHA.119.040205.

90. de Abajo FJ, García Rodríguez LA. Risk of upper gastrointestinal bleeding and perforation associated with low-dose aspirin as plain and enteric-coated formulations. BMC Clin Pharmacol. 2001;1:1–1. https://doi.org/10.1186/1472-6904-1-1.

91. Bhatt DL, Grosser T, Dong JF, et al. Enteric coating and aspirin nonresponsiveness in patients with type 2 diabetes mellitus. J Am Coll Cardiol. 2017;69(6):603–12. https://doi.org/10.1016/j.jacc.2016.11.050.

92. Rothwell PM, Cook NR, Gaziano JM, et al. Effects of aspirin on risks of vascular events and cancer according to bodyweight and dose: analysis of individual patient data from randomised trials. Lancet. 2018;392(10145):387–99. https://doi.org/10.1016/S0140-6736(18)31133-4.

93. Murphy S, McCarthy CP, McEvoy JW. Aspirin for the primary prevention of cardiovascular disease: weighing up the evidence. Am J Med. 2019;132(9):1007–8. https://doi.org/10.1016/j.amjmed.2019.02.025.

94. Nelson MR, Doust JA. Primary prevention of cardiovascular disease: new guidelines, technologies and therapies. Med J Aust. 2013;198(11):606–10. https://doi.org/10.5694/mja12.11054.

95. National Institute for Health and Care Excellence. Scenario: Antiplatelet treatment for primary prevention of cardiovascular disease (CVD). https://cks.nice.org.uk/topics/antiplatelet-treatment/management/primary-prevention-of-cvd/. Accessed 20 Sept 2021.

96. Wein T, Lindsay MP, Gladstone DJ, et al. Canadian Stroke Best Practice Recommendations, seventh edition: acetylsalicylic acid for prevention of vascular events. CMAJ. 2020;192(12):E302–e311. https://doi.org/10.1503/cmaj.191599.

97. American Diabetes Association. 10. Cardiovascular disease and risk management: standards of medical care in diabetes—2021. Diabetes Care. 2021;44(Suppl 1):S125. https://doi.org/10.2337/dc21-S010.

98. U.S. Preventive Services Task Force. Aspirin use to prevent cardiovascular disease: preventive medication (Draft Evidence Review); 2021

99. Antithrombotic Trialists Collaboration. Aspirin in the primary and secondary prevention of vascular disease: collaborative meta-analysis of individual participant data from randomised trials. Lancet. 2009;373(9678):1849–60. https://doi.org/10.1016/S0140-6736(09)60503-1.

100. Jones WS, Mulder H, Wruck LM, et al. Comparative effectiveness of aspirin dosing in cardiovascular disease. N Engl J Med. 2021;384(21):1981–90. https://doi.org/10.1056/NEJMoa2102137.

101. Jacobsen AP, Raber I, McCarthy CP, et al. Lifelong aspirin for all in the secondary prevention of chronic coronary syndrome. Circulation. 2020;142(16):1579–90. https://doi.org/10.1161/CIRCULATIONAHA.120.045695.

102. Cao D, Chandiramani R, Chiarito M, Claessen BE, Mehran R. Evolution of antithrombotic therapy in patients undergoing percutaneous coronary intervention: a 40-year journey. Eur Heart J. 2021;42(4):339–51. https://doi.org/10.1093/eurheartj/ehaa824.

103. Giacoppo D, Matsuda Y, Fovino LN, et al. Short dual antiplatelet therapy followed by P2Y12 inhibitor monotherapy vs. prolonged dual antiplatelet therapy after percutaneous coronary intervention with second-generation drug-eluting stents: a systematic review and meta-analysis of randomized clinical trials. Eur Heart J. 2020;42(4):308–19. https://doi.org/10.1093/eurheartj/ehaa739.

104. O'Donoghue ML, Murphy SA, Sabatine MS. The safety and efficacy of aspirin discontinuation on a background of a P2Y(12) inhibitor in patients after percutaneous coronary intervention: a systematic review and meta-analysis. Circulation. 2020;142(6):538–45. https://doi.org/10.1161/circulationaha.120.046251.

105. Choi KH, Song YB, Lee JM, et al. Clinical usefulness of PRECISE-DAPT score for predicting bleeding events in patients with acute coronary syndrome undergoing percutaneous coronary intervention. Circ Cardiovasc Interv. 2020;13(5):e008530. https://doi.org/10.1161/CIRCINTERVENTIONS.119.008530.

106. Chiarito M, Sanz-Sánchez J, Cannata F, et al. Monotherapy with a P2Y(12) inhibitor or aspirin for secondary prevention in patients with established atherosclerosis: a systematic review and meta-analysis. Lancet. 2020;395(10235):1487–95. https://doi.org/10.1016/s0140-6736(20)30315-9.

107. Collet J-P, Thiele H, Barbato E, et al. 2020 ESC Guidelines for the management of acute coronary syndromes in patients presenting without persistent ST-segment elevation: the Task Force for the management of acute coronary syndromes in patients presenting without persis-

tent ST-segment elevation of the European Society of Cardiology (ESC). Eur Heart J. 2020; https://doi.org/10.1093/eurheartj/ehaa575.

108. Ibanez B, James S, Agewall S, et al. 2017 ESC Guidelines for the management of acute myocardial infarction in patients presenting with ST-segment elevation: the Task Force for the management of acute myocardial infarction in patients presenting with ST-segment elevation of the European Society of Cardiology (ESC). Eur Heart J. 2017;39(2):119–77. https://doi.org/10.1093/eurheartj/ehx393.

109. Levine GN, Bates ER, Bittl JA, et al. 2016 ACC/AHA guideline focused update on duration of dual antiplatelet therapy in patients with coronary artery disease: a report of the American College of Cardiology/American Heart Association Task Force on clinical practice guidelines. Circulation. 2016;134(10):e123–55. https://doi.org/10.1161/CIR.0000000000000404.

110. Wallentin L, Becker RC, Budaj A, et al. Ticagrelor versus clopidogrel in patients with acute coronary syndromes. N Engl J Med. 2009;361(11):1045–57. https://doi.org/10.1056/NEJMoa0904327.

111. Wiviott SD, Braunwald E, McCabe CH, et al. Prasugrel versus clopidogrel in patients with acute coronary syndromes. N Engl J Med. 2007;357(20):2001–15. https://doi.org/10.1056/NEJMoa0706482.

112. Eikelboom JW, Mehta SR, Anand SS, Xie C, Fox KA, Yusuf S. Adverse impact of bleeding on prognosis in patients with acute coronary syndromes. Circulation. 2006;114(8):774–82. https://doi.org/10.1161/circulationaha.106.612812.

113. Roe MT, Goodman SG, Ohman EM, et al. Elderly patients with acute coronary syndromes managed without revascularization. Circulation. 2013;128(8):823–33. https://doi.org/10.1161/CIRCULATIONAHA.113.002303.

114. Savonitto S, Ferri LA, Piatti L, et al. Comparison of reduced-dose prasugrel and standard-dose clopidogrel in elderly patients with acute coronary syndromes undergoing early percutaneous revascularization. Circulation. 2018;137(23):2435–45. https://doi.org/10.1161/circulationaha.117.032180.

115. Gimbel M, Qaderdan K, Willemsen L, et al. Clopidogrel versus ticagrelor or prasugrel in patients aged 70 years or older with non-ST-elevation acute coronary syndrome (POPular AGE): the randomised, open-label, non-inferiority trial. Lancet. 2020;395(10233):1374–81. https://doi.org/10.1016/s0140-6736(20)30325-1.

116. Cuisset T, Deharo P, Quilici J, et al. Benefit of switching dual antiplatelet therapy after acute coronary syndrome: the TOPIC (timing of platelet inhibition after acute coronary syndrome) randomized study. Eur Heart J. 2017;38(41):3070–8. https://doi.org/10.1093/eurheartj/ehx175.

117. Eikelboom JW, Connolly SJ, Bosch J, et al. Rivaroxaban with or without aspirin in stable cardiovascular disease. N Engl J Med. 2017;377(14):1319–30. https://doi.org/10.1056/NEJMoa1709118.

118. Mega JL, Braunwald E, Wiviott SD, et al. Rivaroxaban in patients with a recent acute coronary syndrome. N Engl J Med. 2012;366(1):9–19. https://doi.org/10.1056/NEJMoa1112277.

119. Michniewicz E, Mlodawska E, Lopatowska P, Tomaszuk-Kazberuk A, Malyszko J. Patients with atrial fibrillation and coronary artery disease - double trouble. Adv Med Sci. 2018;63(1):30–5. https://doi.org/10.1016/j.advms.2017.06.005.

120. Hansen ML, Sørensen R, Clausen MT, et al. Risk of bleeding with single, dual, or triple therapy with warfarin, aspirin, and clopidogrel in patients with atrial fibrillation. Arch Intern Med. 2010;170(16):1433–41. https://doi.org/10.1001/archinternmed.2010.271.

121. van Rein N, Heide-Jørgensen U, Lijfering WM, Dekkers OM, Sørensen HT, Cannegieter SC. Major bleeding rates in atrial fibrillation patients on single, dual, or triple antithrombotic therapy. Circulation. 2019;139(6):775–86. https://doi.org/10.1161/circulationaha.118.036248.

122. Hindricks G, Potpara T, Dagres N, et al. 2020 ESC Guidelines for the diagnosis and management of atrial fibrillation developed in collaboration with the European Association of Cardio-Thoracic Surgery (EACTS): the Task Force for the diagnosis and management of

atrial fibrillation of the European Society of Cardiology (ESC) Developed with the special contribution of the European Heart Rhythm Association (EHRA) of the ESC. Eur Heart J. 2020; https://doi.org/10.1093/eurheartj/ehaa612.

123. January CT, Wann LS, Calkins H, et al. 2019 AHA/ACC/HRS focused update of the 2014 AHA/ACC/HRS guideline for the management of patients with atrial fibrillation: a report of the American College of Cardiology/American Heart Association Task Force on Clinical Practice Guidelines and the Heart Rhythm Society in Collaboration With the Society of Thoracic Surgeons. Circulation. 2019;140(2):e125–51. https://doi.org/10.1161/CIR.0000000000000665.

124. Kleindorfer DO, Towfighi A, Chaturvedi S, et al. 2021 Guideline for the prevention of stroke in patients with stroke and transient ischemic attack: a guideline from the American Heart Association/American Stroke Association. Stroke. 2021;52(7):e364–467. https://doi.org/10.1161/STR.0000000000000375.

125. Fonseca AC, Merwick Á, Dennis M, et al. European Stroke Organisation (ESO) guidelines on management of transient ischaemic attack. Eur Stroke J. 2021;6(2):CLXIII–CLXXXVI. https://doi.org/10.1177/2396987321992905.

126. Wang Y, Wang Y, Zhao X, et al. Clopidogrel with aspirin in acute minor stroke or transient ischemic attack. N Engl J Med. 2013;369(1):11–9. https://doi.org/10.1056/NEJMoa1215340.

127. Johnston SC, Easton JD, Farrant M, et al. Clopidogrel and aspirin in acute ischemic stroke and high-risk TIA. N Engl J Med. 2018;379(3):215–25. https://doi.org/10.1056/NEJMoa1800410.

128. Johnston SC, Amarenco P, Denison H, et al. Ticagrelor and aspirin or aspirin alone in acute ischemic stroke or TIA. N Engl J Med. 2020;383(3):207–17. https://doi.org/10.1056/NEJMoa1916870.

129. Wang Y, Johnston C, Bath PM, et al. Clopidogrel with aspirin in High-risk patients with Acute Non-disabling Cerebrovascular Events II (CHANCE-2): rationale and design of a multicentre randomised trial. Stroke Vasc Neurol. 2021;6(2):280–5. https://doi.org/10.1136/svn-2020-000791.

130. Ding L, Peng B. Efficacy and safety of dual antiplatelet therapy in the elderly for stroke prevention: a systematic review and meta-analysis. Eur J Neurol. 2018;25(10):1276–84. https://doi.org/10.1111/ene.13695.

131. Dawson J, Merwick Á, Webb A, Dennis M, Ferrari J, Fonseca AC. European Stroke Organisation expedited recommendation for the use of short-term dual antiplatelet therapy early after minor stroke and high-risk TIA. Eur Stroke J. 2021;6(2):CLXXXVII–CXCI. https://doi.org/10.1177/23969873211000877.

132. Pan Y, Elm JJ, Li H, et al. Outcomes associated with clopidogrel-aspirin use in minor stroke or transient ischemic attack: a pooled analysis of Clopidogrel in High-Risk Patients With Acute Non-Disabling Cerebrovascular Events (CHANCE) and Platelet-Oriented Inhibition in New TIA and Minor Ischemic Stroke (POINT) Trials. JAMA Neurol. 2019;76(12):1466–73. https://doi.org/10.1001/jamaneurol.2019.2531.

133. Diener HC, Bogousslavsky J, Brass LM, et al. Aspirin and clopidogrel compared with clopidogrel alone after recent ischaemic stroke or transient ischaemic attack in high-risk patients (MATCH): randomised, double-blind, placebo-controlled trial. Lancet. 2004;364(9431):331–7. https://doi.org/10.1016/s0140-6736(04)16721-4.

134. Benavente OR, Hart RG, McClure LA, Szychowski JM, Coffey CS, Pearce LA. Effects of clopidogrel added to aspirin in patients with recent lacunar stroke. N Engl J Med. 2012;367(9):817–25. https://doi.org/10.1056/NEJMoa1204133.

135. Aboyans V, Ricco J-B, Bartelink M-LEL, et al. 2017 ESC guidelines on the diagnosis and treatment of peripheral arterial diseases, in collaboration with the European Society for Vascular Surgery (ESVS): document covering atherosclerotic disease of extracranial carotid and vertebral, mesenteric, renal, upper and lower extremity arteries. Endorsed by: the European Stroke Organization (ESO) The Task Force for the Diagnosis and Treatment of Peripheral Arterial Diseases of the European Society of Cardiology (ESC) and of the

European Society for Vascular Surgery (ESVS). Eur Heart J. 2018;39(9):763–816. https://doi.org/10.1093/eurheartj/ehx095.

136. Gerhard-Herman MD, Gornik HL, Barrett C, et al. 2016 AHA/ACC guideline on the management of patients with lower extremity peripheral artery disease: executive summary: a report of the American College of Cardiology/American Heart Association Task Force on Clinical Practice Guidelines. Circulation. 2017;135(12):e686–725. https://doi.org/10.1161/CIR.0000000000000470.

137. Navarese EP, Wernly B, Lichtenauer M, et al. Dual vs single antiplatelet therapy in patients with lower extremity peripheral artery disease; a meta-analysis. Int J Cardiol. 2018;269:292–7. https://doi.org/10.1016/j.ijcard.2018.07.009.

138. Franklin SS, Larson MG, Khan SA, et al. Does the relation of blood pressure to coronary heart disease risk change with aging? The Framingham Heart Study. Circulation. 2001;103(9):1245–9. https://doi.org/10.1161/01.cir.103.9.1245.

139. Saklayen MG, Deshpande NV. Timeline of history of hypertension treatment. Front Cardiovasc Med. 2016;3:3–3. https://doi.org/10.3389/fcvm.2016.00003.

140. Goldring W, Chasis H. Antihypertensive drug therapy; an appraisal. Arch Intern Med. 1965;115:523–5. https://doi.org/10.1001/archinte.1960.03860170005002.

141. Tsimploulis A, Sheriff HM, Lam PH, et al. Systolic-diastolic hypertension versus isolated systolic hypertension and incident heart failure in older adults: Insights from the Cardiovascular Health Study. Int J Cardiol. May 15 2017;235:11–6. https://doi.org/10.1016/j.ijcard.2017.02.139.

142. Oliveros E, Patel H, Kyung S, et al. Hypertension in older adults: assessment, management, and challenges. Clin Cardiol. 2020;43(2):99–107. https://doi.org/10.1002/clc.23303.

143. Pierdomenico SD, Pierdomenico AM, Coccina F, Porreca E. Prognosis of masked and white coat uncontrolled hypertension detected by ambulatory blood pressure monitoring in elderly treated hypertensive patients. Am J Hypertens. 2017;30(11):1106–11. https://doi.org/10.1093/ajh/hpx104.

144. Bobrie G, Chatellier G, Genes N, et al. Cardiovascular prognosis of "masked hypertension" detected by blood pressure self-measurement in elderly treated hypertensive patients. JAMA. 2004;291(11):1342–9. https://doi.org/10.1001/jama.291.11.1342.

145. Lewington S, Clarke R, Qizilbash N, Peto R, Collins R. Age-specific relevance of usual blood pressure to vascular mortality: a meta-analysis of individual data for one million adults in 61 prospective studies. Lancet. 2002;360(9349):1903–13. https://doi.org/10.1016/s0140-6736(02)11911-8.

146. Musini VM, Tejani AM, Bassett K, Puil L, Wright JM. Pharmacotherapy for hypertension in adults 60 years or older. Cochrane Database Syst Rev. 2019;(6) https://doi.org/10.1002/14651858.CD000028.pub3.

147. Hughes D, Judge C, Murphy R, et al. Association of blood pressure lowering with incident dementia or cognitive impairment: a systematic review and meta-analysis. JAMA. 2020;323(19):1934–44. https://doi.org/10.1001/jama.2020.4249.

148. Alsarah A, Alsara O, Bachauwa G. Hypertension management in the elderly: what is the optimal target blood pressure? Heart Views. 2019;20(1):11–6. https://doi.org/10.4103/HEARTVIEWS.HEARTVIEWS_28_18.

149. Wright JT, Fine LJ, Lackland DT, Ogedegbe G, Dennison Himmelfarb CR. Evidence supporting a systolic blood pressure goal of less than 150 mmHg in patients aged 60 years or older: the minority view. Ann Intern Med. 2014;160(7):499–503. https://doi.org/10.7326/M13-2981.

150. James PA, Oparil S, Carter BL, et al. 2014 Evidence-based guideline for the management of high blood pressure in adults: report from the panel members appointed to the Eighth Joint National Committee (JNC 8). JAMA. 2014;311(5):507–20. https://doi.org/10.1001/jama.2013.284427.

151. Rahman F, McEvoy JW. The J-shaped curve for blood pressure and cardiovascular disease risk: historical context and recent updates. Curr Atheroscler Rep. 2017;19(8):34. https://doi.org/10.1007/s11883-017-0670-1.
152. Vidal-Petiot E, Ford I, Greenlaw N, et al. Cardiovascular event rates and mortality according to achieved systolic and diastolic blood pressure in patients with stable coronary artery disease: an international cohort study. Lancet. 2016;388(10056):2142–52. https://doi.org/10.1016/s0140-6736(16)31326-5.
153. Boshuizen HC, Izaks GJ, van Buuren S, Ligthart GJ. Blood pressure and mortality in elderly people aged 85 and older: community based study. BMJ. 1998;316(7147):1780–4. https://doi.org/10.1136/bmj.316.7147.1780.
154. Mattila K, Haavisto M, Rajala S, Heikinheimo R. Blood pressure and five year survival in the very old. BMJ. 1988;296(6626):887–9. https://doi.org/10.1136/bmj.296.6626.887.
155. Dillon P, Smith SM, Gallagher PJ, Cousins G. Association between gaps in antihypertensive medication adherence and injurious falls in older community-dwelling adults: a prospective cohort study. BMJ Open. 2019;9(3):e022927. https://doi.org/10.1136/bmjopen-2018-022927.
156. Tinetti ME, Han L, Lee DS, et al. Antihypertensive medications and serious fall injuries in a nationally representative sample of older adults. JAMA Intern Med. 2014;174(4):588–95. https://doi.org/10.1001/jamainternmed.2013.14764.
157. Beckett NS, Connor M, Sadler JD, Fletcher AE, Bulpitt CJ. Orthostatic fall in blood pressure in the very elderly hypertensive: results from the hypertension in the very elderly trial (HYVET) - pilot. J Hum Hypertens. 1999;13(12):839–40. https://doi.org/10.1038/sj.jhh.1000901.
158. Butt DA, Mamdani M, Austin PC, Tu K, Gomes T, Glazier RH. The risk of hip fracture after initiating antihypertensive drugs in the elderly. Arch Intern Med. 2012;172(22):1739–44. https://doi.org/10.1001/2013.jamainternmed.469.
159. Stroup-Benham CA, Markides KS, Black SA, Goodwin JS. Relationship between low blood pressure and depressive symptomatology in older people. J Am Geriatr Soc. 2000;48(3):250–5. https://doi.org/10.1111/j.1532-5415.2000.tb02642.x.
160. Shimbo D, Barrett Bowling C, Levitan EB, et al. Short-term risk of serious fall injuries in older adults initiating and intensifying treatment with antihypertensive medication. Circ Cardiovasc Qual Outcomes. 2016;9(3):222–9. https://doi.org/10.1161/circoutcomes.115.002524.
161. Kahlaee HR, Latt MD, Schneider CR. Association between chronic or acute use of antihypertensive class of medications and falls in older adults. A systematic review and meta-analysis. Am J Hypertens. 2018;31(4):467–79. https://doi.org/10.1093/ajh/hpx189.
162. Oates DJ, Berlowitz DR, Glickman ME, Silliman RA, Borzecki AM. Blood pressure and survival in the oldest old. J Am Geriatr Soc. 2007;55(3):383–8. https://doi.org/10.1111/j.1532-5415.2007.01069.x.
163. Amery A, Birkenhäger W, Brixko P, et al. Mortality and morbidity results from the European Working Party on High Blood Pressure in the Elderly trial. Lancet. 1985;1(8442):1349–54. https://doi.org/10.1016/s0140-6736(85)91783-0.
164. Coope J, Warrender TS. Randomised trial of treatment of hypertension in elderly patients in primary care. BMJ. 1986;293(6555):1145–51. https://doi.org/10.1136/bmj.293.6555.1145.
165. Perry HM Jr, Smith WM, McDonald RH, et al. Morbidity and mortality in the Systolic Hypertension in the Elderly Program (SHEP) pilot study. Stroke. 1989;20(1):4–13. https://doi.org/10.1161/01.str.20.1.4.
166. Vogt TM, Ireland CC, Black D, Camel G, Hughes G. Recruitment of elderly volunteers for a multicenter clinical trial: the SHEP pilot study. Control Clin Trials. 1986;7(2):118–33. https://doi.org/10.1016/0197-2456(86)90028-0.
167. Hulley SB, Feigal D, Ireland C, Kuller LH, Smith WM. Systolic Hypertension in the Elderly Program (SHEP). The first three months. J Am Geriatr Soc. 1986;34(2):101–5. https://doi.org/10.1111/j.1532-5415.1986.tb05476.x.

168. Hulley SB, Furberg CD, Gurland B, et al. Systolic Hypertension in the Elderly Program (SHEP): antihypertensive efficacy of chlorthalidone. Am J Cardiol. 1985;56(15):913–20. https://doi.org/10.1016/0002-9149(85)90404-7.

169. SHEP Cooperative Research Group. Prevention of stroke by antihypertensive drug treatment in older persons with isolated systolic hypertension: final results of the Systolic Hypertension in the Elderly Program (SHEP). JAMA. 1991;265(24):3255–64. https://doi.org/10.1001/jama.1991.03460240051027.

170. SHEP Cooperative Research Group. Rationale and design of a randomized clinical trial on prevention of stroke in isolated systolic hypertension. The Systolic Hypertension in the Elderly Program (SHEP) Cooperative Research Group. J Clin Epidemiol. 1988;41(12):1197–208. https://doi.org/10.1016/0895-4356(88)90024-8.

171. Charlesworth CJ, Peralta CA, Odden MC. Functional status and antihypertensive therapy in older adults: a new perspective on old data. Am J Hypertens. 2016;29(6):690–5. https://doi.org/10.1093/ajh/hpv177.

172. Dahlöf B, Lindholm LH, Hansson L, Scherstén B, Ekbom T, Wester PO. Morbidity and mortality in the Swedish Trial in Old Patients with Hypertension (STOP-Hypertension). Lancet. 1991;338(8778):1281–5. https://doi.org/10.1016/0140-6736(91)92589-t.

173. Dahlöf B, Hansson L, Lindholm LH, Scherstén B, Ekbom T, Wester PO. Swedish Trial in Old Patients with Hypertension (STOP-Hypertension) analyses performed up to 1992. Clin Exp Hypertens. 1993;15(6):925–39. https://doi.org/10.3109/10641969309037082.

174. MRC Working Party. Medical Research Council trial of treatment of hypertension in older adults: principal results. MRC Working Party. BMJ. 1992;304(6824):405–12. https://doi.org/10.1136/bmj.304.6824.405.

175. Gong L, Zhang W, Zhu Y, et al. Shanghai trial of nifedipine in the elderly (STONE). J Hypertens. 1996;14(10):1237–45. https://doi.org/10.1097/00004872-199610000-00013.

176. Staessen JA, Fagard R, Thijs L, et al. Randomised double-blind comparison of placebo and active treatment for older patients with isolated systolic hypertension. Lancet. 1997;350(9080):757–64. https://doi.org/10.1016/S0140-6736(97)05381-6.

177. Amery A, Birkenhäger W, Bulpitt CJ, et al. Syst-Eur. A multicentre trial on the treatment of isolated systolic hypertension in the elderly: objectives, protocol, and organization. Aging (Milano). 1991;3(3):287–302. https://doi.org/10.1007/bf03324024.

178. Liu L, Wang JG, Gong L, Liu G, Staessen JA. Comparison of active treatment and placebo in older Chinese patients with isolated systolic hypertension. Systolic Hypertension in China (Syst-China) Collaborative Group. J Hypertens. 1998;16(12 Pt 1):1823–9. https://doi.org/10.1097/00004872-199816120-00016.

179. Bulpitt CJ, Beckett NS, Cooke J, et al. Results of the pilot study for the Hypertension in the Very Elderly Trial. J Hypertens. 2003;21(12):2409–17. https://doi.org/10.1097/00004872-200312000-00030.

180. Bulpitt CJ, Fletcher AE, Amery A, et al. The Hypertension in the Very Elderly Trial (HYVET). Rationale, methodology and comparison with previous trials. Drugs Aging. 1994;5(3):171–83. https://doi.org/10.2165/00002512-199405030-00003.

181. Bulpitt C, Fletcher A, Beckett N, et al. Hypertension in the Very Elderly Trial (HYVET): protocol for the main trial. Drugs Aging. 2001;18(3):151–64. https://doi.org/10.2165/00002512-200118030-00001.

182. Beckett NS, Peters R, Fletcher AE, et al. Treatment of hypertension in patients 80 years of age or older. N Engl J Med. 2008;358(18):1887–98. https://doi.org/10.1056/NEJMoa0801369.

183. Warwick J, Falaschetti E, Rockwood K, et al. No evidence that frailty modifies the positive impact of antihypertensive treatment in very elderly people: an investigation of the impact of frailty upon treatment effect in the HYpertension in the Very Elderly Trial (HYVET) study, a double-blind, placebo-controlled study of antihypertensives in people with hypertension aged 80 and over. BMC Med. 2015;13:78. https://doi.org/10.1186/s12916-015-0328-1.

184. JATOS Study Group. Principal results of the Japanese trial to assess optimal systolic blood pressure in elderly hypertensive patients (JATOS). Hypertens Res. 2008;31(12):2115–27. https://doi.org/10.1291/hypres.31.2115.

185. Jatos Study Group. The Japanese Trial to Assess Optimal Systolic Blood Pressure in Elderly Hypertensive Patients (JATOS): protocol, patient characteristics, and blood pressure during the first 12 months. Hypertens Res. 2005;28(6):513–20. https://doi.org/10.1291/hypres.28.513.
186. Ogihara T, Saruta T, Rakugi H, et al. Target blood pressure for treatment of isolated systolic hypertension in the elderly: valsartan in elderly isolated systolic hypertension study. Hypertension. 2010;56(2):196–202. https://doi.org/10.1161/hypertensionaha.109.146035.
187. Ogihara T, Saruta T, Matsuoka H, et al. Valsartan in elderly isolated systolic hypertension (VALISH) study: rationale and design. Hypertens Res. 2004;27(9):657–61. https://doi.org/10.1291/hypres.27.657.
188. Wei Y, Jin Z, Shen G, et al. Effects of intensive antihypertensive treatment on chinese hypertensive patients older than 70 years. J Clin Hypertens. 2013;15(6):420–7. https://doi.org/10.1111/jch.12094.
189. Williamson JD, Supiano MA, Applegate WB, et al. Intensive vs standard blood pressure control and cardiovascular disease outcomes in adults aged ≥75 years: a randomized clinical trial. JAMA. 2016;315(24):2673–82. https://doi.org/10.1001/jama.2016.7050.
190. Garrison SR, Kolber MR, Korownyk CS, McCracken RK, Heran BS, Allan GM. Blood pressure targets for hypertension in older adults. Cochrane Database Syst Rev. 2017;(8) https://doi.org/10.1002/14651858.CD011575.pub2.
191. Drazen JM, Morrissey S, Campion EW, Jarcho JA. A SPRINT to the finish. N Engl J Med. 2015;373(22):2174–5. https://doi.org/10.1056/NEJMe1513991.
192. Jones DW, Weatherly L, Hall JE. SPRINT: what remains unanswered and where do we go from here? Hypertension. 2016;67(2):261–2. https://doi.org/10.1161/hypertensionaha.115.06723.
193. Esler M. SPRINT, or false start, toward a lower universal treated blood pressure target in hypertension. Hypertension. 2016;67(2):266–7. https://doi.org/10.1161/HYPERTENSIONAHA.115.06735.
194. Chellingsworth M, Beevers DG. The treatment of hypertension in the elderly. Postgrad Med J. 1986;62(723):1–5. https://doi.org/10.1136/pgmj.62.723.1.
195. Messerli FH, Sulicka J. Correspondance: treatment of hypertension in the elderly. N Engl J Med. 2008;359(9):971–4. https://doi.org/10.1056/NEJMc081224.
196. Grassi G, Quarti-Trevano F, Casati A, Dell'Oro R. Threshold and target for blood pressure lowering in the elderly. Curr Atheroscler Rep. 2016;18(12):70. https://doi.org/10.1007/s11883-016-0627-9.
197. Bress AP, Tanner RM, Hess R, Colantonio LD, Shimbo D, Muntner P. Generalizability of SPRINT results to the U.S. adult population. J Am Coll Cardiol. 2016;67(5):463–72. https://doi.org/10.1016/j.jacc.2015.10.037.
198. The Accord Study Group. Effects of intensive blood-pressure control in type 2 diabetes mellitus. N Engl J Med. 2010;362(17):1575–85. https://doi.org/10.1056/NEJMoa1001286.
199. Perkovic V, Rodgers A. Redefining blood-pressure targets—SPRINT starts the marathon. N Engl J Med. 2015;373(22):2175–8. https://doi.org/10.1056/NEJMe1513301.
200. Margolis KL, Palermo L, Vittinghoff E, et al. Intensive blood pressure control, falls, and fractures in patients with type 2 diabetes: the ACCORD trial. J Gen Intern Med. 2014;29(12):1599–606. https://doi.org/10.1007/s11606-014-2961-3.
201. Kjeldsen SE, Mancia G. The un-observed automated office blood pressure measurement technique used in the SPRINT study points to a standard target office systolic blood pressure <140 mmHg. Curr Hypertens Rep. 2017;19(1):3. https://doi.org/10.1007/s11906-017-0700-y.
202. Myers MG, Godwin M, Dawes M, Kiss A, Tobe SW, Kaczorowski J. Measurement of blood pressure in the office. Hypertension. 2010;55(2):195–200. https://doi.org/10.1161/HYPERTENSIONAHA.109.141879.
203. Benetos A, Petrovic M, Strandberg T. Hypertension management in older and frail older patients. Circ Res. 2019;124(7):1045–60. https://doi.org/10.1161/CIRCRESAHA.118.313236.
204. Ambrosius WT, Sink KM, Foy CG, et al. The design and rationale of a multicenter clinical trial comparing two strategies for control of systolic blood pressure: the Systolic

Blood Pressure Intervention Trial (SPRINT). Clin Trials. 2014;11(5):532–46. https://doi.org/10.1177/1740774514537404.

205. Wright JT, Whelton PK, Reboussin DM. Correspondance: A randomized trial of intensive versus standard blood-pressure control. N Engl J Med. 2016;374(23):2290–5. https://doi.org/10.1056/NEJMc1602668.

206. Pfeffer M. Correspondance: A randomized trial of intensive versus standard blood-pressure control. N Engl J Med. 2016;374(23):2290–5. https://doi.org/10.1056/NEJMc1602668.

207. Baffour-Awuah B, Dieberg G, Pearson MJ, Smart NA. Blood pressure control in older adults with hypertension: a systematic review with meta-analysis and meta-regression. Int J Cardiol Hypertens. 2020;6:100040. https://doi.org/10.1016/j.ijchy.2020.100040.

208. Delgado J, Masoli JAH, Bowman K, et al. Outcomes of treated hypertension at age 80 and older: cohort analysis of 79,376 individuals. J Am Geriatr Soc. 2017;65(5):995–1003. https://doi.org/10.1111/jgs.14712.

209. Gueyffier F, Bulpitt C, Boissel JP, et al. Antihypertensive drugs in very old people: a subgroup meta-analysis of randomised controlled trials. INDANA Group. Lancet. 1999;353(9155):793–6. https://doi.org/10.1016/s0140-6736(98)08127-6.

210. Kostis JB. Treating hypertension in the very old. N Engl J Med. 2008;358(18):1958–60. https://doi.org/10.1056/NEJMe0801709.

211. Benetos A, Bulpitt CJ, Petrovic M, et al. An expert opinion from the European Society of Hypertension-European Union Geriatric Medicine Society Working Group on the management of hypertension in very old, frail subjects. Hypertension. 2016;67(5):820–5. https://doi.org/10.1161/hypertensionaha.115.07020.

212. Bejan-Angoulvant T, Saadatian-Elahi M, Wright JM, et al. Treatment of hypertension in patients 80 years and older: the lower the better? A meta-analysis of randomized controlled trials. J Hypertens. 2010;28(7):1366–72. https://doi.org/10.1097/hjh.0b013e328339f9c5.

213. Morley JE. Systolic hypertension should not be treated in persons aged 80 and older until blood pressure is greater than 160 mmHg. J Am Geriatr Soc. 2013;61(7):1197–8. https://doi.org/10.1111/jgs.12322_1.

214. Sheppard JP, Burt J, Lown M, et al. Effect of antihypertensive medication reduction vs usual care on short-term blood pressure control in patients with hypertension aged 80 years and older: the OPTIMISE randomized clinical trial. JAMA. 2020;323(20):2039–51. https://doi.org/10.1001/jama.2020.4871.

215. Chobanian AV. SPRINT results in older patients: how low to go? JAMA. 2016;315(24):2669–70. https://doi.org/10.1001/jama.2016.7070.

216. Vetrano DL, Palmer KM, Galluzzo L, et al. Hypertension and frailty: a systematic review and meta-analysis. BMJ Open. 2018;8(12):e024406. https://doi.org/10.1136/bmjopen-2018-024406.

217. Zhang XE, Cheng B, Wang Q. Relationship between high blood pressure and cardiovascular outcomes in elderly frail patients: a systematic review and meta-analysis. Geriatr Nurs. 2016;37(5):385–92. https://doi.org/10.1016/j.gerinurse.2016.05.006.

218. Liu P, Li Y, Zhang Y, Mesbah SE, Ji T, Ma L. Frailty and hypertension in older adults: current understanding and future perspectives. Hypertens Res. 2020;43(12):1352–60. https://doi.org/10.1038/s41440-020-0510-5.

219. Bromfield SG, Ngameni C-A, Colantonio LD, et al. Blood pressure, antihypertensive polypharmacy, frailty, and risk for serious fall injuries among older treated adults with hypertension. Hypertension. 2017;70(2):259–66. https://doi.org/10.1161/HYPERTENSIONAHA.116.09390.

220. Odden MC, Peralta CA, Haan MN, Covinsky KE. Rethinking the association of high blood pressure with mortality in elderly adults: the impact of frailty. Arch Intern Med. 2012;172(15):1162–8. https://doi.org/10.1001/archinternmed.2012.2555.

221. Pajewski NM, Williamson JD, Applegate WB, et al. Characterizing frailty status in the systolic blood pressure intervention trial. J Gerontol A. 2016;71(5):649–55. https://doi.org/10.1093/gerona/glv228.

222. Bowling CB, Lee A, Williamson JD. Blood pressure control among older adults with hypertension: narrative review and introduction of a framework for improving care. Am J Hypertens. 2021;34(3):258–66. https://doi.org/10.1093/ajh/hpab002.
223. Mühlbauer V, Dallmeier D, Brefka S, Bollig C, Voigt-Radloff S, Denkinger M. The pharmacological treatment of arterial hypertension in frail, older patients—a systematic review. Dtsch Arztebl Int. 2019;116(3):23–30. https://doi.org/10.3238/arztebl.2019.0023.
224. Boockvar KS, Song W, Lee S, Intrator O. Hypertension treatment in US long-term nursing home residents with and without dementia. J Am Geriatr Soc. 2019;67(10):2058–64. https://doi.org/10.1111/jgs.16081.
225. Vu M, Schleiden LJ, Harlan ML, Thorpe CT. Hypertension management in nursing homes: review of evidence and considerations for care. Curr Hypertens Rep. 2020;22(1):8. https://doi.org/10.1007/s11906-019-1012-1.
226. Onder G, Landi F, Fusco D, et al. Recommendations to prescribe in complex older adults: results of the CRIteria to assess appropriate Medication use among Elderly complex patients (CRIME) project. Drugs Aging. 2014;31(1):33–45. https://doi.org/10.1007/s40266-013-0134-4.
227. Law MR, Morris JK, Wald NJ. Use of blood pressure lowering drugs in the prevention of cardiovascular disease: meta-analysis of 147 randomised trials in the context of expectations from prospective epidemiological studies. BMJ. 2009;338:b1665. https://doi.org/10.1136/bmj.b1665.
228. Kjeldsen SE, Stenehjem A, Os I, et al. Treatment of high blood pressure in elderly and octogenarians: European Society of Hypertension statement on blood pressure targets. Blood Press. 2016;25(6):333–6. https://doi.org/10.1080/08037051.2016.1236329.
229. Williams B, Mancia G, Spiering W, et al. 2018 ESC/ESH guidelines for the management of arterial hypertension: the Task Force for the management of arterial hypertension of the European Society of Cardiology (ESC) and the European Society of Hypertension (ESH). Eur Heart J. 2018;39(33):3021–104. https://doi.org/10.1093/eurheartj/ehy339.
230. Whelton PK, Carey RM, Aronow WS, et al. 2017 ACC/AHA/AAPA/ABC/ACPM/AGS/APhA/ASH/ASPC/NMA/PCNA Guideline for the prevention, detection, evaluation, and management of high blood pressure in adults: a report of the American College of Cardiology/American Heart Association Task Force on Clinical Practice Guidelines. Hypertension. 2018;71(6):e13–e115. https://doi.org/10.1161/HYP.0000000000000065.
231. National Institute for Health and Care Excellence. Hypertension in adults: diagnosis and management. nice.org.uk/guidance/ng136. Accessed 24 May 2021.
232. Unger T, Borghi C, Charchar F, et al. 2020 International Society of Hypertension Global Hypertension practice guidelines. Hypertension. 2020;75(6):1334–57. https://doi.org/10.1161/HYPERTENSIONAHA.120.15026.
233. Rabi DM, McBrien KA, Sapir-Pichhadze R, et al. Hypertension Canada's 2020 comprehensive guidelines for the prevention, diagnosis, risk assessment, and treatment of hypertension in adults and children. Can J Cardiol. 2020;36(5):596–624. https://doi.org/10.1016/j.cjca.2020.02.086.
234. Harrap SB, Lung T, Chalmers J. New blood pressure guidelines pose difficult choices for Australian physicians. Circ Res. 2019;124(7):975–7. https://doi.org/10.1161/CIRCRESAHA.118.314637.
235. Gabb GM, Mangoni AA, Anderson CS, et al. Guideline for the diagnosis and management of hypertension in adults—2016. Med J Aust. 2016;205(2):85–9. https://doi.org/10.5694/mja16.00526.
236. Qaseem A, Wilt TJ, Rich R, Humphrey LL, Frost J, Forciea MA. Pharmacologic treatment of hypertension in adults aged 60 years or older to higher versus lower blood pressure targets: a clinical practice guideline from the American College of Physicians and the American Academy of Family Physicians. Ann Intern Med. 2017;166(6):430–7. https://doi.org/10.7326/m16-1785.

Atherosclerotic Cardiovascular Disease Prevention in the Older Adult: Part 2

Ella Murphy, Marie Therese Cooney, and John W. McEvoy

1 Cholesterol

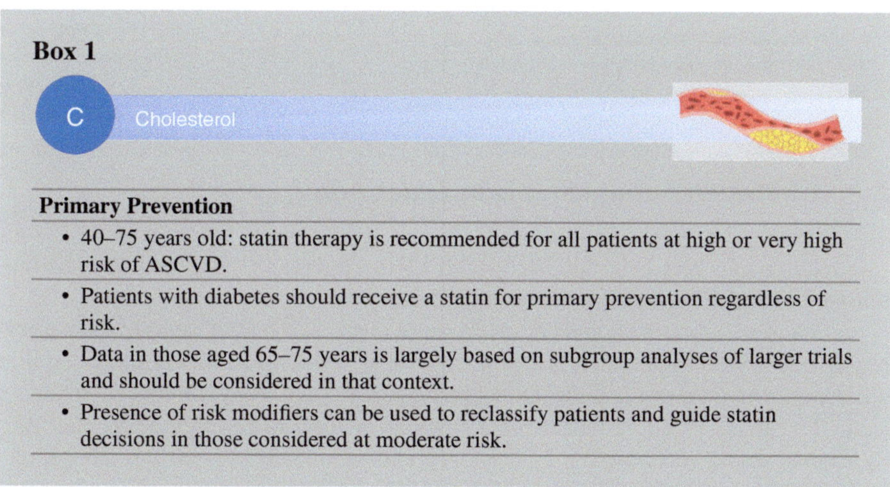

Primary Prevention

- 40–75 years old: statin therapy is recommended for all patients at high or very high risk of ASCVD.
- Patients with diabetes should receive a statin for primary prevention regardless of risk.
- Data in those aged 65–75 years is largely based on subgroup analyses of larger trials and should be considered in that context.
- Presence of risk modifiers can be used to reclassify patients and guide statin decisions in those considered at moderate risk.

E. Murphy · J. W. McEvoy (✉)
University Hospital Galway and SAOLTA University Health Care Group, Galway, Ireland

National University of Ireland School of Medicine, Galway, Ireland

National Institute for Prevention and Cardiovascular Health, National University of Ireland Galway, Galway, Ireland
e-mail: johnwilliam.mcevoy@nuigalway.ie

M. T. Cooney
St Vincent's University Hospital, Dublin, Ireland

School of Medicine, University College Dublin, Dublin, Ireland

© The Author(s), under exclusive license to Springer Nature Switzerland AG 2023
T. M. Leucker, G. Gerstenblith (eds.), *Cardiovascular Disease in the Elderly*, Contemporary Cardiology, https://doi.org/10.1007/978-3-031-16594-8_2

- Patients >75 years old have been largely underrepresented in major lipid trials. Currently, evidence would suggest that statins offer at least some benefit, but all guidelines emphasise an individualised clinical assessment and risk discussion.
- There is little guidance around what to do once a patient, who is already taking a statin, reaches a more advanced age or develops comorbidities. Given the lack of evidence currently available for benefit in primary prevention adults over the age of 80 years, revaluation of the risk-benefit ratios as patients become older seems pragmatic.

Secondary Prevention

- Statin therapy is recommended in the context of secondary prevention of ASCVD for all age groups.
- SAMS are more common with higher dose statin therapy and become more common with increased co-morbidities.
- Moderate intensity, as opposed to high-intensity statins, may be more appropriate for certain patient groups (e.g., those with co-morbidities or more advanced age).
- Ezetimibe and PCSK-9 inhibitors can be added to statin therapy as required for those failing to meet LDL targets.
- To date, no randomised trials examining statin prescription in the context of either primary or secondary prevention have included a validated measure of frailty.

1.1 Cholesterol and ASCVD in Older Adults

The relationship between cholesterol and its lipoproteins (LDL, very low-density lipoprotein and HDL) and cardiovascular disease is well known. The role of LDL-C in particular as a dominant and causal driver of atherosclerotic disease in the general population is well established [1]. While the relative risks of ASCVD appear similar per 1 mmol/L increase in LDL-C at older ages, the absolute benefits of reducing LDL-C increase [2–5]. A recent meta-analysis of lipid-lowering therapy trial data by Gencer et al., included 21,492 primary and secondary prevention older adults over the age of 75 years (mean age 79 years) [4]. They observed a 26% relative risk reduction in major vascular events for every 1 mmol/L reduction in LDL-C cholesterol (Rate ratio 0.74; 95% CI 0.61–0.89; $p = 0.0019$) over a median follow-up period of 2.2–6 years. Similarly, relative risk reductions in cardiovascular death, myocardial infarction, stroke and coronary revascularisation were 15%, 20%, 27% and 20% respectively for each 1 mmol/L reduction in LDL-C. Notably, the risk reductions in those over 75 years were comparable to those in patients younger than 75 years (p for interaction 0.37), suggesting that even the oldest old benefit from a reduction in LDL-C. In keeping with this, Mortensen et al. also demonstrated that the relative risk of developing an MI or ASCVD in those with high LDL-C levels compared to lower LDL-C levels was similar in primary prevention adults aged 70–100 compared to those aged 50–59 years [6]. Furthermore, they observed 2.5 myocardial infarctions per 1000 patient years for every 1 mmol/L increase in LDL-C in those aged 80–100 years, compared to 0.5 myocardial infarctions for those aged

50–59 years for the same LDL increase. Thus, the absolute benefits of reducing LDL-C in older patients is greater. For example, the estimated number needed to treat (NNT) for 5 years (using a moderate intensity statin), to prevent one MI was 80 in those aged 80–100 years, compared to 439 for those aged 50–59 years.

1.2   Elevated Cholesterol and All-Cause Mortality

While an elevated cholesterol level has been clearly associated with an increased risk of ASCVD, its association with all-cause mortality in older patients has generated significant debate, particularly within observational data. While some studies have failed to find any association between cholesterol and all-cause mortality, others have been contradictory, reporting both positive and inverse relationships, particularly among persons over 80 years old [3, 7, 8]. More recently, U-shaped relationships between LDL-C levels and all-cause mortality have also been reported; In other words, both low and high levels of LDL-C may be associated with increased mortality in the elderly [9, 10]. For example, following a multivariable adjusted analysis, Johannsen et al. reported that the concentration of LDL-C associated with the lowest risk of all-cause mortality was 3.6 mmol/L (140 mg/dL) in those not receiving lipid-lowering therapies, compared to 2.3 mmol/L (89 mg/dL) in those who were receiving lipid-lowering therapies, both of which are well above the target recommended by most preventive guidelines [9]. Some experts have used these observational findings, suggesting increased risk for death at very low levels of LDL-C, to argue against the use of statins among the elderly- especially given the paucity of randomized data in older adults.

The association of lower levels of cholesterol and increased mortality may be due to reverse causation. Low cholesterol and LDL-C levels may be a marker of poor health, poor nutritional status and frailty, all of which increase the risk of mortality in older adults [11–13]. Supporting this theory, Johannsen et al. demonstrated that those with lower LDL-C levels are more likely to have co-morbidities and that the association between all-cause mortality and lower LDL-C levels was reduced following adjustment for these baseline comorbidities (ASCVD, cancer, COPD or <5 years of follow up) [9]. However, other analyses have reported an increased risk for death with lower total cholesterol levels despite adjustment for comorbidities (e.g., obesity, hypertension, diabetes) and markers of frailty (physical inactivity, mobility limitation and cognitive impairment) [11, 14].While the latter analyses question whether reverse causality is the sole explanation for the U-shaped association of LDL-C with death, it is possible that these analyses were unable to fully adjust for all possible factors contributing to reverse causation, thereby resulting in residual confounding.

Other potential theories for this U-shaped observational relationship include that lipids and lipoproteins play a protective role in the setting of inflammation and so lower levels may make older patients more vulnerable to inflammatory processes and infections [11]. Higher LDL-C levels have also been inversely associated with cancer [7].

However, the findings from observational data of an inverse relationship between LDL-C and mortality are not supported by the recent meta-analysis of randomized trial data by Gencer et al., where they observed no increased risk of all-cause mortality (risk ratio per 1 mmol/L reduction in LDL-C; 0.93; 95% CI 0.84–1.02) in primary and secondary prevention patients >75 years treated with lipid-lowering therapies (either statin or non-statin), compared to those who received placebo or usual care [4]. As such, unlike in meta-analyses of younger samples, Gencer et al. did not find that LDL-C lowering reduced mortality. The authors did find that LDL-C lowering in this elderly sample did reduce fatal and non-fatal CVD. The mean achieved LDL across included studies was between 1 mmol/L (40 mg/dL) and 3.2 mmol/L (123.8 mg/dL), suggesting that lowering LDL to these levels is safe in this age group.

1.3   Laboratory Measurement of Cholesterol

Contrary to previous guidelines, current guidelines suggest that a non-fasting lipid profile is reasonable for most patients [15, 16]. This offers significant benefits for older patients who now no longer need to routinely fast prior to attending for the test. The exceptions, where a fasting sample is recommended, is in the setting of hypertriglyceridemia or suspected familial hyperlipidemia. Caution should be exerted when LDL-C levels are <1.8 mmol/L as the commonly used Friedewald equation can become less reliable at these levels, particularly in non-fasting samples [17]. The Martin/Hopkins method is a useful alternative in this setting, and also performs better in the setting of hypertriglyceridemia. Measurement of apolipoprotein B can be used as an alternative to LDL-C or can be used to refine risk in those at intermediate risk [16].

1.4   Primary Prevention Lipid-Lowering Therapy

The benefits of lipid-lowering therapy, particularly in those over the age of 75 years, are particularly controversial in the primary prevention of CVD. We will therefore discuss the topic across three different age groups (those 40 to ≤65, those 66–75 years and, those >75 years), focusing primarily on the latter two groups. These categories, while somewhat arbitrary, have been chosen to facilitate discussion of current guidelines and to support discussion of clusters of evidence available within each category. Improved dietary habits and increased exercise remain as first-line interventions for all patients, with pharmacological treatment recommended in appropriately selected individuals.

1.4.1 Primary Prevention Lipid-Lowering Therapy in Those Aged 40–65

Patients up to the age of 65 years, without a history of ASCVD but with elevated risk due to the presence of ASCVD risk factors, have been well represented in high-quality primary prevention statin trials that have consistently demonstrated an overwhelming benefit of statins in this cohort in reducing all-cause cardiovascular events in these patients [18] (Table 1). The quality of available data in this age cohort is reflected in the consensus among major guidelines in providing either a class I or strong recommendation for statin therapy for those deemed at very high or high risk for ASCVD in this age group [15, 16, 19, 20]. In fact, the AHA/ACC also recommend a minimum of a moderate intensity statin for all patients with diabetes mellitus aged 40–75 years, regardless of estimated 10-year risk [15]. For those patients deemed at borderline or intermediate/moderate risk, risk modifiers and coronary artery calcium scoring are recommended to guide decisions [15, 16, 19]. Ezetimibe and PCSK-9 inhibitors can be added on as required in those failing to reach appropriate LDL-C treatment goals on statin therapy alone [15, 16].

1.4.2 Primary Prevention Lipid-Lowering Therapy in Those Aged 65–75

Most of the data on patients nearing the age of 75 has been extrapolated from exploratory subgroup analyses of larger trials (see bottom portion of Table 1). Interpretation of this data, therefore, comes with the caveat that these analyses are likely underpowered and may therefore fail to detect small differences in outcomes between groups. Significantly, however, there appears to be little difference in the benefit between the old and young in most analyses.

A post-hoc analysis of the ALLHAT-LLT trial (Antihypertensive and Lipid-Lowering Treatment to Prevent Heart Attack Trial—Lipid Lowering Trial) found no reduction in all-cause mortality (140 events vs 130 events; HR 1.08; 95% CI 0.85–1.37; $p = 0.55$), cardiovascular mortality (64 events vs 62 events; HR 1.02; 95% CI 0.72–1.45; $p = 0.91$) or stroke (44 events vs 42 events; HR 1.03; 95% CI 0.68–1.57; $p = 0.89$), in the subgroup of participants aged 65–74 years who received pravastatin 40 mg compared to usual care [26]. These findings were in keeping with those younger than 65 years. This subgroup of patients aged 65–74 represented a relatively small percentage of the overall population (21%, or 2141 of the trial population). There was a significant crossover between the two study groups, with 29% of those in the usual care group taking a statin by year 6, compared to 77.9% in the pravastatin group, which may have diminished potential between-group differences.

The subsequent CARDS trial randomised patients with type 2 diabetes and at least one additional ASCVD risk factor, to either atorvastatin 10 mg daily or placebo. 1129 (40%) of the trial population were aged 65–75 years [31]. In contrast to ALLHAT-LLT, a subgroup analysis of CARDS participants between 65–75 years of

Table 1 Statin trials enrolling predominantly primary prevention older adults

	WOSCOPS [21, 22]	AFCAPS/ TexCAPS [23, 24]	ALLHAT-LLT [25, 26] [a]	PROSPER [27] [a] Mixture of primary and secondary prevention	ASCOT-LLA [28, 29] [a] Mixture of primary and secondary prevention	CARDS [30, 31]	MEGA [32, 33]	JUPITER [34]	HOPE-3 [35]
Year	1995	1998	2002	2002	2003	2004	2006	2008	2016
Trial Design	Double-blind, randomised, placebo-controlled trial	Randomised, double-blind, placebo-controlled trial	Multicentre, randomised, nonblinded trial	Double blind, randomised, placebo controlled, multicentre trial	Multicentre, international, prospective, randomised, open, blinded endpoint (PROBE), factorial trial	Multi-centre, randomised, double-blinded, placebo-controlled trial	Prospective, open labelled, blinded-endpoint, trial	Randomised, double blinded, placebo controlled, multicentre trial	Pragmatic, multicentre, international, double blind, randomised, placebo controlled, 2x2 factorial trial
Country	Scotland	USA (Texas)	513 primarily community based North American clinical centres	Scotland, Ireland and the Netherlands	Denmark, Iceland, Finland, Norway, Sweden, UK and Ireland	132 centres in UK and Ireland	Japan	26 countries (Europe, North America, South America, Africa, Asia)	21 countries (South America, North America, Australia, Asia, Europe, Africa)
Intervention	Pravastatin (40 mg daily)	Lovastatin (20-40 mg daily) plus diet	Pravastatin (40 mg daily)	Pravastatin (40 mg daily)	Atorvastatin (10 mg daily)	Atorvastatin (10 mg daily)	Diet plus pravastatin (mean dose 8.3 mg)	Rosuvastatin 20 mg daily	Rosuvastatin 10 mg daily
Control	Placebo	Placebo plus diet	Usual care	Placebo	Placebo	Placebo	Diet only	Placebo	Placebo
No of participants	6595	6605	10,355	5804 3239 (55.8%) primary prevention adults	10,305 (8834, 85.7% = no previous vascular disease)	2838	7832	17,802	12,705
Population	Hypercholesterolemic men (LDL >4.5 mmol/L)	Normal or mildly elevated LDL-C or TC, and reduced HDL	Stage 1 or 2 HTN with at least 1 additional CHD risk factor (14.2% had a history of CHD)	Secondary prevention adults OR primary prevention adults with at least 1 CVD risk factor. Total cholesterol 4-9 mmol/L	Hypertensive patients with at least three CVD risk factors with serum cholesterol ≤6.5 mmol/L	Type 2 diabetics with at least one CV risk factor	Hypercholesterol-emic patients	LDL <3.4 mmol/L Hs-CRP ≥2 mg/L	At least 1 CV risk factor

Proportion of secondary prevention patients	Primary prevention patients only	Primary prevention patients only	History of CHD = 14.2%	History of MI = 13.35% History of stroke or TIA = 11.2% History of PCI and CABG = 4.1% History of vascular disease = 44.2%	Previous stroke or TIA = 9.7% Peripheral vascular disease = 5% Other relevant cardiovascular disease = 3.8%	Primary prevention patients only	Primary prevention patients only	Primary prevention patients only	Primary prevention patients only
Age range	45–64	Men 45–73 Women 55–73	≥55 (whole cohort)	70–82 (whole cohort)	40–79	40–75	Men 40–70 Postmenopausal women 40–70	Men ≥50 Women ≥60	Men ≥55 or Women ≥65 Or women ≥60 with ≥2 risk factors
Age (years)	Mean 55.2	58	Mean 66.4	Mean 75.4 (whole cohort)	Mean 63	Mean 61.65	Mean 58	Median 66	Mean 65.75
Reported age categories of relevance to older persons	≥65 = 0	≥65 = 21%	≥65 and without history of ASCVC = 28%	≥70 = 100%	>60 = 63.75% >70 = 23.44% Whole cohort	60–70 years: 50% >70 years: 12%	23% ≥65 years	65 to <70 years: 26% ≥70 years: 32%[b]	65 to <70 years: 28% ≥70 years: 24%[b]
≥75 years of age	0	0	Without history of CHD = 7%	>75 = 2355 (41%)	>75 = 896 (9%)	>75 = 42 (1%)	0	>75 = 2176 (12%)	>75 = 1088 (8%)
Female	0%	15%	48.8%	51.7%	18.8%	32%	68.5%	38.2%	46.25%
Follow up	Mean 4.9 years	Mean 5.2 years	Mean 4.8 years	Mean 3.2 years	Median 3.3 years	Median 3.9 years	Mean 5.3 years	Median 1.9 years	Median 5.6 years

(continued)

Table 1 (continued)

Main trial outcomes

Primary outcome	Composite of non-fatal MI or death from coronary heart disease as a first event 174 vs 248 events (risk reduction 31%; 95% CI 14–43; $p < 0.001$)	First acute major coronary event (sudden cardiac death, fatal and non-fatal MI and unstable angina) 6.8 per 1000 person years vs 10.9 per 1000 person years (Relative risk 0.63, 95% CI 0.50–0.79; $p < 0.001$)	All-cause mortality 631 events vs 641 (relative risk 0.99; 95% 0.89–1.11; $p = 0.88$)	Composite of coronary heart disease death (definite or suspected), definite plus suspected nonfatal MI, and fatal plus nonfatal stroke Whole cohort: 14.1% vs 16.2% (HR 0.85; 95% CI 0.74–0.97; $p = 0.014$) Primary prevention patients only (no. 3239); 11.4% vs 12.1%; HR 0.94; 95% CI 0.77–1.15	Composite of nonfatal MI plus fatal CHD **Whole cohort:** 6 per 1000 patient years vs 9.4 per 1000 patient years (HR 0.64; 95% CI 0.50–0.83; $p = 0.0005$) **No previous vascular disease (no. 8834)** 5.5 per 1000 patient years vs 9.1 per 1000 patient years (HR 0.61; 95% CI 0.46–0.81; $p = 0.0005$)	Composite (deaths from acute MI, other acute CHD deaths, nonfatal MI, revascularization procedures, unstable angina, resuscitated cardiac arrest or stroke) 5.8% vs 9% (HR 0.63; 0.48–0.83; $p = 0.001$)	Coronary heart disease (fatal and nonfatal MI, angina, cardiac and sudden death, and coronary revascularisation) HR 0.67; 95% CI 0.49–0.91; $p = 0.01$	First major cardiovascular event (nonfatal MI, nonfatal stroke, hospitalisation for unstable angina, an arterial revascularisation procedure, or confirmed death from CV causes) 0.77 per 100 person years vs 1.36 per 100 person years (HR 0.56; 95% CI 0.46–0.69; $p < 0.00001$)	First co-primary outcome (death from CV causes, nonfatal MI, or nonfatal stroke): 3.5% vs 4.8% (HR 0.76; 95% CI 0.64–0.91; $p = 0.002$) Second co-primary outcome (first co-primary outcome, resuscitated cardiac arrest, heart failure, and revascularisation): 4.4% vs 5.7% (HR 0.75; 95% CI 0.64–0.88; $p < 0.001$)
All-cause mortality	106 events vs 135 events (Risk reduction 22%; 95% CI 0–40; $p = 0.051$)	NR	See primary outcome	Whole cohort: 10.3% vs 10.5% (HR 0.97; 95% CI 0.83–1.14; $p = 0.74$) Primary prevention cohort: Relative risk 0.96; 95% CI 0.88–1.04	**Whole cohort:** 11.1 per 1000 patient years vs 12.8 per 1000 patient years (HR 0.87; 95% CI 0.71–1.06; $p = 0.1649$)	4.3% vs 5.8% (HR 0.73; 95% CI 0.52–1.01; $p = 0.059$)	HR 0.72; 95% CI 0.51–1.01; $p = 0.055$	1 per 100 person years vs 1.25 per 100 person years (HR 0.80; 95% CI 0.67–0.97; $p = 0.02$)	5.3% vs 5.6% (HR 0.93; 95% CI 0.80–1.08; $p = 0.32$)

	WOSCOPS	AFCAPS/TexCAPS [36]	ALLHAT-LLT [26]	PROSPER	ASCOT-LLA	CARDS [37]	MEGA [36, 38]	JUPITER [39]	HOPE-3 [40][b]
Myocardial infarction	Definite nonfatal MI 143 events vs 204 events (risk reduction 31%; 95% CI 15–45; $p < 0.001$)	3.3 per 1000 person years vs 5.6 per 1000 person years (relative risk 0.60; 95% CI 0.43–0.83; $p = 0.002$)	NR	Whole cohort: Nonfatal MI; 7.7% vs 8.7% (HR 0.86; 95% CI 0.72–1.03; $p = 0.10$) Primary prevention cohort: Relative risk 0.91; 95% CI 0.72–1.14	NR	Fatal MI: 8 vs 20 events Nonfatal MI: 25 vs 41 events (first events)	HR 0.52; 95% CI 0.29–0.94; $p = 0.03$	0.17 per 100 patient years vs 0.37 per 100 patient years (HR 0.46; 95% CI 0.30–0.70; $p = 0.0002$)	0.7% vs 1.1% (HR 0.65; 95% CI 0.44–0.94)
Stroke	46 events vs 51 events (risk reduction 11%; 95% CI −33 to 40; $p = 0.57$)	NR	209 events vs 231 events (relative risk 0.91; 95% CI 0.75–1.09; $p = 0.31$)	Whole cohort: 4.7% vs 4.5% (HR 1.03; 95% CI 0.81–1.31; $p = 0.81$) c Primary prevention cohort; relative risk 1.03; 95% CI 0.73–1.45	Whole cohort: 5.4 per 1000 patient years vs 7.4 per 1000 patient years (HR 0.73; 95% CI 0.56–0.96; $p = 0.0236$)	1.5% vs 2.8% (HR 0.52; 95% CI 0.31–0.89)	HR 0.83; 95% CI 0.57–1.21; $p = 0.33$	0.18 per 100 patient years vs 0.34 per 100 patient years (HR 0.52;95% CI 0.41–0.72; $p < 0.0001$)	1.1% vs 1.6% (HR 0.70; 95% CI 0.52–0.95)
Death from CVD	All cardiovascular causes 50 vs 73 (risk reduction 32%; 95% CI 3–53; $p = 0.033$)	1 per 1000 person years vs 1.4 per 1000 person years	295 events vs 300 events (relative risk 0.99; 95% CI 0.84–1.16; $p = 0.91$)	CHD deaths 3.3% vs 4.2% (HR 0.76; 95% CI 0.58–0.99; $p = 0.043$)	Whole cohort: 4.4 per 1000 patient years vs 4.9 per 1000 patient years (HR 0.90; 95% CI 0.66–1.23; $p = 0.5066$)	NR	NR	NR	2.4% vs 2.7% (HR 0.89; 95% CI 0.72–1.11)

Post hoc subgroup analyses and data extracted from meta-analyses patients ≥ 65 (only primary prevention adults)

	WOSCOPS	AFCAPS/TexCAPS [36]	ALLHAT-LLT [26] (including primary prevention only)	PROSPER	ASCOT-LLA	CARDS [37]	MEGA [36, 38]	JUPITER [39]	HOPE-3 [40][b]
Subgroup	No participants > = 65	≥65 years	≥65 years	All patients ≥70 years	≥65 years	65–75 years	≥65 years	≥70 years	≥70

(continued)

Table 1 (continued)

Number of patients	All patients <65	1416 (21%)	2867	All patients ≥70 years	4445	1129 (40%)	1812 (23%)	5695 (32%)	3086 (24%)
Main outcome	All patients <65	NR	All-cause mortality 195 events vs 233 events; HR 1.18; 95% CI 0.97–1.42; $p = 0.09$ 65–74 years; 141 vs 130 events; HR 1.08; 95% CI 0.85–1.37; $p = 0.55$ ≥75 years; 92 vs 65 events; HR 1.34; 95% CI 0.98–1.84; $p = 0.07$	All patients ≥70 years	Major adverse cardiovascular event (MI, stroke, coronary revascularisation, sudden cardiac death, angina) Relative risk 0.82; 95% CI 0.73–0.93	Composite of major cardiovascular events (above) 7.2% vs 11.1% (relative risk −38%; 95% CI -58 to −8; $p = 0.017$)	Major adverse cardiovascular event (MI, stroke, coronary revascularisation, sudden cardiac death, angina) Relative risk 0.66 (95% CI 0.38–1.17)	First major cardiovascular event (above) 1.22 per 100 person years vs 1.99 per 100 person years; HR 0.61; 95% CI 0.46–0.82; $p < 0.001$	Composite of nonfatal MI, nonfatal stroke or CV death 1.25 per 100 person years vs 1.5 per 100 person years HR 0.83; 95% CI 0.64–1.07
All-cause mortality	All patients <65	Relative risk 1.01; 95% CI 0.64–1.58	See primary outcome	All patients ≥70 years	Relative risk 0.97; 95% CI 0.77–1.22	7% vs 8.8% (Relative risk −22%; 95% CI −49 to 18; $p = 0.245$)	Relative risk 0.71 (95% CI 0.41–1.22)	1.63 per 100 person years vs 2.04 per 100 person years; HR 0.80; 95% CI 0.62–1.04; $p = 0.090$	NR
MI	All patients <65	Relative risk 0.38; 95% CI 0.18–0.82	Relative risk 0.81; 95% CI 0.67–0.99	All patients ≥70 years	Relative risk 0.63; 95% CI 0.45–0.89	Fatal MI: 0.3% vs 2.2% Nonfatal MI 1.9% vs 3.9% (first event)	NR	0.27 per 100 person years vs 0.50 per 100 person years; HR 0.55; 95% CI 0.31–1.00; $p = 0.034$	NR

| Stroke | All patients <65 | NR | Stroke (fatal and nonfatal) 71 vs 65 events; HR 1.06; 95% CI 0.76–1.49; $p = 0.72$ | All patients ≥70 years | Relative risk 0.80; 95% CI 0.58–1.11 | 2.3% vs 4.3% (relative risk, −49%; 95% CI −74 to 0; $p = 0.051$) | Relative risk 0.44 (95% CI 0.21–0.91) | 0.35 per 100 person years vs 0.64 per 100 person years; HR 0.55; 95% CI 0.33–0.93; $p = 0.023$ | NR |

MI myocardial infarction, *CI* confidence interval, *NR* not reported, *HR* hazard ratio, *CV* cardiovascular, *CVD* cardiovascular disease, *LDL* low density lipoprotein, *CHD* coronary heart disease

[a] Included both primary and secondary prevention patients

[b] Taken from the meta-analysis by Ridker et al. [40]

[c] There was an apparent reduction in TIAs (2.7% vs 3.5%; HR 0.75; 95% CI 0.55–1.00; $p = 0.051$). The observed stroke rate was 4.5% which was about half of that expected, therefore caution when interpreting these results

age demonstrated a 38% relative risk reduction in major cardiovascular events (composite of deaths from acute MI, other acute CHD deaths, nonfatal MI, revascularisation procedures, unstable angina, resuscitated cardiac arrest or stroke) (7.2% vs 11.1%; relative risk −38%; 95% CI -58 to −8. Absolute risk reduction, 3.9%; p = 0.017) [37]. This reduction was almost identical to that observed in those <65 years (relative risk −37%; 95% CI -57 to −7; p = 0.019); however, the absolute risk reduction in major cardiovascular events was greater in older patients (3.9% vs 2.7%), reflecting their increased risk of events. These significantly positive findings may reflect an increased benefit in diabetic patients. Similar to ALLHAT-LLT, there was no significant reduction in all-cause mortality in those ≥65 or <65 years.

The MEGA trial investigators randomised hypercholesterolemic (total cholesterol 5.69–6.98 mmol/L) Japanese primary prevention adults to diet or diet plus pravastatin (10–20 mg daily) [32]. They found that those aged 60 or older who received pravastatin had a numerically greater relative reduction in the occurrence of coronary heart disease (fatal and nonfatal MI, angina, cardiac and sudden death and a coronary revascularisation procedure) compared to those younger than 60 receiving pravastatin (HR 0.59, 95% CI 0.40–0.88 vs HR 0.81, 95% CI 0.49–1.32; p for interaction 0.34). Similarly, a subgroup analysis of the HOPE-3 trial reported that the benefit of rosuvastatin (10 mg daily) in preventing the composite outcome of nonfatal MI, nonfatal stroke or cardiovascular death, was similar in those >65.3 years (HR 0.75; 95% CI 0.61–0.93) compared to those ≤65.3 years (HR 0.78; 95% CI 0.59–1.05) who had at least one cardiovascular risk factor [35].

There has been only one trial to date that has shown a significant reduction in all-cause mortality (p = 0.02) in primary prevention adults who received treatment with statins: the JUPITER (Justification for the Use of Statins in Primary Prevention: an Intervention Trial Evaluating Rosuvastatin) trial [34]. This double-blinded randomised controlled trial aimed to assess the benefits of treatment of rosuvastatin (20 mg daily) compared to placebo, in primary prevention adults with normal or low cholesterol levels but relatively elevated high-sensitivity C-reactive protein (hsCRP) levels. A post-hoc secondary subgroup analysis of the main trial, which included 5695 patients who were 70 years or older, demonstrated a significant 30% relative reduction in a composite of MI, stroke and all-cause mortality (HR 0.70; 95% CI 0.56–0.87; p = 0.001), in those treated with rosuvastatin, compared to placebo [39]. Relevantly, the observed benefits of statin therapy were consistent with those seen in younger patients (50–69 years).

Since publication, however, the JUPITER trial has come under some criticism [41–43]. The trial was terminated early after a median of 1.9 years of follow up and although the reason for early termination was cited as being due to a highly significant reduction in morbidity and mortality, pre-specified stopping rules were not published in detail in the study protocol. Focusing on hard endpoints, such as fatal and nonfatal MI and stroke, the trial was discontinued after only 240 events such events [41]. Finally, the all-cause mortality curves were beginning to converge as the trial was ended, raising the question as to whether the difference between groups would have disappeared if the follow-up period of the trial had been longer [41].

A meta-analysis by Savarese et al., focussing on adults ≥65 years (mean age 73 years) with no prior history of CV disease, included trials that compared statin use to placebo [36]. They reported a 39.9% reduced risk of MI (relative risk; 0.606; 95% CI 0.434–0.847; $p = 0.003$) and 23.8% reduction in stroke risk (relative risk 0.762; 95% CI 0.626–0.926; $p = 0.006$) for a mean LDL reduction of 0.69 mmol/L. From this, they estimated that the NNT for 1 year to prevent 1 event was 24 for MI and 42 for stroke. In contrast, all-cause mortality, and cardiovascular death were not significantly reduced, at least in the short term (mean follow-up 3.5 years). A similar meta-analysis by Teng et al. also included trials of patients ≥65 (mean age 72.7 years) where statin therapy was compared to placebo or usual care, with the same mean follow up of 3.5 years [38]. They confirmed similar findings, with a significant reduction in MACEs (relative risk 0.82; 95% CI 0.74–0.92; I^2–71.5%) and no reduction in all-cause mortality (relative risk 0.96; 95% CI 0.88–1.04, $I^2 = 0$). Similar to Savarese et al., they noted a 26% reduction in total MI (relative risk 0.74; 95% CI 0.61–0.90) and significantly also in nonfatal MI (RR 0.75; 95% CI 0.59–0.94). In contrast, however, they concluded that statins did not reduce the risk of fatal stroke (relative risk 0.76; 95% CI 0.24–2.45), nonfatal stroke (relative risk 0.76; 95% CI 0.53–1.11) or total stroke (relative risk 0.85; 95% CI 0.68–1.06). A potential reason for the lack of concordance with Savarese et al's findings, is that the respective analyses included different trials. While both analyses included data from ASCOT-LLA [28], CARDS [31], MEGA [32] and, PROSPER [27], Teng et al. included data from the ALLHAT-LLT [25] trial in their analysis on stroke (weight: 22.50%), while Savarese et al. included data from the JUPITER [34] trial (weight: 17.55%). The most recent meta-analysis by Ridker et al. combined the results of the JUPITER and HOPE-3 trials and described a net benefit of rosuvastatin compared to placebo in preventing ASCVD "hard" events (composite of nonfatal MI, nonfatal stroke or cardiovascular death) across the different age strata; <65 (HR 0.75; 95% CI 0.57–0.97), 65–<70 (HR 0.51; 95% CI 0.38–0.69) and ≥70 (HR 0.74; 95% CI 0.61–0.91) [40].

Overall, statins appear to be of benefit in primary prevention for at risk adults up to the age of 75, bearing in mind that many trials were of a short duration of follow up and a significant portion of trial data for those over the age of 65 has been extrapolated from post hoc subgroup analyses. All guidelines offer a class I or strong recommendation for statin therapy for those deemed at very high or high risk for ASCVD in this age group [15, 16, 19, 20]. For those deemed at borderline or intermediate risk, risk modifiers and coronary artery calcium scoring are recommended to guide decisions.

1.4.3 Primary Prevention Lipid-Lowering Therapy in Those Over 75 Years

Limited inclusion of those ≥75 years in cholesterol-lowering trials [26–28, 31, 35, 39], coupled with recent observational data yielding conflicting results, has created a real challenge for the preventive community when faced with decisions surrounding statin use for primary prevention in this age group. The only statin trial to date designed to include a significant number of patients over the age of 75 was the Prospective Study of Pravastatin in the Elderly at Risk (PROSPER) trial [27]. This included a mixture of primary (3239; 56%) and secondary (2565; 44%) prevention patients with a mean age of 75.4 years (41% >75 years) [18]. Primary prevention adults were required to have at least one CVD risk factor to be considered for inclusion. When considering the study population as a whole (i.e., both primary and secondary prevention patients), treatment with pravastatin 40 mg daily, compared to placebo, significantly lowered the risk of cardiovascular events; a composite outcome of definite or suspected CHD death, definite or suspected nonfatal MI and fatal and nonfatal stroke (14.1% vs 16.2%; HR 0.85; 95% CI 0.74–0.97; $p = 0.014$) over a mean follow up of 3.2 years. The authors also observed a 24% relative risk reduction in coronary heart disease deaths (3.3% vs 4.2%; HR 0.76; 95% CI 0.58–0.99; $p = 0.043$). However, though there was no evidence for statistical interaction, when primary prevention patients only were considered there was no significant reduction in the primary outcome (HR 0.94; 95% CI 0.77–1.15) or the secondary outcomes of the trial. The fact that the trial was not powered to detect a significant effect in each subgroup, may offer one explanation for this lack of observed benefit in the older primary prevention cohort [44]. These findings are in keeping with a subgroup analysis of the ALLHAT-LLT trial, where daily pravastatin failed to demonstrate any major benefit, compared to usual care, in preventing major CV events, such as CV death, CHD death, heart failure, fatal or nonfatal stroke in 726 primary prevention patients ≥75 years old (7% of the trial population) [26].

A meta-analysis by the Cholesterol Treatment Trialists' Collaboration (CTC) has corroborated these findings, combining all trial data (from both primary and secondary prevention adults) in those >75 that compared those who received statin therapy to control/less intense statin therapy [18]. There was a net benefit of statin therapy in reducing major vascular events in those >75 years (mean age 78.8) with a prior history of vascular disease, with a 15% proportional risk reduction per 1 mmol/L decrease in LDL cholesterol (756 events vs 845 events; rate ratio 0.85; 99% CI 0.73–0.98). This statistically significant benefit was not observed in adults >75 years without a history of vascular disease (295 events vs 308 events; rate ratio 0.92; 99% CI 0.73–1.16), though the confidence intervals include the possibility of a benefit and overlap with the findings of participants with a history of vascular disease. The authors also noted a borderline significant trend towards smaller proportional risk reductions with increasing age ($p_{trend} = 0.05$) in primary prevention patients. As has been the case with most trials, older patients, those with frailty, and functional or cognitive decline have been underrepresented in trial data.

Somewhat at odds with statin meta-analysis subgroup data from persons over 75, a recent non-statin trial, the Ezetimibe Lipid-Lowering Trial On Prevention of Atherosclerosis in 75 or Older (EWTOPIA) 75 trial, compared ezetimibe (10 mg daily) to usual care in hypercholesterolemic Japanese patients ≥75 years (mean age 80.6 years), without a history of CAD, and reported favourable results [45]. Over 86.7% of participants had at least one CV risk factor. Over a median follow up period of 4.1 years the investigators reported a significant reduction in the primary outcome (composite of sudden cardiac death, fatal/nonfatal MI, coronary revascularisation, or fatal/nonfatal stroke), cardiac events (HR 0.60; 95% CI 0.37–0.98; $p = 0.039$) and coronary revascularisation (HR 0.38; 95% CI 0.18–0.79; $p = 0.007$) in the ezetimibe group compared to those assigned to usual care (HR 0.66; 95% CI 0.50–0.86; $p = 0.002$). Similar to the statin trials, they found no significant reduction in stroke (HR 0.78; 95% CI 0.55–1.11; $p = 0.17$) or all-cause mortality (HR 1.09; 95% CI 0.89–1.34; $p = 0.43$).

It is clear that those over the age of 75 years have been underrepresented in clinical trials, with all data to date coming from post hoc subgroup analyses with trials excluding co-morbid patients. To add to the uncertainty, and as noted above, several recent observational studies have reported mixed findings that, at times, have been at odds with the available trial data; particularly in relation to observed reductions in all-cause mortality in those treated with statins. For example, in favor of statins, a recent retrospective cohort study that included 326,981 US veterans aged 75 and older (mean age 81.1 years) without a history of ASCVD, found that statin use, compared to no statin use, was associated with a lower risk of all-cause mortality, cardiovascular mortality and ASCVD (defined as time to first MI or ischemic stroke or CABG/PCI) over a mean follow up of 6.8 years [46]. Significantly, the reductions in both all-cause mortality and CV mortality remained consistent even in those over the age of 90 or with dementia. The authors observed no reduction in ischemic stroke (HR 0.98; 95% CI 0.96–1.01; $p = 0.20$). In concordance with these favorable results, the SCOPE-75 study and Jun et al. observed a reduction in all cause-mortality in Korean populations [47, 48]. SCOPE-75, a retrospective, propensity score matched observational study, found that statin users over the age of 75 years (median age 78 years) had lower rates of major CVD (HR 0.59; 95% CI 0.41–0.85; $p = 0.005$) and all-cause mortality compared (HR 0.65; 95% CI 0.34–0.93; $p = 0.02$) to non-statin users over a median period of 5.2 years [47]. On subgroup analysis, the association of statins with a decrease in all-cause mortality was more pronounced in diabetic patients (HR 0.28; 95% CI 0.11–0.71), compared to non-diabetics (HR 0.79; 95% CI 0.43–1.48). Significantly, Jun et al. noted that the benefits of statin use appeared to increase with time, with no observed benefit observed within the first year of starting treatment. Other groups have observed that the benefit of statins in primary prevention adults ≥75 years are only seen in those with other modifiable ASCVD risk factors (diabetes, currently being dispensed antihypertensive therapy, antiplatelet agents or anticoagulants) [49]. This is worth noting because, while the majority of adults over 75 years have either hypertension or other CVD risk factor or are elevated risk by CVD risk calculators, a small fraction of this older population remain healthy and without CVD risk factors. Further supporting the benefit of statins among the elderly, a population-based cohort study including 120,173 French primary prevention adults, suggested that statin discontinuation in those ≥75 years may be associated with a 33% increased risk of hospitalisation for cardiovascular events [50]. However, these results are subject to potential confounding, in that is possible that those who discontinued the statins had poorer health or were frailer and thus more likely to require hospitalisation for reasons other than statin discontinuation.

While the potential benefit of statin therapy on all-cause mortality in older adults has also been reported in other observational studies [51], the observational data for statins in adults over 75 years have been mixed, as noted above. A recent retrospective cohort study by Ramos et al., including 46,864 primary prevention adults 75 years or older in Spain, found that statins were not associated with reduced ASCVD or all-cause mortality in those without diabetes, over a median follow-up of 7.7 years (IQR 7.2–8 years) [52]. The authors did note a benefit in those with diabetes aged 75–84 years, with a 24% relative reduction in ASCVD (HR 0.76; 95% CI 0.65–0.89) and 15% relative reduction in all-cause mortality (HR 0.84; 95% CI 0.75–0.94). These benefits were reduced in those aged 85 years and above (ASCVD: HR 0.82; 95% CI 0.53–1.26; all-cause mortality: HR 1.05; 95% CI 0.86–1.28) and disappeared completely in nonagenarians, suggesting that statin benefit was limited to those <85 years old. The sample size of those ≥85 with diabetes was limited (1239 patients) in this study, and so lacked statistical power and may in part be responsible for the lack of observed effect in this group, but the effect of diminishing benefits with increased age is in keeping with that observed in the PROSPER trial and in the meta-analysis by Gencer et al. Similarly, the accentuated benefit in diabetics is in keeping with the SCOPE-75 study and other previous data in older diabetic patients [47, 53].

The question remains, why have there been differences within the observational data and differences between trials and observational data? One reason could be differing inclusion criteria. For example, the above analysis by Ramos et al. excluded patients with cancer, dementia, paralysis, those receiving dialysis, and those in residential care. This is in contrast to the work by Orkaby et al., who specifically included those with cancer, dementia and paralysis in an attempt to achieve a more representative population [54]. Orkaby et al. included a predominantly male population (97.3% of included veterans were male) and found that statin use was associated with an 18% lower risk of all-cause mortality, HR 0.82 (95% CI 0.69–0.98).

The open question as to whether statins are of value in elderly primary prevention adults will be further addressed in the STAin therapy for Reducing Events in the Elderly trial (STAREE) trial, which is aiming to recruit 18,000 primary prevention adults aged 70 years or more, in order to assess whether treatment with 40 mg atorvastatin daily compared with placebo will prolong the length of a disability-free life in these patients (NCT02099123). This is the first primary prevention statin trial designed specifically around an older population. Unfortunately, as the recruitment age starts at 70, it is likely that this trial will add little substantial data to those >80 years with multiple comorbidities [55]. The use of placebo in this trial reflects the uncertainty surrounding benefit. French investigators are concurrently aiming to evaluate the cost/effectiveness ratio of station cessation in those 75 years and older as part of the SITE (Statins In the Elderly) trial (NCT02547883).

Guideline Recommendations

Compared to the class I recommendations in younger adults, the ESC provides a class IIb recommendation for primary prevention adults 75 and above who are considered at high risk or above, emphasising the importance of a risk-benefit discussion with the patient [16]. The AHA provides a similar class IIb recommendation for statin therapy for those >75 who are diabetic, providing a recommendation for an individualised clinical assessment and risk discussion for those >75 without diabetes [15]. In contrast, the NICE guideline recommends statin treatment in those with a 10% 10-year risk of CVD up to the age of 84 [20]. They also recommend consideration of atorvastatin 20 mg for patients aged 85 or older, taking into account potential benefits from lifestyle modifications, informed patient preference, comorbidities, polypharmacy, general frailty and life expectancy. A summary of recommendations is provided in Box 1.

1.5   Secondary Prevention Lipid-Lowering Therapy

Unlike in primary prevention, the benefit of cholesterol-lowering therapies, particularly statins, are well established in the setting of secondary prevention. Lifestyle measures remain a fundamental adjunct to all pharmacological treatments in secondary prevention.

1.5.1   Statins in Secondary Prevention

The Cholesterol Treatment Trialists' Collaboration (CTC) have recently provided an updated meta-analysis of randomised evidence on the effects of statin therapy across 6 different age groups: 55 years or younger, 56–60 years, 61–65 years, 66–70 years, 71–75 years, and older than 75 years [18]. The analysis included 186,854 primary and secondary prevention patients, with 14,483 (7%) over the age of 75 years at the time of randomisation. They reported that treatment with a statin or more intensive statin regimen compared to control or a less intensive statin regimen resulted in a 21% relative reduction in major vascular events for every 1 mmol/L reduction in LDL-C (HR 0.79; 95% CI 0.77–0.81). Significantly, they observed independently significant risk reductions in each of the age subgroups, even in those over 75 years (HR 0.87; 95% CI 0.77–0.99). Considering only secondary prevention patients, statins led to significant reductions in major vascular events that were again, similar across all 6 age groups, including those over 75 years (HR 0.85; 95%

CI 0.73–0.98), suggesting that statins continue to offer benefit with increasing age in the setting of secondary prevention.

Previous studies have shown that statins do not reduce major vascular events in those with moderate or severe heart failure, or those undergoing dialysis for renal failure (see references 16–20 in CTC). Interestingly, most of the patients included in these trials were older.

1.5.2 Non-statin Therapy in Secondary Prevention

Ezetimibe is the most commonly prescribed non-statin cholesterol-lowering agent and is currently recommended as a first-line alternative for those who cannot tolerate statin therapy or who fail to achieve adequate LDL-C levels despite maximally tolerated statin doses. The IMPROVE-IT trial demonstrated that a combination of simvastatin-ezetimibe was superior to simvastatin monotherapy in reducing cardiovascular events (death from CVD, a major coronary event or nonfatal stroke) in patients (mean age 63.6 years) following an acute coronary syndrome (absolute risk reduction of 2%; HR 0.936; 95% CI 0.89–0.99; $p = 0.016$) [56]. The authors also observed a significant reduction in myocardial infarction and stroke. Cardiovascular deaths and all-cause mortality were similar across both groups. A subsequent pre-specified secondary analysis compared those aged <65 (10,173 or 56.1%), to those aged 65–75 (5173 or 28.5%) and those ≥75 (2798 or 15.4%) [57]. When compared to simvastatin monotherapy, the simvastatin-ezetimibe combination conferred greater absolute risk reductions in the primary endpoint in those ≥75 years (7-year Kaplan Meier event rates of 38.9% vs 47.6%; HR 0.80; 95% CI 0.70–0.90) compared to those younger than 75. The numbers needed to treat to prevent 1 primary endpoint event by treatment with simvastatin-ezetimibe was 11(95% CI 2–23) for those ≥75 compared to 125(95% CI 113 to infinity) for those <75. Unlike statins, ezetimibe has relatively few associated adverse events, making it an attractive alternative for older adults at risk of adverse events. In recognition of the above, the latest AHA/ACC guidelines suggest that it may be reasonable to add ezetimibe to moderate intensity statin therapy in those ≥75 years of age, where high intensity therapy would otherwise be indicated (i.e., secondary prevention) but is not tolerated, provided the LDL-C remains ≥1.8 mmol/L [15].

PCSK9 inhibitors have emerged as a potent adjunctive therapy to statins in reducing LDL-C and major cardiac events. The FOURIER trial included 27,256 patients (mean age 63 years. 22.6% >69 years) with a history of ASCVD [58]. Patients were randomised to either evolocumab or matching placebo and followed for a median of 26 months. Treatment with evolocumab resulted in a 15% relative risk reduction in major cardiovascular events (composite of cardiovascular death, myocardial infarction, stroke, hospitalisation for unstable angina, or coronary revascularisation) compared to placebo (1344 events vs 1563 events; HR 0.85; 95% CI 0.79–0.92; $p < 0.001$). The authors also observed significant reductions in MI, stroke and coronary revascularisation individually. There was no observed benefit in cardiovascular mortality. Subsequent subgroup analysis confirmed that evolocumab significantly reduced LDL-C levels across all age groups. Reductions in the primary endpoint were also sustained across all age groups with no significant differences in efficacy between those <56, 56 to ≤63, 63 to ≤69 years or >69 years old [59]. Most recently, age-stratified outcomes from the ODYSSEY OUTCOMES trial showed that the addition of the PCSK9 inhibitor alirocumab to maximum tolerated statin therapy, reduced the primary composite endpoint of coronary heart disease death, nonfatal MI, ischemic stroke, unstable angina requiring hospitalisation, compared to placebo in both younger and older patients with a recent ACS [60]. 5084 (26.9%) of patients were ≥65 years, 1007 (5.3%) aged ≥75 years and 42 (0.2%) 85 years or older. Alirocumab reduced the risk of the primary endpoint by 22% in those aged 65 years or older (Kaplan-Meier at 3 years: 12.9% vs 16.8%; HR 0.78; 95% CI 0.68–0.91), compared to 11% in those younger than 65 years (Kaplan-Meier at 3 years; 8.8% vs 9.7%; HR 0.89; 95% CI 0.80–1.00; $p_{interaction} = 0.19$). Alirocumab also decreased the rate of the primary outcome in those >=75 and those <75 years compared to placebo, however, this was not a pre-specified analysis and included relatively few patients. As expected, the risk of MACE increased with advancing age, leaving a greater absolute risk reduction in those ≥65 compared to younger patients ($p = 0.015$). The NNT for 3 years to prevent one primary composite outcome decreased with increasing age; 43 at age 45 years, 26 at age 75 years and 12 at age 85 years. Excess cost remains one barrier to physician prescribing these drugs. While PCSK-9 inhibitors may be a promising option to lower LDL-C levels there are practical considerations that become relevant in older patients. There may be limitations in practicality of delivering a subcutaneous injection; patients may not be able to self-administer and may not be able to travel to get them administered.

1.5.3 Guideline Lipid Lowering Therapy in Secondary Prevention

In secondary prevention, the AHA/ACC offer a class I recommendation for high intensity statin therapy in those ≤75 with a history of ASCVD [15]. In contrast, they give only a class IIa recommendation for moderate or high-intensity statin therapy in those over the age of 75. They also add the recommendation that this decision be made in the context of consideration of adverse effects, drug-drug interactions, as well as patient frailty and patient preferences. In contrast, the ESC recommends that treatment remains the same in younger and older patients in the setting of secondary prevention, recommending lipid-lowering therapy in all patients with LDL ≥1.4 mmol/L or 55 mg/dL (Cholesterol mmol/l × 38.67 = mg/dl) [16]. So too do the NICE guidelines [20].

1.6 Special Considerations in Older Adults

1.6.1 Adverse Events of Statins

Current trial data suggest that statins are generally well tolerated in older adults, however with important caveats [18, 36, 38]. Data are limited in those >75, and particularly in those >80 years old. It should also be remembered that those enrolled in clinical trials are generally a healthier population than patients often encountered in routine clinical practice, and so trial results may not be directly applicable to the older patient in a general clinic [6].

One of the most common adverse effects reported with statin use are statin-associated muscle symptoms (SAMS). [61] These represent a spectrum of outcomes ranging from myalgias to myositis and rarely rhabdomyolysis. Advanced age, female sex, physical disability, renal impairment and a lower BMI are all risk factors for the development of SAMS [61]. Higher statin doses also make these side effects more likely. Despite this, a meta-analysis by Iwere et al. included data on 18,845 patients aged 65 or older who had been either randomised to receive a statin or placebo, and did not report any increased risk in SAMS [62]. As such, and despite common perceptions, trial data on statin use from older and younger populations consistently question whether the association between statin use and SAMS is causal. Furthermore, Iwere et al. did not observe any significantly increased risk of myalgia (OR 1.03; 95% CI 0.90–1.17; $p = 0.66$) or rhabdomyolysis in those assigned to statin treatment (OR 2.93; 95% CI 0.30–28.18; $p = 0.35$). This is in contrast to data from observational studies, where myopathy was reported more frequently in those assigned to statins (OR 2.63; 95% CI 1.50–4.61), albeit it with significant heterogeneity between studies ($I^2 = 98.2\%$) [63].

As statins are metabolised by the cytochrome P450 system of isoenzymes, there is a significant potential for increased adverse effects when patients are co-prescribed a medication that competes for catabolism by this system. This becomes an important consideration in the setting of polypharmacy, particularly in older adults. Examples of statin drug-drug interactions include non-dihydropyridine calcium channel blockers, macrolide antibiotics, ranitidine, fibrates, and amiodarone.

There have also been concerns that statin use increases the risk of haemorrhagic stroke in patients with a prior history of ischemic stroke. However, the absolute risk is very small and the net benefit of statins in reducing ischemic stroke and other vascular events, generally outweighs the risk [64].

Although the exact mechanism is currently unclear, statin therapy has also been shown to modestly increase the risk of developing newly diagnosed diabetes, with an estimated hazard ratio of approximately 1.1 for moderate intensity statin and 1.2 for high intensity statin therapy for 5 years, equating to an absolute risk of about 0.2% per year in major trials [64]. This risk seems to be predominately confined to patients who already have multiple risk factors for the condition, and the risk seems to be higher in older women [65].

While there have been previous concerns that statin use may be associated with cognitive impairment and dementia, a number of recent meta-analyses do not support these concerns [66].

1.6.2   Statins in Frail Older Adults

To date, no randomised trials examining statin prescription in the context of either primary or secondary prevention have included a validated measure of frailty. A meta-analysis by Hale el al, included observational data on 153,082 older adults living with frailty, and while they reported a lower mortality among patients who were prescribed a statin in the context of secondary prevention there was no data on primary prevention adults, and insufficient data to conclude whether statins reduces ASCVD in frail older adults [67]. Further research is required in this area to establish a risk benefit relationship of lipid lowering therapies in this patient cohort.

1.6.3 Role for Deprescribing Statins

As it stands, the majority of statin prescribing in older adults happens in the context of secondary prevention, even in those over 80 years old [68]. However, as comorbidities and frailty increase with age, in tandem with a more limited life expectancy, the question remains whether there is an age at which statins could, or even should, be discontinued i.e., where the risks of treatment now outweigh the benefits (see Fig. 1). While guidelines place a particular emphasis on a patient centred approach when initiating statins in the oldest old, there is little guidance around what to do once a patient, who is already taking a statin, reaches a more advanced age or develops comorbidities. Given the lack of evidence currently available for benefit in primary prevention for adults over the age of 80, revaluation of the risk-benefit ratios as patients become older seems pragmatic. In fact, statin deprescribing is already happening, and as one might expect, it appears to be more common with

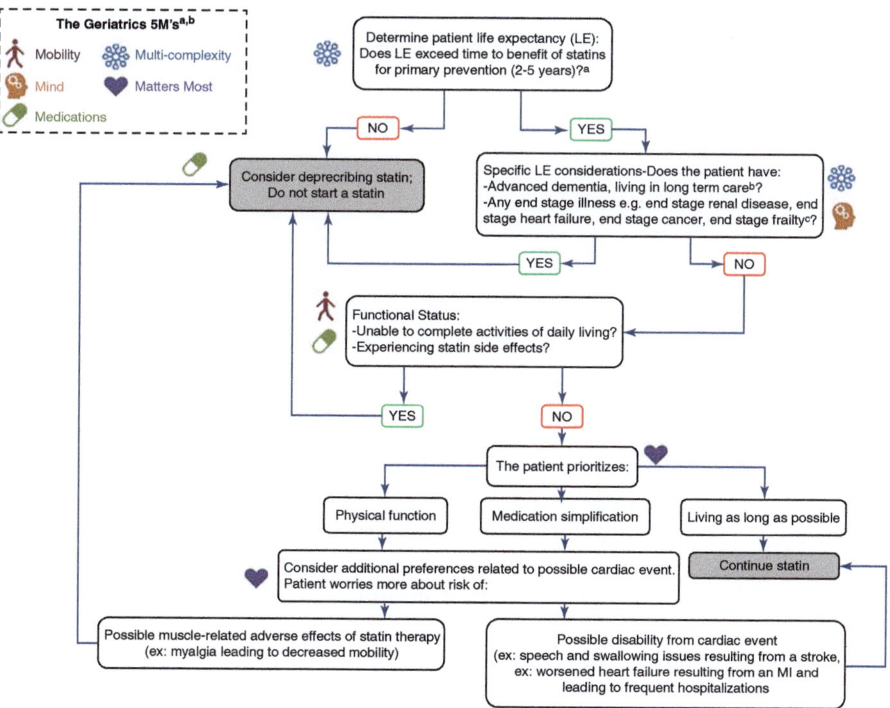

Fig. 1 Deprescribing statins. Need permission (this figure is obtained from a Springer publication) from 10.1007/s40266-019-00673-w

increasing age and in the setting of primary prevention [69]. Data from a small, randomised trial, support statin discontinuation in patients who have advanced and life-limiting illnesses [70]. Further work is required in this area to help proactively identify older patients where risk-benefit ratios shift and where statin deprescribing may become appropriate.

2 Cigarette Smoking

Box 2

- Consider smoking status a vital sign.
- Smoking cessation continues to confer benefits, even in those 80 years and older.
- As such, smoking cessation is recommended in all patients.
- Use both motivational interviewing and pharmacotherapy as part of a patient tailored smoking cessation programme.
- Nicotine replacement therapies, bupropion, and varenicline are all potential pharmacological interventions.
- Electronic nicotine delivery systems (e-cigarettes) are currently not recommended as part of smoking cessation programmes.

2.1 *Benefits of Cessation in the Older Adult*

The link between cigarette smoking and the development of atherosclerotic cardiovascular disease is well established with the 10 year fatal CVD risk approximately doubled in smokers compared to non-smokers [71]. While the rates of cigarette smoking in the population are declining overall, the deleterious consequences of smoking occur disproportionately in older patients due to the cumulative adverse effects of smoking over the years [72]. Smokers over the age of 60 years continue to have a twofold increased risk of acute coronary events and a 1.5-fold increased risk of stroke events compared to non-smokers [73]. Although smoking cessation at older ages cannot reverse all of the accumulated harm from years of smoking, cessation continues to be of benefit in those with increased chronological age, even when aged 80 and older [74, 75]. Follow up from the British Male Doctors study, suggested that those who quit smoking at age 60 years, gained 3 years of life expectancy compared to those who continued to smoke [76], with similar results seen in a US population [77]. Likewise, an observational meta-analysis by Mons et al. reported that cardiovascular mortality was significantly reduced in those over 60 who quit smoking within 5 years, compared to those who continued smoking [73]. Despite the fact that older smokers are less likely to attempt smoking cessation, those who are motivated and do attempt cessation are more likely to be successful [78–80]. This may in part be due to the fact that older patients are more likely to avail of smoking cessation assistance [78]. And thus, the major take home point when considering older aged smokers is to avoid the fatalistic misperception that there is "no point" in tackling smoking cessation with more advanced age [81].

2.2 Smoking Cessation Interventions

Despite the benefits of cessation, evidence-based tobacco cessation treatments are underutilised in older adults, and so there is significant scope to improve cessation measures in such patients [82]. There is an increasing awareness of this need to include older adults in cessation programmes, with the National Cancer Institute's campaign "smokefree60+" targeting such groups. In an attempt to prioritise the importance of smoking cessation as a preventive measure, the AHA now also recommends recording tobacco use as a vital sign at each visit [83].

All guidelines now support a dual-pronged approach to smoking cessation in all adults, regardless of age, using a combination of motivational interviewing and pharmacotherapy [83, 84]. All smokers should receive cessation counselling at every healthcare encounter. There is a particular impetus for smoking cessation around the time of diagnosis of CVD event, often leaving cardiologists uniquely posed to act when known diagnoses are established. In addition to clinician counselling, there are now multiple helplines available, for example in America through the National Cancer institute and Smokefree.gov, where patients can access trained counsellors that are valuable adjuncts for those working in busy clinical settings.

There are currently 7 FDA-approved cessation medications and most of which have the advantage of having relatively few major side effects. Both short (gum, lozenge, nasal spray, inhaler) and long-acting nicotine replacement therapies (NRT) like patches can be used as initial starting measures and have been shown to increase the rate of quitting by up to 50–70% [85]. Bupropion, an atypical antidepressant, has been shown to be as effective as NRT [86]. Bupropion increases a patient's seizure risk, affecting approximately 1 in 1000 users, so it should therefore be avoided in patients with a propensity for seizure. Varenicline remains the most effective pharmacological adjunct to smoking cessation, with potentiated effects when used in combination with NRT [87]. Initial concerns of an increase in suicidal ideation following the initiation of varenicline were not substantiated in the EAGLES study [88]. The most common adverse events observed in those taking varenicline are nausea and sleep disturbances [89]. Importantly, varenicline has not been demonstrated to be unsafe when used in persons with recent acute coronary syndrome. As varenicline is almost exclusively renally excreted it requires dose adjustment once the estimated creatinine clearance drops below 30ml/min, and so a history of CKD in older adults becomes a relevant consideration when commencing such pharmacotherapy.

While the introduction of Electronic Nicotine Delivery Systems (ENDS) (often called e-cigarettes) was initially hoped to provide a safer alternative to tobacco smoking, there is evidence suggesting potential adverse CV effects, with no long term outcome data available [90–92]. ENDS are therefore currently not recommended as part of a smoking cessation programme [83].

3 Diabetes

> **Box 3**
>
> **D** Diabetes
>
> - A target HbA1c of <7% is recommended in an otherwise well older patient, with a long-life expectancy.
> - Consider more lenient targets in those with functional impairment, frailty, limited life expectancy or those with multiple comorbidities.
> - For older patients residing in a nursing home, those with a limited life expectancy or those with certain chronic conditions, the aim should be to minimise the symptoms related to hyperglycaemia, rather than aiming for a target HbA1c.
> - Where tight glycaemic control is difficult or impossible, addressing other ASCVD risk factors more intensively can add significant benefit.
> - Metformin remains the first-line drug in older adults with type 2 diabetes.
> - Where possible, avoid drugs that increase the risk of hypoglycaemia (e.g., sulphonylureas).

Both type 1 diabetes mellitus and type 2 diabetes mellitus and pre-diabetes are independent risk factors for ASCVD [93]. Furthermore, CVD is the leading cause of death in diabetic patients. It is estimated that almost a quarter of those aged 65 years and older in the US have diabetes, with a further quarter reaching a diagnosis of pre-diabetes [94]. The overlap of older age, diabetes and other ASCVD risk factors, such as hypertension, mean that the risks for microvascular and macrovascular diabetic complications are also heightened in this population cohort, making diabetes and pre-diabetes a key target in our preventive efforts.

3.1 *Diagnosis and Screening of Diabetes in Older Adults*

The American Diabetes Association (ADA) recommends screening for diabetes in all adults over the age of 45 years, with repeat testing every 3 years or sooner if a patient has multiple additional risk factors [95]. In contrast, Canadian guidelines recommend individualised screening in older adults, acknowledging that screening for diabetes in those over the age of 80 is unlikely to be beneficial [96]. This is supported by data from a large Swedish registry, including over 200,000 patients with type 2 diabetes and over one million controls, which found that a diagnosis of type 2 diabetes at age 65 years resulted in a median loss of 2 years of life, in contrast to no accelerated loss of life if diagnosed after the age of 80 [97]. Relevantly, a new diagnosis of type 2 diabetes after the age of 80 years, resulted in an adjusted mortality risk of <1.0 for both CVD mortality and non-CVD mortality, with risks for other outcomes significantly attenuated also. For nonagenarians, the only outcome for which the risk was higher in those with new type 2 diabetes vs controls was stroke [97]. This data questions the value of screening for diabetes in those over 80, particularly where comorbidities are present. It also highlights the relevance of reassessing whether intensive glycemia treatment goals are appropriate in those over the age of 80 with a new diagnosis of diabetes, particularly if they are asymptomatic.

Outside of a clear clinical diagnosis (i.e., a patient in a hyperglycaemic crisis or classic symptoms of hyperglycaemia and a random glucose ≥200 mg/dL or ≥11.1 mmol/L) a diagnosis of diabetes can be established with a fasting plasma glucose of ≥126 mg/dL (7.0 mmol/L), a glucose of ≥200 mg/dL (11.1 mmol/L) 2 h post oral glucose tolerance test, or a serum HbA1c level of ≥6.5% (48 mmol/mol) [95]. While these cut-offs remain consistent across guidelines, it is worth nothing that HbA1c levels have been shown to increase with age by an estimated 0.1–0.2% per decade, even in non-diabetic patients [98–100]. Given the potential discordance between fasting plasma glucose levels and HbA1c levels in older patients, Canadian guidelines make the recommendation that a diagnosis of diabetes should ideally be based on a combination of 2 different tests in older adults, particularly where the HbA1c level is modestly elevated [96, 101].

Guidelines also recommend routine assessment for evidence of microalbuminuria in all diabetic patients in order to help identify patients at risk of diabetic nephropathy or at high risk of future CVD events who may benefit from more intensive treatment strategies [102, 103].

3.2 Glycaemic Targets in Older Adults: The Background

Given the association of hyperglycaemia with both microvascular and macrovascular complications, the seemingly rational hypothesis is that achieving a near euglycemic state should minimise the complications associated with diabetes. However, while there is a significant body of evidence confirming that intensive glucose control benefits microvascular endpoints, the relationship between intensive glucose lowering and the reduction in incidence and/or progression of macrovascular complications is less clear [104].

One of the first landmark trials to explore glycaemic targets was the Diabetes Control and Complications Trial (DCCT) [105]. This historical trial demonstrated that patients with type 1 diabetes with more intensive insulin regimens (achieving a mean HbA1c 7.4%) could delay the onset of microvascular complications compared to those who aimed for more lenient control (mean HbA1c 9.1%) [105]. Interestingly; however, the investigators observed no significant reduction in CV events over the 6.5-year follow-up period. A subsequent follow-up study, which collected data on the same participants followed for a mean of 17 years, did however show a benefit, with 0.38 cardiovascular events per 100 patient years occurring in the intensive group, compared to 0.80 per 100 patient years in the control group ($p = 0.007$) suggesting early glycaemic control may take some time to manifest benefits in macrovascular disease [106]. The DCCT trial inspired a host of subsequent trials with a focus on glycaemic control to reduce ASCVD in patients with type 2 diabetes (Table 2).

One of the first trials to compare the effect of more intensive glycaemic control to less stringent control on cardiovascular outcomes in type 2 diabetic patients was the UK Prospective Diabetes Study (UKPDS) [108]. This trial enrolled almost 4000 non-overweight patients (mean age 53 years), and found that maintaining more intensive glycaemic control with either a sulphonylurea or insulin (to a median HbA1c level of 7%), was superior in the prevention of microvascular complications, compared to conventional care (median HbA1c 7.9%) in those with a new diagnosis of type 2 diabetes [108]. While there were reductions in the occurrence of myocardial infarction (relative risk 0.84; 95% CI 0.71–10; $p = 0.052$), and the incidence of CV mortality (relative risk 0.80; 95% CI 0.71–1.00; $p = 0.052$) in those assigned to intensive control, these findings were not statistically significant. There was also no reduction observed in the occurrence of stroke (relative risk 1.11; 95% CI 0.81–1.51; $p = 0.52$). By contrast, a separate arm of the UKPDS trial enrolled overweight patients, who were primarily assigned to metformin, and reported a reduction in MI (relative risk 0.61; 95% CI 0.41–0.89; $p = 0.01$), all-cause mortality (relative risk 0.64; 95% CI 0.45–0.91; $p = 0.011$) and cardiovascular mortality (relative risk 0.5; 95% CI 0.23–1.09; $p = 0.02$) with stricter glycaemic targets (mean end of trial Hba1c of 7.4% in the intensive group vs 8% in the conventional group) [109].

A 10-year post-trial follow-up of the UKPDS showed that, despite an early loss of differences in HbA1c levels between groups within 1-year post-trial completion, the observed benefits for any diabetes-related endpoint and microvascular disease were maintained—an effect now frequently referred to as "the legacy effect" [125]. This observation of a maintained benefit over time has also been observed by others [126, 129]. A 5-year post-trial follow-up of the ACCORD trial, demonstrated a similar sustained benefit of intensive glycaemic control, despite diminishing differences in glycaemic control between groups, with a consistent reduction in nonfatal MI (HR 0.84; 95% CI 0.72–0.96; $p = 0.02$) [129].

There was a second interesting observation at the UKPDS 10-year follow-up. Similar to the DCCT trial follow-up study, there was an emergence of a significant post-trial reduction in myocardial infarction (Risk ratio 0.85; 95% CI 0.74–0.97; $p = 0.01$) and death from any cause (risk ratio; 0.87; 95% CI 0.79–0.96; $p = 0.007$) in the those assigned to the sulphonylurea/insulin intensive arm at the 10-year mark, despite no observed reduction during the active trial period [125]. The Veterans Affair Diabetes trial (VADT), observed similar effects. In this trial a HbA1c of 6.9% was achieved in the intensive group during the trial period compared to 8.4% in the

Table 2 Summary of main trials comparing intensive vs conventional glycaemic control in patients with type 2 diabetes

	Kumamoto [107]	UKPDS [108]	UKPDS [109] (metformin)	VA CSDM [110, 111]	Bagg et al. [112]	Becker et al. [113, 114]	Steno-2 [115, 116]	PROactive [117, 118]	ADVANCE trial [119]	ACCORD [120]	IDA [121]	VADT [122, 123]	Akari [124]
	1995	1998	1998	1999	2001	2003	2003	2005	2008	2008	2009	2009	2012
Study design	Randomised control trial	Multicentre randomised controlled trial	Multicentre randomised controlled trial	Multicentre randomised controlled trial	Randomised, control trial	Randomised control trial	Open label parallel group, randomised trial – multiple interventions	Multicentre, randomised, double blind, placebo-controlled outcome trial	Multicentre, factorial, randomised controlled trial	Multicentre, factorial, randomised controlled trial	Randomised controlled trial	Open label, randomised controlled trial	Randomised, controlled trial – multiple interventions
Number of participants	110	3867	753	153	43	214	160	5238	11,140	10,251	102	1791	1173
Population	Type 2 diabetic patients who had been treated with 1 or 2 daily injections of intermediate acting insulin	Patients aged 25–65 years with newly diagnosed diabetes with a fasting plasma glucose >6 mmol/L	Patients aged 25–65 years with newly diagnosed diabetes with a fasting plasma glucose >6 mmol/L who were overweight (>120% ideal bodyweight)	Men between the ages of 40–69 years, with diabetes for 15 years or less and on max dose of sulfonylurea and/or any dose of insulin	Type 2 diabetics <15 years duration with a HbA1c >8.9%	Diabetic patients aged 40–75 years	Diabetes with a urine albumin excretion rate of 30–300 mg/24 h	Patients with type 2 diabetes, aged 35–75 years with a HbA1c >6.5%, despite management of diabetes with diet alone or with oral blood glucose lowering agents	Type 2 diabetes diagnosed at age 30 years or older, ≥55 years of age at time of study entry, a history of major macrovascular or microvascular disease or at least one other risk factor for vascular disease	Type 2 diabetes and a HbA1c of > = 7.5% between the ages of 40–79 years with cardiovascular disease OR those between 55 and 79 years with evidence of significant atherosclerosis, albuminuria, left ventricular hypertrophy or at least 2 additional risk factors for CVD	Type 2 diabetic patients undergoing PCI for coronary artery disease	Veterans >=41 years old with a centrally measured HbA1c > =7.5% (or else local HbA1c > =8.3%) maximum dose of at least one oral agent and/or daily insulin injections	Type 2 diabetic patients aged 65–85 years, HbA1c > =7.9% or HbA1c > =7.4% with at least one of the following (BMI > =25, BP > =130/85, cholesterol > = 200 mg/dL, triglycerides > = 150 mg/dL and HDL-C < 40 mg/dL

(continued)

Table 2 (continued)

Exclusion	Retinopathy, urinary albumin > = 300 mg/24 h, serum creatinine > = 1.5 mg/dL, diabetic somatic or autonomic neuropathy severe enough to require treatment, age > =70 years, severe medical conditions	Ketonuria >3 mmol/L, serum creatinine >175 µmol/L, MI in the previous year, current heart failure or angina, more than one major vascular event, retinopathy requiring laser treatment, malignant hypertension, uncorrected endocrine disorder, occupation that precluded insulin therapy, severe concurrent illness that would limit life or require extensive systemic treatment, inadequate understand-ing; and unwillingness to enter the study	Ketonuria >3 mmol/L, serum creatinine >175 µmol/L, MI in the previous year, current heart failure or angina, more than one major vascular event, retinopathy requiring laser treatment, malignant hypertension, uncorrected endocrine disorder, occupation that precluded insulin therapy, severe concurrent illness that would limit life or require extensive systemic treatment, inadequate understanding; and unwillingness to enter the study	Diabetes >15 years duration, more than one MI previously, class III or IV angina refractory to medical therapy, NYHA class III or IV HF refractory to medical therapy, TIA within the last year, CVA in last 6 months or a CVD with more than a minor functional deficit, malignancies or other life threatening disease if likely to cause death within 7 years, history of hypoglycaemic reactions with LOC, creatinine >1.6 mg/Dl, uncooperative or unreliable, any underlying condition that the physician feels may prevent adherence to the protocol	Age > 75 years or < 40 years, BMI >40, current diastolic BP >100 mmHg, creatinine >0.16 mmol/L, any severe concurrent illness, left ventricular failure, MI or unstable angina in the past 6 months prior to enrolment	Carcinoma, other comorbidities preventing 3 monthly vistis to the study centre or seriously impairing well being, language problems or GP objected to participants of patient because of psychological problems	Age older than 65 years or younger than 40 years, a stimulated serum C peptide <600pmol/L 6 mins after injection of 1 mg glucagon, pancreatic insufficiency or diabetes secondary to pancreatitis, alcohol abuse, non-diabetic kidney disease, malignancy or life threatening disease with death probable within 4 years	Patients currently using pioglitazone or any other TZD, any signs of type 1 diabetes, insulin as the sole therapy for diabetes, planned revascularisation, symptomatic heart failure, leg ulcers, gangrene, or pain at rest, haemodialysis or significantly impaired hepatic function	Definite indication for, or contraindica-tion to, any of the study treatments, or a definite indication for long term insulin therapy at the time of study entry	Frequent or recent serious hypoglycaemia events, unwillingness to do home glucose monitoring or inject insulin, a BMI >45, creatinine >1.5 mg/dL or other serious illness	Acute MI wihtin 48 h, inability to participate for physical or psychological reasons, residency outside the hospital catchment areas	Any condition that would preclude a participant from receiving intensive treatment or completing the trial, CHA class III or IV angina, NYHA class III or IV HF, stroke, MI, invasive revascularisation within the past 6 months, BMI > =40, serum creatinine >1.6 mg/dL, hepatic dysfunction, type 1 diabetes, autonomic neuropathy, living alone without access to a person who can assist in an emergency, unable to self care or has a severe illness, + others	Recent (<6 months) MI, or stroke, acute or serious illness, aphasia and severe dementia

Interven-tion	Multiple insulin injection therapy group (administered insulin 3 or more times daily – rapid acting insulin at each mealtime and intermediate acting insulin at bedtime. Aim: FPG <140 mg/dL, 2 h post prandial <200 mg/dL, HbA1c <7% and mean amplitude of glycaemic excursions (MAGE) <100 mg/dL	Intensive treatment with insulin or sulphonyl-urea aiming for a fasting plasma glucose <6 mmol/L (in addition to a pre meal glucose 4-7 mmol/L in those on insulin)	Intensive treatment with metformin ± insulin ± sulphonylurea aiming for a fasting plasma glucose <6 mmol/L (in addition to a pre meal glucose 4-7 mmol/L in those on insulin)	HbA1c 4% to 6.1% with a stepwise treatment approach (insulin ± glipizide)	Premeal capillary readings of 4-7 mmol/L and 2 h post meal glucose levels of <10 mmol/L. A target HbA1c <7% at the end of 2 weeks Stepwise approach to treatment: first with oral hypoglycemic agents before commencing insulin	Strict fasting capillary glucose (<6.5 mmol/L)	HbA1c <6.5% Other: BP <130/80, light to moderate exercise for at least 30 min 3–5 times a week, smoking cessation courses, total daily fat intake <30% of daily intake and saturated fatty acids <10% of daily intake	Add on of pioglitazone to existing therapy to maintain a HbA1c <6.5%	Intensive control group aiming for a targe A1c level of ≤6.5% using gliclazide MR	Target HbA1c <6%	HbA1c <6.5%, FBC 5-7 mmol/L and blood glucose pre-meals of <10 mmol/L Treatment with TDS fast acting insulin and long acting insulin at bedtime	Absolute reduction of 1.5% points in HbA1c as compared to the standard treatment group	HbA1c <6.9% Other targets: BMI <25, SBP <130, DBP <85, HDL-c > 40 mg/dL, serum triglycerides <150 mg/dL, total serum cholesterol <180 mg/dL
Control	Conventional insulin therapy (1 or 2 daily injections of intermediate acting insulin) Aim: FPG as close to <140 mg/dL with no symptoms of hyperglycaemia or hypoglycaemia	Conventional treatment with diet to achieve a FPG <15 mmol/L without symptoms of hyperglycaemia Drugs were added if patients had hyperglycaemic symptoms or had a fasting plasma glucose >15 mmol/L	Conventional treatment with diet to achieve a FPG <15 mmol/L without symptoms of hyperglycaemia Drugs were added if patients had hyperglycaemic symptoms or had a fasting plasma glucose >15 mmol/L	Standard treatment – avoiding excessive hyperglycaemia and maintaining good general medical care (HbA1c <13%, or 2 SDs above mean diabetic values in participating centres, ketonuria, or hypoglycaemia). Usually 1 insulin injection/day	Avoid symptomatic hyperglycaemia and fortnightly fasting capillary glucose tests >17 mmol/L	Less strict fasting capillary glucose target (<8.5 mmol/L)	Conventional treatment by their general practitioners – target HbA1c <7.5%	Placebo	Standard control group – A1c target defined based on local guidelines	Target HbA1c 7% to 7.9%	Continued ongoing glucose lowering treatment, with any change in medication at the discretion of their physician	Target HbA1c of 8–9% and preventing symptoms of glycosuria, hypoglycaemia and ketonuria	Continued their baseline treatment for diabetes, hypertension or dyslipidaemia without a specific treatment goal
Follow-up	6 years	Median 10 years	Median 10.7 years	24 months	20 weeks	Mean 22 months	Mean 7.8 years	34.5 months	Median 5 years	Mean 3.5 years		Median 5.6 years	Mean 6 years
Age	Mean 49 years	Mean 53.3 years	Mean 53 years	Mean 60 years	Mean 56 years	Mean 63.3 years	Mean 55.1 years	Mean 62 years	Mean 66 years	Mean 62.2 years	Median 64 years	Mean 60.4 years	Mean 71.8 years

(continued)

Table 2 (continued)

Sex	48% female	40% female	54% female	100% male	56% female	51% female	26% female	34% female	42.5% female	38% female	25% female	3% female	54% female
Intervention HbA1c	Mean 7.2%	HbA1c 7%	HbA1c 7.4%	Mean 7.3%	Mean 8.02%	7.2%	7.9%	Mean 7%	HbA1c 6.5%	Median 6.4%	Mean 6.3%	Median 6.9%	Mean 7.7%
Control HbA1c	Mean 9.4%	HbA1c 7.9%	HbA1c 8%	Mean 9.4%	Mean 10.23%	7.4%	9%	Mean 7.6%	HbA1c 7.3%	Median 7.5%	Mean 6.6$	Median 8.4%	Mean 7.8%
Primary outcome	Microvascular complications Worsening retinopathy (13.4% vs 38%; $p = 0.007$) Worsening nephropathy (9.6% vs 30%; $p = 0.005$)	Any diabetes related endpoint (relative risk 0.88; 95% CI 0.79–0.99; $p = 0.029$) Diabetes related death (relative risk 0.90; 95% CI 0.73–1.11; $p = 0.34$)	Any diabetes related endpoint (relative risk; 0.68; 95% CI 0.53–0.87; $p = 0.0023$) Diabetes related death (relative risk 0.58; 95% CI 0.37–0.91; $p = 0.017$)	Change in prevalence of peripheral neuropathy No statistically significant difference between groups	Weight change (92.7Kg vs 80.5kg; $p = 0.003$) BMI (32.1 vs 29.4; $p = 0.002$)	Insufficient differences in HbA1c between groups at the end of the trial so data was reanalysed data to assess if lowering HbA1c would result in changes of various CV risk factors Triglycerides, total cholesterol, BP and ACR improved with decreasing HbA1c	Composite of death from CV causes, nonfatal MI, nonfatal stroke, revascularisation and amputation Unadjusted HR: 0.47; 95% CI 0.24–0.73; $p = 0.008$ Adjusted HR: 0.47; 95% CI 0.22–0.74; $p = 0.01$	Composite outcome: Time from randomisation to first occurrence of any of the following events (all-cause mortality, nonfatal MI, ACS, cardiac intervention, stroke, major leg amputation, bypass surgery or revascularisation in the leg) HR 0.90; 95% CI 0.80–1.02; $p = 0.095$	Composite of macrovascular events and composite of microvascular events HR 0.90; 95% CI 0.82–0.98; $p = 0.01$)	Composite of nonfatal MI, nonfatal stroke, or death from cardiovascular causes (HR, 0.9; 95% CI 0.78–1.04; $p = 0.16$)	Rate of restenosis after PCI (41% vs 44%; $p = 0.8$)	Composite of any major CV event (MI, stroke, new or worsening CCF, amputation for ischemic diabetic gangrene, invasive intervention for CAD or PVD, and CV death) HR 0.88; 95% CI 0.74–1.05; $p = 0.14$)	Composite of death due to diabetes, death unrelated to diabetes, coronary vascular events, stroke, total diabetes related events, and all events (death unrelated to diabetes as well as all events related to diabetes) $P = 0.2239$
Microvascular complications	See primary outcome	Relative risk 0.75; 955 CI 0.60–0.93; $p = 0.0099$) Mainly due to a decrease in retinal photocoagulation and microalbuminuria	Relative risk 0.71; 95% CI 0.43–1.19; $p = 0.71$)	–	–	–	Nephropathy (relative risk 0.39; 95% CI 0.17–0.87; $p = 0.003$) Retinopathy (relative risk 0.42; 95% CI 0.21–0.86; $p = 0.02$) Autonomic neuropathy (relative risk 0.37; 95% CI 0.18–0.79; $p = 0.002$) Peripheral neuropathy 1.09; 95% CI 0.54–2.22; $p = 0.66$	–	9.4% vs 10.9% (HR 0.86; 95% CI 0.77–0.97; $p = 0.01$) Mainly due to a reduction in nephropathy	–	–	No significant changes in retinopathy, nephropathy or neuropathy between groups	–

Macrovascular complications	–	Fatal MI (RR 0.94; 95% CI 0.68–1.30; $p = 0.63$ Nonfatal MI (RR 0.79; 95% CI 0.58–1.09; $p = 0.79$), death from PVD (RR 0.28; 95% CI 0.03–2.77; $p = 0.28$) Fatal stroke (RR 1.17; 95% CI 0.54–2.54; $p = 0.60$) Nonfatal stroke (RR 1.07; 95% CI 0.68–1.69; $p = 0.72$)	MI (RR 0.61; 95% CI 0.41–0.89; $p = 0.01$) Stroke (RR 0.59; 95% CI 0.29–1.18; $p = 0.13$) PVD (RR 0.74; 95% CI 0.28–2.09; $p = 0.57$)	–	–	–	Composite primary outcome	Time to first event: Nonfatal MI (HR 0.83; 95% CI 0.65–1.06) Stroke (HR 0.81; 95% CI 0.61–1.07)	10% vs 10.6% (HR 0.94; 95% CI 0.84–1.06; $p = 0.32$)	Nonfatal MI: 3.6% vs 4.6%; HR 0.76; 95% CI 0.62–0.92; $p = 0.004$) Nonfatal stroke: 1.3% vs 1.2%; HR 1.06; 95% CI 0.75–1.50; $p = 0.74$	–	First event: MI 64 events vs 78 events (HR 0.82; 95% CI 0.59–1.14; Stroke (HR 0.78; 95% CI 0.48–1.28)	Nonfatal MI ($p = 0.998$) Fatal MI (0.083) Nonfatal stroke ($p = 0.281$) Fatal stroke ($p = 0.656$)
All-cause mortality	–	Relative risk 0.94; 95% CI 0.80–1.1; $p = 0.44$	Relative risk 0.64; 95% CI 0.45–0.91; $p = 0.011$	–	–	–	–	HR 0.96; 95% CI 0.78–1.18	8.9% vs 9.6% (HR 0.93; 95% CI 0.83–1.06; $p = 0.28$)	5% vs 4%; HR 1.22; 95% CI 1.01–1.46; $p = 0.04$	–	95 events vs 102 events (HR 1.07; 95% CI 0.81–1.42; $p = 0.62$)	–
Cardiovascular mortality	–	Relative risk 0.80; 95% CI 0.71–1.00; $p = 0.052$	Relative risk 0.5; 95% CI 0.23–1.09; $p = 0.02$	–	–	–	7 events vs 7 events (NR)	–	4.5% vs 5.2% (HR 0.88; 95% CI 0.74–1.04; $p = 0.12$)	2.6% vs 1.8%; HR 1.35 (95% CI 1.04–1.76; $p = 0.02$)	–	40 events vs 33 events ($p = 0.29$)	–

(continued)

Table 2 (continued)

Hypogly-caemia	6% (6 patients) vs 4% (4 patients)	Significantly higher in the intensive treatment group	–		Mild to moderate episodes (OR 25.5; 95% CI 4.3–151.4; p < 0.001) No episodes of severe hypoglycaemia occurred in either group	–	Minor hypoglycaemic event (p = 0.50) Major hypoglycaemic event that impaired consciousness or required help from another person (p = 0.12)	–	2.7% vs 1.5% had at least 1 hypoglycae-mic event (HR 1.86; 95% CI 1.42–2.40; p < 0.0001)	Requiring medical assistance; 10.5% vs 3.5% (p < 0.001) Requiring any assistance: 16.2% vs 5.1% (p < 0.001)	–	Significantly increased in the intensive treatment group (p < 0.001)	–
Hospitali-sation	–	–	–	–	–	–	–	–	44.9% vs 42.8% (HR 1.07; 95% CI 1.01–1.13; p = 0.03)	–	–	–	–

Post trial follow completion up studies

Name		UKPDS follow up [125]	UKPDS follow up [125]	–	–	–	Steno-2 follow up [126]	–	ADVANCE-ON [127]	ACCORD [128]	ACCOR-DION [129]	–	VADT [130]	VADT-F [131]	–
Year		**2008**	**2008**	–	–	–	**2008**	–	**2014**	**2011**	**2016**	–	**2015**	**2019**	–
Total follow-up duration from time of trial onset		Median 16.8 years	Median 17.7 years	–	–	–	Mean 13.3 years	–	Median 9.9 years	Mean 5 years	Median 8.8 years	–	Median 9.8 years	Median 13.6 years – 15 years	–
Follow up time outside of trial intervention (observational)		Median 6.8 years	Median 7 years	–	–	–	Mean 5.5 years	–	Median 4.9 years	Mean 1.2 years	~5 years	–	4.2 years	8 years to 9.4 years	–

HbA1c		NS difference between groups ($p = 0.71$)	NS difference between groups ($p = 0.86$)	–	–	–	Intensive: 7.7% Standard: 8%	–	Intensive: 7.2% Standard: 7.4%	Intensive 7.2% Standard: 7.6%	Intensive: 7.8% vs standard: 8%	–	Difference of 0.2%–0.3% between groups	Median 8% in both groups	–
Primary outcome		Any diabetes related endpoint (risk ratio 0.91; 95% CI 0.83–0.99; $p = 0.04$) Diabetes related death (risk ratio 0.83; 95% CI 0.73–0.96; $p = 0.01$)	Any diabetes related endpoint (risk ratio 0.79; 95% CI 0.66–0.95; $p = 0.01$) Diabetes related death (risk ratio 0.70; 95% CI 0.53–0.92; $p = 0.01$)	–	–	–	All cause mortality (HR 0.54; 95% CI 0.32–0.89; $p = 0.02$)	–	All cause mortality (HR 1.00; 95% CI 0.92–1.08; $p = 0.91$) Major macrovascular events (a composite of nonfatal MI, nonfatal stroke or death from any CV cause) (HR 1.00; 95% CI 0.92–1.08; $p = 0.93$)	Composite of cardiovascular death, nonfatal MI, or nonfatal stroke HR 0.91 (95% CI 0.81–1.03; $p = 0.12$)	Composite of cardiovascular death, nonfatal MI, or nonfatal stroke (HR 0.95; 95% CI 0.87–1.04; $p = 0.27$)	–	Time to first major CV event (a composite of heart attack, stroke, new or worsening CCF, death from CV causes, or amputation for ischemic gangrene) 253 events vs 288 events (HR 0.83; 95% CI 0.70–0.99; $p = 0.04$)	Time to first major CV event (composite of nonfatal MI, nonfatal stroke, new or worsening CCF, death from CV causes or amputation for ischemic gangrene) (HR 0.91; 95% CI 0.78–1.06; $p = 0.23$)	

(continued)

Table 2 (continued)

Outcome															
Microvascular complications		Risk ratio 0.76; 95% CI 0.64–0.89; $p = 0.001$	Risk ratio 0.84; 95% CI 0.60–1.17; $p = 0.31$	–	–	–	Diabetic nephropathy (relative risk 0.44; 95% CI 0.25–0.77; $p = 0.004$) Progression of diabetic retinopathy (RR 0.57; 95% CI 0.37–0.88; $p = 0.01$) Progression autonomic neuropathy (RR 0.53; 95% CI 0.34–0.81; $p = 0.004$)	–	HR 0.92; 95% CI 0.80–1.05; $p = 0.23$	–	–	–	–	–	–
Macrovascular complications		MI (risk ratio 0.85; 95% CI 0.74–0.97; $p = 0.01$) Stroke (risk ratio 0.91; 95% CI 0.73–1.13; $p = 0.39$) PVD (risk ratio 0.88; 95% CI 0.56–1.19; $p = 0.001$)	MI (risk ratio 0.67; 95% CI 0.51–0.89; $p = 0.005$) Stroke (risk ratio 0.80; 95% CI 0.50–1.27; $p = 0.35$) PVD (risk ratio 0.63; 95% CI 0.32–1.27; $p = 0.19$)	–	–	–	Cardiovascular events (HR 0.41; 95% CI 0.25–0.67; $p < 0.001$)	–	MI (HR 1.02; 95% CI 0.89–1.19; $p = 0.75$) Stroke (HR 1.01; 95% CI 0.89–1.15; $p = 0.82$)	Nonfatal MI 1.18% vs 1.42% (HR 0.82; 95% CI 0.70–0.96; $p = 0.01$)	Nonfatal MI (HR 0.84; 95% CI 0.72–0.98; $p = 0.02$) Nonfatal stroke (HR 0.84; 95% CI 0.66–1.07; 0.16)	–	Nonfatal MI 103 events vs 119 events (HR 0.85; 95% CI 0.65–1.11) Non fatal stroke (HR 0.98; 95% CI 0.71–1.36)	Nonfatal MI 136 events vs 146 events (HR 0.91; 95% CI 0.72–1.44) Nonfatal strokes: 102 events vs 102 events (HR 0.96; 95% CI 0.73–1.27)	–
All-cause mortality		Risk ratio 0.87; 95% CI 0.79–0.96; $p = 0.007$	Risk ratio 0.73; 95% CI 0.59–0.89; $p = 0.002$	–	–	–	See primary outcome	–	See primary outcome	HR 1.19 (95% CI 1.03–1.38, $p = 0.02$)	HR 1.01 (95% CI 0.92–1.11; $p = 0.91$)	–	HR 1.05; 95% CI 0.89–1.25; $p = 0.54$	HR 1.02; 95% CI 0.88–1.18	–
CV mortality		–	–	–	–	–	HR 0.43; 95% CI 0.19–0.94; $p = 0.04$	–	HR 0.97 (95% CI 0.86–1.10; $p = 0.63$)	0.74% vs 0.57%; HR 1.29; 95% CI 1.04–1.06; $p = 0.02$)	HR 1.20; 95% CI 1.03–1.40; $p = 0.02$	–	HR 0.88; 95% CI 0.64–1.20; $p = 0.42$	HR 0.94; 95% CI 0.73–1.20	–

standard group (mean age 60.4 years) [122]. After a median follow-up of 5.6 years, there was no observed reduction in time to first major CV event (HR 0.88; 95% CI 0.74–1.05; $p = 0.14$). A subsequent observational follow-up approximately 4 years after trial completion (median 9.8 years since the trial began), noted that while the difference in HbA1c between groups had reduced to approximately 0.2–0.3%, there was now a 17% lower risk of primary CV events (HR 0.83; 95% CI 0.70–0.99; $p = 0.04$) in those who had received intensive therapy, compared to those who had been assigned to the standard group during the active trial period, suggesting a modest long term cardiovascular benefit of more intensive glycaemic control [130]. These delayed benefits on CV outcomes may have significant implications when considering a time to benefit for older patients.

There have also been concerns that excessive glycaemic control may cause harm. The ACCORD trial included over 10,000 type 2 diabetic patients and was terminated 17 months prior to the scheduled end of study, following an unexpected increase in both all-cause mortality (5% vs 4%; HR 1.22; 95% CI 1.01–1.46; $p = 0.04$) and cardiovascular mortality (2.6% vs 1.8%; HR 1.35; 95% CI 1.04–1.76; $p = 0.02$) in those assigned to the intensive treatment arm [120]. There was, however, a significant reduction in the occurrence of nonfatal MI (HR 0.76; 95% CI 0.62–0.92; $p = 0.004$). The target HbA1c in this trial was tight at <6% in the intensive arm, with a median end of trial HbA1c of 6.4% in the intensive group, compared to 7.5% in the standard treatment arm. Follow-up studies of trial participants out to 8.8 years confirmed persistence of an increased risk of CV mortality, but with a neutral effect on all-cause mortality long term, despite diminished differences in HbA1c levels between groups (At 8.8 years: HbA1c of 7.8% in those who had been assigned intensive treatment vs 8% in those assigned to conventional care) [128, 129]. Of note, observational data suggest a link between hypoglycemic episodes and myocardial injury (detected using high-sensitivity troponin) and ASCVD events [132, 133].

Several meta-analyses have been conducted in an attempt to further elucidate if intensive glucose lowering confers a benefit in reducing cardiovascular events in type 2 diabetic patients [134–138]. Considering these, it appears that lowering patients' HbA1c by an average of 1% has a limited benefit on all-cause mortality, results in an approximate 10% reduction in the risk of microalbuminuria and a 15–20% reduction in the incidence of nonfatal MI [139]. There are however several important caveats to consider when applying this data to older patients. Firstly, most of the trials to date have almost exclusively recruited younger patients (Table 2), with limited data on those over the age of 70 years, meaning that we have insufficient trial data to guide decisions on best glycaemic targets in older patients. Secondly, a consistent trade-off noted in intensive treatment arms across all trials was the increased risk of hypoglycaemia, which can have heightened deleterious effects in older patients and so remains a key consideration when making an individualised risk benefit decision for a patient. And finally, patients assigned to intensive interventions were closely followed and monitored during the conduct of trials. As an example, in the Action in Diabetes and Vascular Disease: Preterax and Diamicron Modified Release Controlled Evaluation (ADVANCE) trial the intensive group had an average of 31 study visits over the 5 years compared to 11 for the standard treatment group [119]. These extensive follow up regimens may not be practical or feasible if attempting to achieve similar targets for community-dwelling older adults, and less frequent follow-ups may make intensive regimens unsafe.

While we do not currently have adequate trial data to guide decision making on glycaemic targets in older adults, there have been several large observational studies that appear to support a more lenient approach to glycaemic control in this population. A large retrospective cohort study by Huang et al. including over 70,000 patients 60 years or older (mean age of 71 years, with 14.6% over the age of 80 years) with type 2 diabetes demonstrated that the risk of developing chronic microvascular complications and chronic cardiovascular events increased in a stepwise fashion with each unit increase in HbA1c above 6% (42 mmol/mol) [140]. In contrast, there was a U shaped relationship between HbA1c and mortality, suggesting that HbA1c levels <6% or $\geq$ 10% (86 mmol/mol) were associated with increased mortality risks [140]. From this observation they recommended an optimum HbA1c of below 8% (64 mmol/mol) in older patients but with a caution that a level < 6% was associated with increased mortality risk. This is in keeping with data from ACCORD and from the NHANES III study which also found that a HbA1c >8% in those $\geq$65 years was associated with elevated all-cause mortality and cardiovascular mortality [141]. Others have reported similar findings with elevated mortality at both extreme ends of HbA1c even in younger patients, leading to suggestions that guidelines should also include a minimum HbA1c value, although no guideline to date has provided a specific recommendation to this effect [142].

While the focus of management of type 2 diabetes has historically been predominantly glucocentric, it has been recently been highlighted that this approach may require a paradigm shift, moving away from a largely solitary focus on intense glycaemic control, and instead concentrating on ensuring adequate and equitable access to diabetes care, individualising glycaemic targets to patients' goals and circumstances, minimising complications of the disease itself but also of treatment effects, as well as improving quality of life [143]. This is further supported by the fact that recent cardiovascular outcome trials have demonstrated that microvascular and macrovascular complications can be meaningfully improved with certain antidiabetic medications that appear to primarily act via novel glucose lowering therapies, with most trials achieving significant improvements in CV outcomes with mean HbA1c levels between 7–8% (Table 3).

3.3 Glycaemic Targets in Older Adults: Guideline Recommendations

Contemporary guidelines generally advocate for a patient-centred approach when making decisions surrounding care in diabetes. Reflecting the lack of clear evidence, a discordance remains as to what the optimal glycaemic target should be in older adults. In general, guidelines recommend that the approach to managing diabetes in an otherwise well older patient with an anticipated long-life expectancy should be largely similar to younger patients, with most agreeing on a target HbA1c of <7% in these patients (Table 4). However, there is increasing recognition that

Table 3 Recent major trials CVOT following treatment with novel glucose-lowering therapies in patients with type 2 diabetes

	RECORD [144]	EXAMINE [145]	SAVOR-TIMI [146]	AleCardio [147]	EMPA-REG [148]	ELIXA [149]	TESCOS [150]	LEADER [151]	SUSTAIN-6 [152]	CANVAS [153]	DEVOTE [154]	EXSCEL [155]	HARMONY [156]	CARMELINA [157]	DECLARE-TIMI [158]	REWIND [159]	CAROLINA [160]	PIONEER-6 [161]	VERTIS-CV [162]	SCORED [163]
Year	2009	2013	2013	2014	2015	2015	2015	2016	2016	2017	2017	2017	2018	2019	2019	2019	2019	2019	2020	2021
Trial	Multicentre, randomised, open-label trial	Multicentre, randomised, double-blind, placebo-controlled trial	Multi-centre, randomised, double-blind, placebo-controlled trial	Multicentre, randomised, double-blind, placebo-controlled trial Terminated early due to increase rates of safety end points	Multicentre, randomised, double-blind, placebo-controlled trial	Multicentre, randomised, double-blind, placebo-controlled trial	Multicentre, randomised, double-blind, placebo-controlled trial	Multicentre, double-blind, placebo-controlled trial	Randomised, double blind, multicentre, placebo-controlled	Randomised, double blind, multicentre, placebo-controlled	Randomised, double-blind, controlled trial	Pragmatic, multicentre, randomised, double-blind, placebo-controlled, trial	Multicentre, double blind, randomised, placebo-controlled trial	Multicentre, randomised, double-blind, placebo-controlled trial	Randomised, double-blind, multicentre, placebo-controlled trial	Multicentre, randomised, double blind, placebo-controlled trial	Multicentre randomised, double blind, active controlled trial	Multicentre, randomised, double blind, placebo-controlled trial	Multicentre, randomised, double blind, randomised control trial	Multicentre, randomised, double-blind, placebo-controlled trial Trial ended early due to loss of funding
Trial design	Non-inferiority	Non-inferiority	Superiority	Superiority	Non-inferiority	Non-inferiority	Non-inferiority	Non-inferiority	Non-inferiority	Non-inferiority	Non-inferiority	Non-inferiority	Non-inferiority	Non-inferiority	Non-inferiority	Superiority	Non-inferiority	Non-inferiority	Non-inferiority	Non-inferiority
Drug class of intervention	TZD	DPP-4 inhibitor	DPP4-inhibitor	Agonist of peroxisome proliferator-activated receptor a and y	SGLT-2 inhibitor	GLP-1 agonist	DPP4-inhibotr	GLP-1 agonist	GLP-1 agonists	SGLT-2 inhibitor	Ultra-long-acting insulin analogue	GLP-1 agonists	GLP-1 agonists	DPP4 inhibitor	SGLT-2 inhibitor	GLP-1 agonists	DPP-4 inhibitor	GLP-1 agonists	SGLT-2 inhibitor	SGLT-2 inhibitor
Number	4447	5380	16,492	7226	7020	6068	14,523 (analysed)	9340	3297	10,142	7637	14,752	9463	6979	17,160	9901	6033	3183	8246	10,584
Population	Age 40–75 years, on a max tolerated dose of metformin or a sulfonylurea monotherapy and a HbA1c >7–9%	Type 2 diabetes with a HbA1c 6.5–11% (or 7–11% if on insulin)and were receiving anti-diabetic therapy (other than a DPP4-inhibitor or GLP-1 agonist) and had an ACS within 15–90 days before randomisation	Type 2 diabetes, HbA1c 6.5–12%, and either a history of established CV disease or multiple risk factors for CV disease	Patients with a new diagnosis of type 2 diabetes or an established diagnosis of type 2 diabetes AND hospitalised for ACS	Type 2 diabetics ≥18 years with established cardiovascular disease and a Hba1c >7% but <9% (or < 10% if they had received a stable dose of glucose-lowering therapy for at least 12 weeks)	Type 2 diabetes who had a MI or who had been hospitalised for unstable within the previous 180 days	Type 2 diabetes >50 years WITH established CV disease WITH a HbA1c 6.5–8% when treated with stable doses of 1 or 2 OHA or insulin	Type 2 diabetes, and with a HbA1c ≥7%, ≥50 years and at least one cardiovascular condition or ≥ 60 years with one or more CV risk factors	Type 2 diabetes and a HbA1c ≥7% ≥50 years old with established CV disease, CCF or CKD, or those ≥60 years with 2 or more CV risk factors	HbA1c ≥7% and ≤ 10.5% ≥30 years old with a history of symptomatic ASCVD or ≥ 50 years with 2 or more CV risk factors	Type 2 diabetics ≥50 years with at least one coexisting CV or renal condition OR ≥ 60 years with at least one CV risk factor AND who were being treated with at least one oral or injectable antihyperglyce-mic agent AND with a HbA1c ≥7% (<7% was accepted if the patient was being treated with at least 20 units of basal insulin per day)	Type 2 diabetic with a HbA1c ≥6.5% and ≤ 10% on one of the following: treatment with up to 3 oral anti-hypogly-caemic agents or insulin therapy	Type 2 diabetics ≥40 years old with an established disease of coronary, cerebrovas-cular or peripheral arterial circulation AND a HbA1c ≥7%	Adults with type 2 diabetes, a HbA1c of 6.5–10% inclusion and a high CV and renal risk	≥40 years with a HbA1c >6.5% but <12% and a creatinine clearance ≥60ml/min with established ASCVD OR multiple risk factors for ASCVD	Type 2 diabetes >50 years with known vascular disease or at risk for vascular disease AND HbA1c < =9.5% on stable doses of glucose lowering drugs	Type 2 diabetic patients ≥40 years and ≤ 85 years AND a HbA1c 6.5–8.5% (or 6.5–7.5% if a patient was on certain predefined AHA) AND at high risk of CV events	≥50 years with established CV disease or CKD, or ≥ 60 with cardiovascu-lar risk factors	Type 2 diabetics >40 years of age with established ASCVD AND a HbA1c level between 7–10.5%	Type 2 diabetes ≥18 years with a HbA1c ≥7% AND CKD (eGFR 25-60ml/min) AND risks for CVD

(continued)

Table 3 (continued)

	RECORD [144]	EXAMINE [145]	SAVOR-TIMI [146]	AleCardio [147]	EMPA-REG [148]	ELIXA [149]	TESCOS [150]	LEADER [151]	SUSTAIN-6 [152]	CANVAS [153]
Year	2009	2013	2013	2014	2015	2015	2015	2016	2016	2017
Main exclusion criteria	Hospitalisation for a major CV event in the 3 months before, planned CV intervention; the presence, history or treatment for heart failure	Type 1 diabetes, unstable cardiac disorders, and dialysis within 14 days before screening	Currently or had received an incretin based therapy within the last 6 months, ESRD and on long-term dialysis, previous renal transplant, or serum creatinine >530umol/L.	Symptomatic heart failure, hospitalisation with heart failure within the previous 12 months, severe peripheral oedema, eGFR <45ml/min, or a fasting triglyceride level > 400 mg/dL	eGFR <30ml/min, uncontrolled hyperglycaemia >240 mg/dL after an overnight fast, liver disease, cancer within the past 5 years, ACS, stroke or TIA within 2 months prior to informed consent, an uncontrolled endocrine disorder (other than diabetes), BMI >45	<30 years, PCI within the previous 15 days, CABG prior to the qualifying event, eGFR <30ml/min, a HbA1c <5% or > 11%	Taken a DPP4 inhibitor, GLP-1 agonist or thiazolidinedione during the preceding 3 months; if they had a history of 2 or more episodes of severe hypoglycaemia during the preceding 12 months, or if the eGFR was <30ml/min	Type 1 diabetes, use of GLP-1 agonists, DPP-4 inhibitors, pramlintide or rapid-acting insulin, familial or personal history of MEN2 or medullary thyroid cancer, ACS or CVA 14 days before screening	Treatment with a DDP4 inhibitor 30 days before screening, or treatment with a GLP-1 agonist 90 days before, a history of an ACS or CVA within 90 days before randomisation, planned revascularisation of a coronary, carotid or peripheral artery, or long-term dialysis	Not on a stable anti-glycaemic regime for at least 8 weeks before screening, fasting fingerpick glucose >15 mmol/L at baseline, history of 1 or more severe hypoglycaemic events within 6 months before screening, MI, unstable angina, CVA or revascularisation procedure within 3 months before screening, NYHA class IV HF, any condition that would make the patient unable to adhere to the initial trial visit schedule and procedures
Intervention	Rosiglitazone plus metformin or sulfonylurea	Alogliptin 6.25-25 mg daily	Saxagliptin 5 mg or 2.5 mg daily	Aleglitazar 150ug daily	Empagliflozin 10 mg or 25 mg daily	Lixisenatide 10-20ug	Sitagliptin 50 mg or 100 mg daily	Liraglutide 1.8 mg (or max dose tolerated)	Semaglutide 0.25 mg increased to 0.5 mg weekly sub cut	Canagliflozin 100 mg or 300 mg daily
Control	Metformin plus sulfonylurea	Placebo	Placebo	Placebo	Placebo	Placebo	Placebo	Placebo	Placebo	Placebo
Follow up duration	Mean 5.5 years	Median 18 months	Median 2.1 years	Median 104 weeks	Median 3.1 years	Median 25 months	Median 3 years	Median 3.8 years	Median 2.1 years	Mean 3.6 years
Mean age	Mean 58.4 years	Median 61 years	Mean 65 years	Mean 61 years	Mean 63 years	Mean 60 years	Mean 65.5 years	Mean 64.3 years	Mean 64.6 years	Mean 63.3 years
Inclusion of older patients	≥60 = 2035 (45.8%)	≥65 years = 1901 (35.5%)	>= 75 = 2330 (14.1%)	>75 = 581 (8%)	≥65 = 3172 (45%) ≥75 = 652 (9.4%)	≥65 = 2043 (33.8%)	≥65 = 7735 (53.9%) ≥75 = 2004 (14%)	≥65 = 7019 (75%) ≥75 = 836 (9%)	≥65 = 1598 (48.5%) ≥75 = 321(9.7%)	–

	DEVOTE [154]	EXSCEL [155]	HARMONY [156]	CARMELINA [157]	DECLARE-TIMI [158]	REWIND [159]	CAROLINA [160]	PIONEER-6 [161]	VERTIS-CV [162]	SCORED [163]
Year	2017	2017	2018	2019	2019	2019	2019	2019	2020	2021
Main exclusion criteria	Planned coronary, carotid or peripheral artery revascularisation, NYHA class IV heart failure, current dialysis or eGFR <30ml/min, ACS or CVA within the previous 60 days, any condition that would make the patient unable to adhere to the initial trial visit schedule and procedures	2 or more episodes of severe hypoglycaemia during the previous 12 months, eGFR <30ml/min, previous treatment with a GLP-1 agonist, personal or family history of medullary thyroid cancer or MEN-2	eGFR <30ml/min, severe gastroparesis, previous pancreatitis or substantial risk factors for pancreatitis, personal or family history medullary carcinoma of the thyroid or MEN2, or current use of a GLP-1 agonist	eGFR <15ml/min or requiring dialysis, type 1 diabetes, treatment with GLP-1 agonist, other DPP4 inhibitors or SGLT-2 inihibitors prior to informed Conseco, life expecacny <5 years for non-CV causes, cancer within the last 3 years, patients considered unreliable concerning the requirements for follow up during the study and/or compliance with the study drug	Previous treatment with an SGLT-2 inhibitor; acute cardiovascular event <8 weeks prior to randomisation, BP >180/100, type 1 diabetes, history of cancer within 5 years, chronic cystitis and/or recurrent UTIs, any conditions that may render the patient unable to complete the study (e.g., NHYA class IV HF), individuals at risk for poor protocol or medication compliance	eGFR <15ml/min, cancer in the previous 5 years, severe hypoglycaemia in the previous year, life expectancy less than 1 year, a coronary or cerebrovascular event within the previous 2 months and plans for revascularisation	Type 1 diabetes, uncontrolled hyperglycaemia (overnight fasting level > 13.3 mmol/L), NYHA class III or IV HF, pre-planned coronary revascularisation within 6 months, ACS ≤6 weeks prior or stroke or TIA ≤3 months prior	Treatment with any GLP-1 agonist, DDP-4 inhibitor or pramlintide within 90 days before screening, NYHA class IV heart failure, planned coronary artery, carotid artery or peripheral artery revascularisation; MI, stroke or hospitalisation for unstable angina or TIA within 60 days before screening; on haemodialysis or eGFR <30ml/min	Type 1 diabetes or ketoacidosis, eGFR <30ml/min	DKA, or nonketotic hyperosmolar coma within 3 months, antihyperglycemic treatment not stable for past 12 weeks, end stage heart failure, planned coronary revascularisation procedures, any SGLT-2 inhibitor <1 months prior to screening, severe disease or short life expectancy, any other conditions (actual or anticipated) that would restrict or limit participation during the study, BP ≥180/110
Intervention	Insulin degludec 1000U once daily	Extended release exenatide 2 mg weekly	Albiglutide 30-50 mg weekly	Linagliptin 5 mg OD	Dapagliflozin 10 mg daily	Dulaglutide 1.5 mg weekly	5 mg linagliptin OD	Oral semaglutide (target dose 14 mg)	5 mg or 15 mg of ertugliflozin	Sotaglifloazin 200 mg or 400 mg OD
Control	Insulin glargine 1000 units OD	Placebo	Placebo	Placebo	Placebo	Placebo	1–4 mg of glimepiride	Placebo	Placebo	Placebo
Follow up duration	Median 1.99 years	Median 3.2 years	Median 1.5 years	Median 2.2 years	4.2 years	Median 5.4 years	Median 6.3 years	Median 15.9 months	Mean 3.5 years	Median 16 months
Mean age	Mean 65 years	Mean 62 years	Mean 64.2 years	Mean 65.9 years	Mean age 64 years	Mean 66.2 years	Mean 64 years	Mean 66 years	Mean 64.4 years	Median 69 years
Inclusion of older patients	10.8% ≥75 years	8.5% ≥75 years	≥65 to <75 years = 3609 (38%) ≥75 = 1140 (12%)	≥65 = 4011 (57%)	≥65 = 7907 (46%) ≥75 = 1096 (6.4%)	≥66 = 2332 (47%)	≥65 = 2975 (49%)	≥65 = 1849 (58%)	≥65 = 4145 (50%) ≥75 = 452 (11%)	≥65 = 7360 (70%)

Female	48%	32%	33%	27%	28.4%	30.7%	29.3%	36%	39.3%	35.8%	37.4%	38%	30.5%	37.1%	37.4%	46.4%	39.9%	31.6%	30.2%	44.9% female
Mean HbA1c end of trial (intervention)	7.5%	7.7%	7.7%	6.8%	7.6%	7.3%	7.1%	7.8%	7.6%	8%	7.5%	7.5%	7.9%	7.7%	7.9%	7%	Weighted average mean difference between groups: 0% (7.1%)	Mean 7.2%	Mean 7.5%	Change in HbA1c from baseline (8.3%): least squares mean − 0.60%
Mean HbA1c end of trial (control)	7.8%	8%	7.9%	7.4%	8%	7.5%	7.4%	8%	7.3%	8.3%	7.5%	7.8%	8.2%	8%	8.1%	7.5%	Weighted average mean difference between groups: 0% (7.2%)	Mean 7.9%	Mean 8.0%	Change in HbA1c from baseline (8.3%): least squares mean − 0.17%
Primary outcome (whole population)	Time to first occurrence of CV hospitalisation or CV death HR 0.99; 95% CI .085–1.16; p = 0.93	Composite of death from CV causes, nonfatal MI, or nonfatal stroke HR 0.96; upper bound of one sided repeater CI < =1.16; p < 0.001 for noninferiority; p = 0.32 for superiority)	Composite of CV death, nonfatal MI, or nonfatal stroke HR 1.00; 95% CI 0.89–1.12; p = 0.99 for superiority; p < 0.001 for noninferiority	Time to CV death, nonfatal MI or nonfatal stroke HR 0.96; 955 CI 0.83–1.11; p = 0.57	Composite of death from CV causes, nonfatal MI (excluding silent MI), or stroke HR 0.86; 95% CI 0.74–0.99; p < 0.001 for noninferiority and p = 0.04 for superiority	Composite of the first occurrence of any of the following: Death from CV causes, nonfatal MI, nonfatal stroke, or hospitalisation for unstable angina HR 1.02; 95% CI 0.89–1.17; p < 0.001 for non-inferiority; p = 0.81 for superiority	Composite of first confirmed event of CV death, nonfatal MI, nonfatal stroke or hospitalisation for unstable angina Per protocol: HR 0.98; 95% CI 0.88–1.09; p < 0.001 for noninferiority Intention to treat: HR; 0.98; 95% CI 0.89–1.08; p = 0.65 for superiority	First occurrence of death from CV causes, nonfatal (including silent) MI or nonfatal stroke HR 0.87; 95% CI 0.78–0.97; p = 0.01	First occurrence of death from CV causes, nonfatal MI, or nonfatal stroke HR 0.74 (95% CI 0.58–0.95) P < 0.001 for non-inferiority, 0.02 for superiority	Composite of death from CV causes, nonfatal MI or nonfatal stroke HR 0.86 (95% CI 0.75–0.97) P < 0.001 for noninferiority; p = 0.02 for superiority	First occurrence of death from CV causes, nonfatal MI or nonfatal stroke HR 0.91 (95% CI 0.78–1.06) P < 0.001 for non-inferiority	First occurrence of any component of composite outcome of death from CV causes, nonfatal MI or nonfatal stroke HR 0.91 (95% CI 0.83–1.00) P < 0.001 for non-inferiority	First occurrence of CVD death, MI or stroke HR 0.78 (95% CI 0.68–0.90; p < 0.0001 for non-inferiority and 0.0006 for superiority)	First occurrence of CV death, nonfatal MI or nonfatal stroke HR 1.02 (95% CI 0.89–1.17; p < 0.001 for noninferiority; p = 0.74 for superiority)	Major cardiovascular event (defined as cardiovascular death, MI or ischemic stroke) HR 0.93 (95% CI 0.84–1.03; p = 0.17) Cardiovascular death or hospitalisation for heart failure (HR 0.83; 95% CI 0.73–0.95; p = 0.005)	First occurrence of any component of composite outcome comprising nonfatal MI, non fata stroke, and death from CV or unknown causes HR 0.88 (95% CI 0.79–0.99; p = 0.026)	First occurrence of CV death, nonfatal MI, or nonfatal stroke HR 0.98; 95% CI 0.84–1.14; p < 0.001 for non-inferiority and p = 0.76 for superiority	First occurrence of death from CV causes, nonfatal MI or nonfatal stroke HR 0.79; 95% CI 0.57–1.11; p < 0.001 for noninferiority	Composite of death from cardiovascular causes, nonfatal MI, or nonfatal stroke HR 0.97; 95% CI 0.85–1.11; p for non-inferiority <0.001	Composite of total number of CV deaths, hospitalisations for HF and urgent visits for HF (changed during the trial due to loss of sponsor as the trial had fewer than planned number of events) HR 0.74; 95% CI 0.63–0.88; p < 0.001
Primary outcome by age	≥60; HR 1.02; 95% CI 0.84–1.23 <60 (HR 0.96; 95% CI 0.74–1.25)	≥65; HR 0.98; 95% CI 0.78–1.24 <65: HR 0.91; 95% CI 0.73–1.13	≥75; HR 0.96; 95% CI 0.75–1.22 <75: HR 1.01; 95% CI 0.89–1.15	–	≥65; HR 0.71; 95% CI 0.59–0.87 <65 years: HR 1.04; 95% CI 0.84–1.29	Not reporter (there is a forest plot but no p values for interaction)	> = 75 years: HR 1.09; 95% CI 0.88–1.35 <75: HR 0.97; 95% CI 0.87–1.08	≥60: HR 0.90; 95% CI 0.79–1.02 <60; HR 0.78; 95% CI 0.62–0.97	≥65 years: HR 0.72; 95% CI 0.51–1.02 <65 years: HR 0.74; 95% CI 0.52–1.05	≥65 years: HR 0.80; 95% CI 0.67–0.95 <65 years: HR 0.91; 95% CI 0.76–1.10	≥75: HR 1.24; 95% CI 0.82–1.88 <75: HR 0.87; 95% CI 0.74–1.02 ≥65: HR 0.97; 95% CI 0.79–1.19 <65: HR 0.84; 95% CI 0.67–1.05	≥75 years: HR 0.82; 95% CI 0.64–1.05 <75: HR 0.93; 95% CI 0.84–1.03 ≥65: HR 0.80; 95% CI 0.71–0.91 <65; HR 1.05; 95% CI 0.92–1.21	≥75 years: HR 0.69; 95% CI 0.48–1.00 ≥65 to <75: HR 0.97; 95% CI 0.78–1.21 <65 years: HR 0.66; 95% CI 0.53–0.82	≥65 years: HR 0.97; 95% CI 0.82–1.15 <65 years: HR 1.11; 95% CI 0.89–1.40	MACE: p value for interaction 0.90	≥66: HR 0.86; 95% CI 0.74–1.00 <66: HR 0.92; 95% CI 0.78–1.09	≥65 years: HR 0.91; 95% CI 0.76–1.10 <65: HR 1.11; 95% CI 0.88–1.41	≥65: HR 1.04; 95% CI 0.68–1.59 <65: HR 0.51; 95% CI 0.29–0.90	CV death, nonfatal MI, nonfatal stroke >=65 (HR 1.03; 95% CI 0.86–1.22) <65 (HR 0.90; 95% CI 0.73–1.10) CV death or HF hospitalisation >=65 (HR 0.89; 95% CI 0.74–1.09) <65 (HR 0.86; 95% CI 0.66–1.11)	≥65: HR 0.79; 95% CI 0.66–0.95 <65: HR 0.60; 95% CI 0.43–0.83

(continued)

Table 3 (continued)

	RECORD [144]	EXAMINE [145]	SAVOR-TIMI [146]	AleCardio [147]	EMPA-REG [148]	ELIXA [149]	TESCOS [150]	LEADER [151]	SUSTAIN-6 [152]	CANVAS [153]
Year	2009	2013	2013	2014	2015	2015	2015	2016	2016	2017
CV death	HR 0.84; 95% CI 0.59–1.18; p = 0.32	HR 0.85; 95% CI 0.66 to 1.10; p = 0.21	HR 1.03; 95% CI 0.87–1.22; p = 0.72	HR 1.15; 95% CI 0.87–1.50; p = 0.32	HR 0.62; 95% CI 0.49–0.77; <0.001	HR 0.98; 95% CI 0.78–1.22; p = 0.85	HR 1.03; 95% CI 0.89–1.19; p = 0.71	HR 0.78; 95% CI 0.66–0.93; p = 0.007	HR 0.98; 95% CI 0.65–1.48; 0.92	HR 0.87; 95% CI 0.72–1.06
Nonfatal MI	Fatal and nonfatal MI (HR 1.14; 95% CI 0.80–1.63; p = 0.47)	HR 1.08; 95% CI 0.88–1.33; p = 0.47	Fatal or nonfatal: HR 0.95; 95% CI 0.80–1.12; p = 0.52	HR 0.89; 95% CI 0.74–1.07; p = 0.22	(Excluding silent MI) HR 0.87; 95% CI 0.70–1.09; p = 0.22	Fatal or nonfatal MI: HR 1.03; 95% CI 0.87–1.22; p = 0.71	Fatal or nonfatal MI (HR 0.95; 95% CI 0.81–1.11; p = 0.49)	HR 0.88; 95% CI 0.75–1.03; p = 0.11	HR 0.74; 95% CI 0.51–1.08; p = 0.12	HR 0.85; 95% CI 0.69–1.05
Nonfatal stroke	Fatal or nonfatal stroke (HR 0.72; 95% CI 0.49–1.06; p = 0.10)	HR 0.91; 95% CI 0.55–1.50; p = 0.71	Ischemic stroke: HR 1.11; 955 CI 0.88–1.39; p = 0.38	HR 0.98; 95% CI 0.66–1.45; p = 0.92	HR 1.24; 95% CI 0.92–1.67; p = 0.16	Fatal or nonfatal stroke: HR 1.12; 95% CI 0.79–1.58; p = 0.54	Fatal or nonfatal stroke (HR 0.97; 95% CI 0.79–1.19; p = 0.76)	HR 0.89; 95% CI 0.72–1.11; p = 0.30	HR 0.61; 95% CI 0.38–0.99; p = 0.04	HR 0.90; 95% CI 0.71–1.15
Hospitalisation for HF	Heart failure (HR 2.10; 95% CI 1.35–3.27; p = 0.0010)	–	3.5% vs 2.8% (HR 1.27; 955 CI 1.07–1.51; p = 0.007)	HR 1.22; 95% CI 0.94–1.59; p = 0.14	HR 0.65; 95% CI 0.50–0.85; p = 0.002	HR 0.96; 95% CI 0.75–1.23; p = 0.75	HR 1.00; 95% CI 0.83–1.20; p = 0.98	HR 0.87; 95% CI 0.73–1.05; p = 0.14	HR 1.11; 95% CI 0.77–1.61; p = 0.57	HR 0.67; 95% CI 0.52–0.87
Hypoglycaemia	0.7% vs 0.3%; p = 0.076	Serious hypoglycaemia (0.7% vs 0.6%; p = 0.86) Any hypoglycaemia (6.7% vs 6.5%; p = 0.74)	Minor hypoglycaemia (14.2% vs 12.5%; p = 0.002) Major hypoglycaemia (2.1% vs 1.7%; p = 0.047)	Hypoglycaemic event (HR 1.60; 95% CI 1.41–1.82; p < 0.001)	Any hypoglycaemic event (27.9% vs 27.8%) Requiring assistance (1.5% vs 1.3%)	16.6% vs 15.2% (p = 0.14) Serious hypoglycaemia episode (16 events vs 37 events)	Severe hypoglycaemia: HR 1.12; 95% CI 0.89–1.40; p = 0.33	Severe hypoglycaemia (2.4% vs 3.3%; p = 0.02)	Severe or symptomatic hypoglycaemic event 0.5 mg (23.1% vs 21.5%) 1 mg (21.7% vs 21%)	Hypoglycaemia (50 events per 1000 patient years vs 46.4 events per 1000 patient years; p = 0.20)

	DEVOTE [154]	EXSCEL [155]	HARMONY [156]	CARMELINA [157]	DECLARE-TIMI [158]	REWIND [159]	CAROLINA [160]	PIONEER-6 [161]	VERTIS-CV [162]	SCORED [163]
Year	2017	2017	2018	2019	2019	2019	2019	2019	2020	2021
CV death	HR 0.96; 95% CI 0.76–1.21; p = 0.71	HR 0.88; 95% CI 0.76–1.02	HR 0.93; 95% CI 0.73–1.19; p = 0.578	HR 0.96: 95% CI 0.81–1.14; p = 0.63	HR 0.98; 95% CI 0.82–1.17	HR 0.91; 95% CI 0.78–1.06; p = 0.21	HR 1; 95% CI 0.81–1.24	HR 0.49; 95% CI 0.27–0.92	HR 0.92; 95% CI 0.77–1.11	HR 0.90; 95% CI 0.73–1.12; p = 0.35
Nonfatal MI	HR 0.85; 95% CI 0.68–1.06; p = 0.15	Fatal or nonfatal: HR 0.97; 95% CI 0.85–1.10	Fatal or nonfatal: HR 0.75; 95% CI 0.61–0.90; p = 0.003	HR 1.15; 95% CI 0.91–1.45; p = 0.23	Fatal or nonfatal MI: HR 0.89; 95% CI 0.77–1.01	HR 0.96; 95% CI 0.79–1.16; p = 0.65)	HR 1.01; 95% CI 0.80–1.28	HR 1.18; 95% CI 0.73–1.90	HR 1.04; 95% CI 0.86–1.27	Fatal or nonfatal (HR 0.68; 95% CI 0.52–0.89)
Nonfatal stroke	HR 0.90; 95% CI 0.65–1.23; p = 0.50	Fatal or nonfatal: HR 0.85; 95% CI 0.70–1.03	Fatal or nonfatal: HR 0.86; 95% CI 0.66–1.14; p = 0.300	HR 0.88; 95% CI 0.63–1.23; p = 0.45	Ischemic stroke: HR 1.01; 95% CI 0.84–1.21	HR 0.76; 95% CI 0.61–0.95; p = 0.017	HR 0.87; 95% CI 0.66–1.15	HR 0.74; 95% CI 0.35–1.57	HR 1.00; 95% CI 0.76–1.32	Fatal or nonfatal (HR 0.66; 95% CI 0.48–0.91)
Hospitalisation for HF	–	HR 0.94; 95% CI 0.78–1.13	–	HR 0.90; 95% CI 0.74–1.08; p = 0.26	HR 0.73; 955 CI 0.61–0.88	Hospitalisations and urgent visits: HR 0.93; 95% CI 0.77–1.12; p = 0.46	HR 1.21; 95% CI 0.92–1.59	HR 0.86; 95% CI 0.48–1.55	HR 0.70; 95% CI 0.54–0.90	Hospitalisations and urgent visits for HF: HR 0.67; 95% CI 0.55–0.82; p < 0.001
Hypoglycaemia	Severe hypoglycaemia (rate ratio; 0.60; 95% CI 0.48–0.76; p < 0.001 for superiority)	Severe hypoglycaemia (3.4% vs 3%)	Severe hypoglycaemia: relative risk 0.56; 95% CI 0.36–0.87	Investigator reporter hypos (29.7% vs 29.4%) Severe events (3% vs 3.1%)	Major hypoglycaemic event (HR 0.68; 95% CI 0.49–0.95; p = 0.02)	Severe hypoglycaemia (1.3% vs 1.5%)	>=1 investigator reported episode (10.6% vs 37.7%) >=1 investigator reported episode of symptomatic hypoglycaemia with plasma glucose <=70 mg/dL or severe hypoglycaemia (6.5% vs 30.9%)	Severe hypoglycaemia (1.4% vs 0.8%)	Severe hypoglycaemia 5 mg (risk difference − .09; 95% CI -2.2–0.3) 15 mg (risk difference − 0.5; 95% CI -1.7–0.7)	Severe hypoglycaemia (1% vs 1%; p = 0.84)

Other significant adverse events																				
Other signifi-cant adverse events	Infections (6.3% vs 7%; p = 0.32) Malignancies (5.7% vs 6.6%; p = 0.20) GI disorders (6% vs 5.3%; p = 0.39) Heart failure (3.7% vs 1.9%; p = 0.003) Fractures (risk ratio 1.57; 95% CI 1.26–1.97; p < 0.001)	Serious adverse event (33.6% vs 35.5%; p = 0.14) Any adverse event (80% vs 78.8%; p = 0.30) Acute pancreatitis (0.4% vs 0.3%; p = 0.50) Chronic pancreatitis (0.4% vs 0.3%; p = 0.50)	Any pancreatitis (0.3% vs 0.3%; p = 0.77) Opportunistic infection (0.3% vs 0.4%; p = 0.06) Cancer (3.9% vs 4.4%; p = 0.15)	Gastrointestinal haemorrhage (HR 1.44; 95% CI 1.03–2.00; p = 0.03) Bone fracture (HR 1.03; 95% CI 0.94–1.80; p = 0.11) Composite renal endpoint (development of ESRD, doubling of serum creatinine, or greater than 50% increase in creatinine leading to study drug discontinua-tion): HR 2.85; 95% CI 2.25–3.60; p < 0.001	Adverse event (91.7% vs 90.2%; p < 0.001) Serious adverse event (42.3% vs 38.2%; p < 0.001) UTI men (9.4% vs 10.5%) UTI women (40.6% vs 36.4%; p < 0.05) Complicated UTI (1.8% vs 1.7%) Genital infection (1.8% vs 6.4%; p < 0.001) Volume depletion (4.9% vs 5.1%)	Any serious adverse event: 20.6% vs 22.1% GI event 2.2% vs 2.7%	Acute pancreatitis: HR 1.93; 95% CI 0.96–3.88; p = 0.07 Cancer: HR 0.91; 95% CI 0.77–1.08; p = 0.27 GI disorder (1.8% vs 1.4%)	Any adverse event (62.3% vs 60.8%; p = 0.12) Acute gallstones disease (3.1% vs 1.9%; p < 0.001) Acute pancreatitis (0.4% vs 0.5%; p = 0.44) Nausea, vomiting or diarrhoea leading to discontinuation of the drug (p < 0.001)	Serious adverse event 0.5 mg (35% vs 39.9%) 1 mg (33.6% vs 36.1%) GI disorder 0.5 mg (50.7% vs 35.7%) 1 mg (52.3% vs 35.2%) Acute pancreatitis 0.5 mg (0.7% vs 0.4%) 1 mg (0.4% vs 1.1%)	Serious adverse events (104.3 events per 1000 patient years vs 120 events per 1000 patient years; p = 0.04) Mycotic genital infection in women (68.8 per 1000 patient years vs 17.5 per 1000 patient years; p < 0.001) Infection o the genitalia in men (34.9 events per 1000 patient years vs 10.8 events per 1000 patient years; p < 0.001) Osmotic diuresis (34.5 per 1000 patient years vs 13.3 per 1000 patient years; p < 0.001) DKA (0.6 per 1000 patient years vs 0.3 per 1000 patient years; p = 0.14)	Serious adverse events (44.2 per 100 patient years vs 49.6 per 100 patient years) All adverse events (44.7 per 100 patient years vs 50.1 per 100 patient years)	Any serious adverse event (16.8% vs 16.6%) Pancreatitis (0.4% vs 0.3%)	Pancreatitis (relative risk 1.43; 95% CI 0.54–3.75; Serious GI events (relative risk 1.06; 95% CI 0.79–1.41)	Any adverse events (77.2% vs 78.1%) Serious adverse events (37% vs 38.5%) Acute pancreatitis (0.3% vs 0.1%) Chronic pancreatitis (0.1% vs 0.1%) All cancer (3.3% vs 3.8%)	Serious adverse event (HR 0.91; 95% CI 0.87–0.95; p < 0.001) Symptoms of volume depletion (HR 1.00; 95% CI 0.83–1.21; p = 0.99) DKA (HR 2.18; 95% CI 1.10–4.30; p = 0.02) UTI (HR 0.93; 95% CI 0.73–1.18; p = 0.54)	Acute pancreatitis (0.5% vs 0.3%; p = 0.11) Serious hepatic event (0.5% vs 0.8%; p = 0.057) Serious GI event (2.4% vs 2.4%; 0.87) First study drug discontinua-tion (42.3% vs 43.8%; p = 0.38)	Serious adverse events (46.6% vs 48.1%) Any adverse event (93.6% vs 95.2%)	GI disorders (6.8% vs 1.6%) Serious adverse events (18.9% vs 22.5%)	UTI 5 mg (risk difference 2.1; 95% CI 0.40–3.7; p = 0.02) UTI 15 mg (risk difference 1.8; 95% CI 0.20–3.5; p = 0.03) Genital mycotic infection in creased in for both doses in both men and women (p < 0.001) UTI 5 mg (risk difference 2.1%; 95% CI 0.4–3.7; p = 0.02) UTI 15 mg (risk difference 1.8; 95% CI 0.2–3.5; p = 0.03)	Diarrhoea (9.5% vs 6%; p < 0.001) Volume depletion (5,3% vs 4%; p = 0.003) Genital mycotic infections (2.4% vs 0.9%; p < 0.001) DKA (0.6% vs 0.3%; p = 0.02)

Table 4 Guideline and professional organization recommendations on glycaemic control

	IAGG, EDWPOP, and International task force of experts in diabetes [171]	American Geriatrics Society [172]	American College of Physicians [167]	Diabetes Canada Clinical Practice Guidelines Expert Committee [96]	Australian Diabetes Society [173, 174]	American Association of Clinical Endocrinology/ American College of Endocrinology [175, 176]	NICE [177, 178]	ADA [95, 168]	ESC/EASD [166, 179]
Year	2012	2013 (note—no longer considered active as more than 5 years out of date)	2018	2018	2015 (for screening)	2020	Updated 2020	2021	2021
Screening	–	–	–	Decisions on screening in older patients should be made on an individual basis Screening is unlikely to be beneficial in those over the age of 80	Only those at high risk of undiagnosed diabetes should be tested. These include a medical condition or ethnic background associated with high risk of diabetes OR an Australian type 2 diabetes risk score of ≥12	≥45 without other risk factors, consider screening younger in those with risk factors Repeat testing every 3 years for those at risk, or consideration for screening annually in those with 2 or more risk factors	Those with high-risk scores using a validated computer based risk assessment tool or self-assessment questionnaire	≥45 years onwards and every 3 years thereafter, with consideration for more frequent testing depending on initial results and risk status	–

HbA1c targets									
In general, a target of 7–7.5% should be aimed for Consider individual co-morbidities, and cognitive and functional status when determining what glucose levels should be agreed with the patient and/or carer	Target should generally be 7.5% to 8% A target of 7% to 7.5% may be appropriate if it can be safely achieved in those who are otherwise healthy and with good functional status Higher targets (8–9%) are appropriate for older adults with multiple co-morbidities, poor health, and limited life expectancy There is potential harm in lowering HbA1c to less than 6.5% in older adults with type 2 diabetes	Clinicians should aim for a HbA1c level between 7% and 8% in most patients with type 2 diabetes Clinicians should consider de-intensifying pharmacologic therapy in patients with type 2 diabetes & a HbA1c level < 6.5% Clinicians should treat patients with type 2 diabetes to minimise symptoms related to hyperglycaemia and avoid targeting a HbA1c level in patients with a life expectancy less than 10 years due to advanced age (≥80 years), residence in a nursing home, or chronic disease (eg dementia, cancer, ESKD, or severe COPD or CHF) because the harm outweigh the benefits	Low risk of hypoglycaemia (i.e., therapy does not include insulin or SU) Functionally independent (CFI 1–3), HbA1c ≤7% Functionally dependent (CFI 4–5) HbA1c <8% Frail and/or with dementia (CFI 6–8) HbA1c <8.5% End of life (CFI 9) HbA1c measurement not recommended. Avoid symptomatic hyperglycaemia or any hypoglycaemia	Individualise the target—commonly ≤53 mmol/mol (7%) but should be reviewed regularly Patients with severe hypoglycaemia— < =8% Diabetes of short duration and no clinical cardiovascular disease • Lifestyle modification ± metformin - < =6%. • Requiring any antidiabetic agents other than metformin or insulin <=6.5%. • Requiring insulin <=7%. Major comorbidities likely to limit life expectancy—symptomatic therapy of hyperglycaemia	HbA1c target ≤6.5% in those without concurrent serious illness and low hypoglycaemic risk HbA1c >6.5%—for patients with concurrent serious illness and at risk for hypoglycaemia Recognise that targets should be individualised on the basis of age, comorbidities and duration of disease, but do not provide specific guidance	Adopt an individualised approach to diabetes care that is tailored to the needs of adults with type 2 diabetes, taking into account their personal preferences, comorbidities, risks from polypharmacy, and their ability to benefit from long-term interventions because of reduced life expectancy Support an aim of 6.5% for those being managed with diet alone or being managed with a single drug not associated with hypoglycaemia For adults on drugs associated with hypoglycaemia, aim for a HbA1c of 7% Consider relaxing the target on a case by case basis in older or frail adults	Older adults who are otherwise healthy with few coexisting chronic illnesses and intact cognitive function and functional status—HbA1c <7.0–7.5% (53–58 mmol/mol) Those with co-existing chronic illnesses, cognitive impairment, or functional dependence should have less strict goals (HbA1c <8–8.5% (64–69 mmol/mol) Very complex/poor health or moderate to severe cognitive impairment or 2+ ADL impairments— avoid reliance on HbA1c. Glucose control decisions should be based on avoiding hypoglycaemia and symptomatic hyperglycaemia	A target of <7% (53 mmol/mol) is recommended for most adults with type 1 or 2 diabetes mellitus For patients with a long duration of DM and in old or frail adults, a less stringent target should be considered A target of ≤6.5% (48 mmol/mol) should be considered in type 2 diabetes if the patient is not frail and does not have ASCVD

ADA American Diabetes Association, *CFI* Clinical Frailty Index, *EASD* European Association for the Study of Diabetes, *EDWPOP* European Diabetes Working Party for Older People, *ESC* European Society of Cardiology, IAGG: International Association of Gerontology and Geriatrics, *NICE* National Institute for Clinical Excellence

rigidly applying similar strategies to functionally impaired, frail, individuals with multiple co-morbidities or a more limited life expectancy may lead to excess harm in these patients, and so various guidelines have recently been published recommending more lenient glycaemic targets for these patients [164–166]. Canadian guidelines have also incorporated a clinical frailty index to guide decisions on glycaemic targets [96]. Similarly, the American College of Physicians recommends minimising the symptoms related to hyperglycaemia, rather than targeting a specific HbA1c, for those residing in a nursing home, those with a life expectancy less than 10 years due to advanced age, or those with certain chronic conditions [167]. For those with very poor health or those nearing the end of life, the focus should shift to the prevention of hypoglycaemia and symptomatic hyperglycemia [168]. Efforts have been made to develop tools that can help to predict life expectancy in older diabetic patients, and may be useful adjuncts in determining risk-benefit ratios [169].

While maintaining good glycaemic control is important in non-frail older patients with diabetes, control of other cardiovascular risk factors, such as hypertension, may result in greater reductions in morbidity and mortality, and, so, when achieving tighter glycaemic control is difficult or not possible, addressing these other ASCVD risk factors more intensively can still add significant benefit [168].

With advancements in technology, continuous glucose monitoring might also afford opportunities to monitor glycaemic control more closely, particularly in older patients at risk of hypoglycaemia. The Wireless Innovation in Seniors with Diabetes Mellitus (WISDM) trial, showed that continuous glucose monitoring in older patients (median age 68 years) with type 1 diabetes, reduced the time spent in hypoglycaemia compared to those with standard monitoring [170]. While the trial only included 203 patients, it does support the relevance of further research in this area in older patients, potentially increasing the safety profile of antidiabetic regimens in higher risk patients.

3.4 Antihyperglycemic Therapies

Lifestyle interventions, as discussed in more detail in later sections in this chapter, remain a critical component in the prevention of ASCVD in all diabetic patients. In particular, early lifestyle intervention in older patients with pre-diabetes, primarily in the form of weight loss and an increase in physical activity, offer a unique preventive opportunity in potentially halting the progression to type 2 diabetes, and, hence, the subsequent requirement for pharmacological interventions and their associated risks [180–182]. All patients with diabetes should receive advice on nutrition [183]. Diabetes self-management programmes that include tailored interventions and psychological support have also been shown to be a useful adjunct in improving diabetic control, adherence to diabetic medications and attendance at retinal screening in older adults [184, 185].

When it comes to adding in medications for diabetic patients, the same principles apply as with all other diagnoses in older patients: one should avoid polypharmacy and try to use simplified treatment regimens (e.g., once daily) where possible [171]. While there have been few RCTs examining metformin use exclusively in older patients with diabetes, it remains the first line medication in most patients with type 2 diabetes [183, 186]. Particular advantages of metformin include its low risk for hypoglycaemia, while its gastrointestinal side effects and contraindications in cases of renal impairment, are potential drawbacks in older patients. There have been questions raised as to the benefit of continuing metformin in those over the age of 80, although overall evidence in this age group is too scarce to guide definitive recommendations [186].

The are several new classes of drugs emerging, which have shown some impressive results in reducing cardiovascular risk, achieving HbA1c levels averaging between 7 and 8%. Additionally since 2008, following the finding that rosiglitazone was linked to an increased risk of CV events and mortality, the FDA mandated that all glucose-lowering drugs must demonstrate cardiovascular safety in post-marketing studies with non-inferiority designs [187]. As a result of these CVOT trials, we have had a rapid increase of data on the effect of new glucose lowering drugs on relevant CV outcomes.

3.4.1 Sodium Glucose Co-transporter 2 (SGLT-2) Inhibitors

SGLT-2 inhibitors are a particularly exciting new class of anti-diabetes drug in the area of preventive cardiology. By inhibiting the sodium dependent glucose transporter (SGLT-2) in the early proximal tubule of the kidney, these medications reduce renal glucose reabsorption, in turn increasing urinary glucose excretion [188]. One of the first CVOTs to assess the impact of SGLT-2 inhibitors was the EMPA-REG trial [148]. Here the investigators demonstrated that empagliflozin, compared to placebo, resulted in a reduction in the primary outcome of death from CV causes, nonfatal MI (excluding silent MI), or nonfatal stroke (HR 0.86; 95% CI 0.74–0.99; $p < 0.001$ for noninferiority and $p = 0.04$ for superiority) as well as a significant reduction in all-cause mortality and hospitalisations for heart failure. Almost 50% of the trial population were ≥ 65 years of age (3172 patients), and on subgroup analysis, the reductions in the primary outcome in the empagliflozin group were greater in those ≥ 65 (HR 0.71; 95% CI 0.59–0.87) compared to those <65 years (HR 1.04; 95% CI 0.84–1.29), with a significant p-value for interaction of 0.01. The subsequent CANVAS trial demonstrated similar results with canagliflozin in reducing CV mortality, nonfatal MI or nonfatal stroke and hospitalisations for heart failure in those with a history of ASCVD or known CV risk factors, again with greater reductions observed in those ≥ 65 years. In the DECLARE-TIMI trial, dapagliflozin also reduced the rate of hospitalisation for heart failure, but the reduction in major CV events failed to reach statistical significance [158]. Recently, the VERTIS-CV trial again showed a reduction in a composite outcome of cardiovascular mortality, nonfatal MI and nonfatal stroke with ertugliflozin, where 50% of the trial population were ≥ 65 years [162]. The most recent trial, SCORED (Effect of Sotagliflozin on Cardiovascular and Renal Events in Patients with Type 2 Diabetes and Moderate

Renal Impairment Who Are at Cardiovascular Risk), was unfortunately terminated early at 16 months follow-up due to loss of funding from the sponsor [163]. Due to fewer than expected event rates, the primary outcome was adjusted prior to data analysis. Despite early termination, they observed a lower risk of the composite primary outcome (deaths from CV causes, hospitalisations for heart failure and urgent visits for heart failure), with sotagliflozin compared to placebo (5.6 vs 7.5 events per 100 patient years; HR 0.74; 95% CI 0.63–0.88; $p < 0.001$) in type 2 diabetics with CKD and increased CV risk. On subgroup analysis, these benefits were continued to those aged 65 and over.

A recent meta-analysis examining SGLT-2 inhibitor use in older patients, confirmed their efficacy in reducing major cardiovascular events in those over 65 years [189]. Significantly the observed reduction in heart failure hospitalisation was greater in those older than 65 compared to younger patients. While those aged 75 years and older were under-represented, the available data does suggest that these patients may see similar benefits.

Given the increased glucose concentration in the urine with SGLT-2 inhibitor use, one of the main side effects that trials have observed is an increased propensity to develop urinary tract infections, as well as mycotic genital infections. The resultant osmotic diuresis also means that potential volume depletion is also a risk that may be particularly relevant in older adults. Some trials have also reported an increased risk for DKA [158, 163].

3.4.2 Glucagon-Like Peptide 1 (GLP-1) Agonists

GLP-1 agonists have also been shown to have significant cardiovascular benefits. A recent CVOT assessing the impact of GLP-1 agonists, was the PIONEER-6 trial [161]. Here, oral semaglutide was non-inferior to placebo in reducing the primary outcome, a composite of death from CV causes, nonfatal MI and nonfatal stroke (HR 0.79; 95% CI 0.57–1.11; $p < 0.001$ for non-inferiority) in type 2 diabetics with either established CVD or with risk factors for CVD (mean age 66 years) over a period of 15.9 months. These results were similar to the previous similar SUSTAIN-6 trial, which found that semaglutide given subcutaneously over a median period of 2.1 years was superior to placebo in reducing the same primary outcome (HR 0.86; 95% CI 0.74–0.99; $p < 0.001$ for noninferiority and 0.04 for superiority) [152]. This lower risk was primarily driven by a significant 39% decrease in the rate of nonfatal stroke (HR 0.61; 95% CI 0.38–0.99; $p = 0.04$) and a non-significant 26% reduction in nonfatal MI (HR 0.74; 95% CI 0.51–1.08; $p = 0.12$). The authors observed no significant difference in the rate of CV death over a follow-up period of 2.1 years. The SUSTAIN-6 group did, however, note an increased risk of heart failure hospitalisations, as well as retinopathy. The latter was particularly notable in the early part of the trial. On subgroup analysis, the reductions in occurrence of the primary outcome were greater for those less than 65 years old in PIONEER-6, while in the SUSTAIN-6 trial those ≥65 conferred a greater benefit.

In the REWIND trial ($N = 9901$, mean age 66.2 years), dulaglutide was superior to placebo in reducing the composite outcome of nonfatal MI, nonfatal stroke and death from CV or unknown causes over a median 5.4 years, a reduction which was largely driven by a 24% reduction in nonfatal stroke (HR 0.76; 95% CI 0.61–0.95; $p = 0.017$) [159]. Albiglutide and exenatide were also found to reduce composite cardiovascular events in the HARMONY and EXSCEL trials respectively [155, 156]. While both trials failed to show a significant reduction in nonfatal stroke, the HARMONY trial did observe a 25% reduction in fatal or nonfatal MI (HR 0.75; 95% CI 0.61–0.90; $p = 0.003$). The earlier LEADER trial demonstrated similar benefits with liraglutide in reducing the rate of first occurrence of death from CV causes, nonfatal MI and nonfatal stroke, as well as independently statistically significant reductions in cardiovascular mortality, all cause mortality and microvascular events [151]. Notably, 75% of those in the LEADER trial were aged 65 years or older, with 9% of the trial population 75 years or older. The short acting GLP-1 agonist, lixisenatide was found to have a neutral effect on CV outcomes compared to placebo in the diabetic patients with a recent ACS [149].

The benefits of GLP-1 agonists in reducing the composite outcome of ASCVD in those aged 65 years and older was confirmed in a recent meta-analysis, reducing the risk by 11% (HR 0.89; 95% CI 0.82–0.96; $I^2 = 48\%$; 6 trials). Cardiovascular mortality was also found to be reduced by 22% (HR 0.78; 95% CI 0.63–0.97; $I^2 = 25\%$; two trials), with reductions in stroke risk (HR 0.80; 95% CI 0.69–0.92; $I^2 = 0\%$; 3 trials) and myocardial infarction (HR 0.85; 95% CI 0.73–0.98; $I^2 = 0\%$; 2 trials) also noted [189]. In addition, although more rigorous research is required, there have been suggestions of potential additional pleiotropic effects of GLP-1 agonists, including modest reductions in cholesterol and blood pressure, that may make this class of drug useful in the setting of polypharmacy [190–192].

In terms of potential drawbacks, gastrointestinal disorders are more common with some GLP-1 agonists and injection site reactions are also more common if these medications are given subcutaneously. Dose reductions with slow up titration of doses may be required in older, more frail adults [191]. While once weekly dosing regimens available for most GLP-1 agonists may be appealing, delivery by subcutaneous injection may not be practical for all older adults.

3.4.3 DPP-4 Inhibitors

There have been several studies that have examined the efficacy and safety of DPP-4 inhibitors in older adults and in those with co-morbidities [193, 194]. Relevantly, DPP-4 inhibitors have been shown to lower HbA1c to the same extent as sulfonylureas, but without the same risk of hypoglycaemia [195]. Linagliptin, in addition to usual care, has been shown to be non-inferior to both placebo plus usual care and glimepiride plus usual care in reducing a composite outcome of CV death, nonfatal MI and nonfatal stroke, in patients with more advanced CKD or at high CV risk respectively, making it a useful option in older patients with renal impairment [157, 160].

There have been trials suggesting an increased risk of hospitalisation for heart failure, particularly with the use of saxagliptin [146]. However, others have found no increased risk of hospitalisation with sitagliptin or linagliptin [150, 157]. Given the uncertainty, guidelines recommend against their use in patients with a known history of heart failure.

3.4.4 Thiazolidinediones

Thiazolidinediones have been shown to maintain glycaemic targets longer when compared to metformin or the sulfonylurea, glyburide, albeit in a younger patient cohort (mean age 57 years), while avoiding the risk of hypoglycemia [196]. However, there are a number of drawbacks associated with thiazolidinedione use in older patients, in particular the increased risk of oedema and heart failure. The RECORD (Rosiglitazone Evaluated for Cardiovascular Outcomes in Oral Agent Combination Therapy for Type 2 Diabetes) trial found a two-fold increased risk of heart failure in those who received rosiglitazone compared with active control (metformin or sulfonylurea) [144]. Significantly, these events resulted in hospitalisation and increased heart failure deaths, meaning that, at least in some cases, thiazolidinedione-associated heart failure is not benign. As a result, rosiglitazone in particular, should be avoided in patients with a history of heart failure. Rosiglitazone should also be used with caution in those at high risk of fractures, particularly in women [144]. Given rosiglitazone's link with an increased risk of stroke, heart failure and all-cause mortality in patients over the age of 65 years, pioglitazone should be ideally used preferentially if considering thiazolidinedione use in older patients [197, 198].

3.4.5 Insulin and Others

There has only been one RCT evaluating the effects of insulin on macrovascular outcomes [199]. While there was an improvement in glycaemic control, there was no benefit for cardiovascular outcomes. A major drawback of insulin use in the older adult is the risk of hypoglycaemia. Administration of insulin therapy also requires good visual and motor skills, as well as good cognitive ability. This may be a barrier to administration in some patients. Where possible, once daily dosing should be used.

Sulfonylureas, particularly long-acting formulations, should be avoided if possible in older patients due to their risk of hypoglycaemia and its associated consequences [200].

4　Diet

Box 4

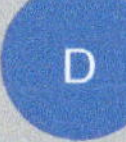

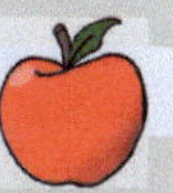

- Both the Mediterranean diet and DASH diet are recommended dietary patterns.
- Dos: diet rich in fruit, vegetables, skinless poultry, fish, unsaturated fats, nuts and whole grains.
- Don'ts: diets high in sugar, salt, trans fats, saturated fats, and red meat.
- Limit daily alcohol consumption to ≤2 drinks (20g/day of alcohol) in men, and ≤1 drink (10g/day of alcohol) for women.
- Both low and high BMIs are associated with increased ASCVD in older adults.
- While the ideal BMI in younger patients is defined as being between 18.5 and 24.9kg/m^2, a slightly higher BMI may be acceptable in older adults.
- An increasing prevalence of sarcopenic obesity, and growing recognition of its link to ASCVD, means there may be a role for measuring grip strength in association with BMI to achieve a more accurate picture of a patient's ASCVD risk.

While maintaining a healthy diet is intuitive for improving general health, most of the evidence for a relationship between diet and ASCVD comes from observational research, with a paucity of high quality, large, randomised trials assessing the impact of diet on hard ASCVD outcomes, particularly in older patients. Much of the evidence discussed below is therefore derived from data in younger patients. However, given the low risks associated with maintaining a healthy diet, as well as the general health benefits gained from maintaining a healthy diet, it would seem reasonable to recommend similar measures for older patients. Additionally, a reduction in salt intake and weight have has been shown to have the added benefit of reducing the requirement of antihypertensive therapy in older adults by up to 30%, thereby reducing the risk of unwanted medication side effects as well as potential polypharmacy [201].

4.1　Benefits of Maintaining a Healthy Diet in Older Adults

One of the key outputs of maintaining a healthy diet is maintaining a healthy body weight. Traditionally, a healthy weight has been defined as a body mass index between 18.5 and 24.9kg/m^2 [202]. An elevated BMI has consistently been shown to be linked to higher all cause and CVD mortality even up to the age of 75 years, albeit with attenuation in associated risk observed with increasing age [203, 204]. Despite this, it has been estimated that two-thirds of those over the age of 65 years in westernised countries have a BMI above the recommended target, meaning we have significant opportunity to improve our preventive efforts in this area [205, 206].

While there is an agreement that an elevated BMI is associated with increased CVD risk, there has been some debate in the literature if the same target range for BMI is appropriate for older adults as is generally targeted in younger adults [207, 208]. Winter et al. recently reported a U-shaped observational relationship between BMI and all-cause mortality in community dwelling adults aged 65 years or older, with the nadir of the curve sitting at a BMI between 24 kg/m^2 and 30.9kg/m^2, raising the question as to whether slightly higher BMIs may be an acceptable target in certain older adults [209]. There are also some limitations to reliance on BMI as the sole measure of weight in older adults as it does not account for changes in body composition with age, specifically the decline in muscle mass and strength, and this potential impact on CVD risk [210]. With a concurrent increase in the prevalence of obesity and an aging population, the prevalence of obesity in the presence of a low muscle mass or strength, also known as sarcopenic obesity, is becoming increasingly recognised as a relevant marker of CVD risk in older adults [211]. A prospective cohort by Stephen et al. included 3366 community-dwelling primary prevention adults and demonstrated that while obesity (determined using waist circumference) and sarcopenia alone were not sufficient to increase CVD risk in these patients, the presence of both i.e., sarcopenic obesity (defined as a high waist circumference and low grip strength) increased the risk of CVD by 23% [212]. There may therefore be a role for assessing grip strength as part of weight assessments in older patients. Measuring a patient's waist circumference can also help unmask increased visceral adiposity and is increasingly recommended as part of the routine assessment [213]. An elevated waist circumference, even in those with a normal BMI, is independently associated with an increased CVD risk. Guidelines currently agree that a normal waist circumference is <40 inches in men or < 35 inches in women, with smaller measures for those of South Asian, Chinese or Japanese ethnicity [83, 214].

4.2   Components of a Healthy Diet

A diet rich in fruit and vegetables, skinless poultry, fish, unsaturated fats, nuts and whole grains remains key to reducing both the risk of cardiovascular disease and all-cause mortality [215–218]. Conversely, diets high in sugar consumption, salt, trans fats, saturated fats and red meat have all been linked to increased CVD events and mortality [217, 219–223]. While single food groups and nutrients have been linked to CV disease, there is now increased attention on studying dietary patterns, as individual dietary components are almost always consumed in combination with strong correlations between each other [224]. While there are numerous dietary patterns globally, probably two of the most commonly encountered in CV literature are the Mediterranean diet (MedDiet) and the DASH diet.

The term "Mediterranean Diet" (MedDiet) began appearing in the literature following a landmark study in the 1980s, which demonstrated that CVD risk varied across countries with different dietary habits [225]. The study by Keys et al., found that there was a lower CHD mortality rate in countries bordering the Mediterranean. While there are some variations in definitions, generally the Mediterranean diet is accepted as a diet where olive oil is the main source of dietary fat, where there is a high intake of plant foods, a low to moderate intake of animal foods and wine in moderation with meals [226]. Since the original work by Keys et al., there have been several meta-analyses examining the effects of adherence to a Mediterranean diet on various CVD risks, with suggestions that such a diet is inversely associated with the risk of developing diabetes and metabolic syndrome, with beneficial effects on blood pressure, triglycerides, LDL-C, body weight and development of heart failure [226–228]. Relevantly, adherence to a Mediterranean diet has also been shown to improve overall survival in those over 70 years, meaning that evaluation of a patient's diet should continue to form a key part of preventive conversations even in older patients [229]. While there was some controversy surrounding the initial published report, data from the PREDIMED trial demonstrated that a Mediterranean diet supplemented with extra-virgin olive oil or a Mediterranean diet supplemented with mixed nuts was superior to a reduced fat diet (control) in preventing major cardiovascular events in those at high risk of CVD [230]. Current guidelines are consistent in recommending a Mediterranean type diet, rich in vegetables, fruits, legumes, nuts, whole grains and fish, while avoiding trans fats and minimising intake of processed meats, carbohydrates and sweetened beverages [83, 84].

The Dietary Approaches to Stop Hypertension (DASH) diet has large overlaps with the MedDiet, including a high intake of fruit and vegetables, legumes, low fat diary, whole grain products, nuts, fish and poultry, with a reduced intake of saturated fat, red and processed meats and sweet beverages [231]. This dietary pattern has been associated with improved blood pressure control and a reduction in CV events [222].

Other dietary patterns, including those low in carbohydrates but high in fat, so called "ketogenic diets," have been associated with short term weight loss in younger patients, at the expense of increased LDL-C [17]. Similarly, diets with very low or very high carbohydrate intake have been associated with an increase in mortality [232]. At present, guidelines do not recommend ketogenic diets for ASCVD reduction.

There have been suggestions that consumption of alcohol in moderation may in fact improve vascular function and reduce the risk of ASCVD, however advice to increase alcohol consumption should be avoided given the other health risks associated with excessive drinking [233]. Daily alcohol consumption should be limited to ≤ 2 drinks (20g/day of alcohol) for men, and ≤ 1 drink (10g/day of alcohol) for women [83, 84].

5   Exercise

Box 5

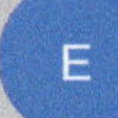
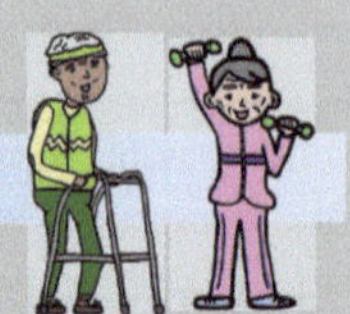

- Regular exercise helps improve weight loss, muscle mass, blood pressure control, cholesterol levels and insulin sensitivity.
- Guideline recommendations are that all adults should engage in at least 150 min of accumulated moderate intensity or 75 min of vigorous intensity aerobic physical activity per week.
- Older adults who cannot reach those targets should be as physically active as their condition allows.
- Any exercise is better than none.
- Sedentary behaviour (defined as all sitting or reclining with low energy expenditure) increases the risk of ASCVD independent of physical activity levels, and thus minimising such behaviour is key.
- Ideally, exercise should include a combination of balance training, aerobic exercises and muscle strengthening activities.
- The FITT-VP principle provides a useful structure for discussing an individualised exercise regime.
- Inclusion of older adults in cardiac rehabilitation programmes remain a key component in the setting of secondary prevention.

Regular physical activity helps improve weight loss, blood pressure control, cholesterol levels and insulin sensitivity, and thus, maintaining a physically active lifestyle remains a critical component in the prevention of ASCVD. Additional benefits of exercise in older adults include anti-inflammatory and anti-thrombotic effects, improved cardiovascular hemodynamics, improved psychological wellbeing, quality of life and decreased risk of falls and injury. Similar to other lifestyle interventions, the benefits of being physically active on balance significantly outweigh any potential risks in most patients. Despite this, it is estimated that more than a quarter of all adults globally are not engaging in enough physical activity [234]. Compounding the issue further, physical activity levels tend to progressively decline with increasing age.

5.1   Recommended Exercise Prescription

There is an inverse dose response relationship between the amount of moderate to vigorous physical activity and incident ASCVD events and death. This dose-response relationship is curvilinear, meaning that those who go from a relatively inactive lifestyle to engaging in mild or moderately physical activity will yield a relatively large risk reduction in CVD outcomes, whereas further increases in physical activity levels beyond this will produce smaller risk reductions [235, 236]. While current guidelines recommend that all adults should engage in at least 150 min of accumulated moderate intensity or 75 min of vigorous-intensity aerobic physical activity per week, the benefits of encouraging older adults who do little or no exercise to engage in any form of physical activity can have substantial health benefits [83, 166, 237]. To realise the full health benefits of being physically active, older adults should ideally includes combination of balance training, aerobic exercises and muscle strengthening activities into their weekly physical activity routine [238]. There is increasing recognition that older adults who cannot reach these targets should be as physically active as their abilities and conditions allow [238, 239]. Those with physical activities well below guideline recommendations continue to observe CVD and general health benefits. Replacing sitting with even light intensity physical activity or standing may provide significant health benefits for patients [240]. Similarly, the addition of only 30 min of normal walking per day for 5 days a week has been associated with a 19% reduction in CHD risk [241]. O'Donovan et al. demonstrated that patients (mean age 58.9 years) who reported 1–2 sessions of moderate- or vigorous intensity leisure time physical activity, which is less than 150 min, per week had a reduced all-cause mortality and CVD mortality as compared to those who were physically inactive [242].

While sedentary behaviour was previously conceptualised as one end of the physical activity spectrum, it is increasingly being recognised as a distinct construct from physical activity. Defined as, all sitting or reclining with low energy expenditure (<1.5 metabolic equivalents), sedentary behaviour has been shown to pose a significant risk for the development of ASCVD, independent of physical activity levels [243–246]. Sedentary behaviour has increased in the last decade, and is highest in older adults, with adults over the age of 60 years estimated to spend 80% of their awake time engaged in sedentary activities [245, 247, 248]. A recent large meta-analysis by Patterson et al., including data from over one million patients, found that self-reported sitting for more than 6–8 h a day was linked to increased CVD mortality, even after adjustment for physical activity levels [244]. Significantly, data from the OPACH study, including 5638 women aged 63–97 years (mean age 78.55 years), found that reducing sedentary time by 1 h per day was associated with a 12% lower risk of CVD (defined as the first occurrence of an MI, revascularisation, hospitalised angina, heart failure, stroke or death attributable to CVD) and a 26% lower risk of heart disease [249]. Increased bouts of time spent in sedentary positions were also associated with increased risk, while short interruptions to sedentary time with light intensity exercise is associated with lower CVD risk. Data from the Canadian Fitness Study observed similar findings; among those who achieve physical activity recommendations, the subgroup who spent more time sitting were at increased risk of CVD mortality compared to those who spent less time sitting [250]. Thus, a key component when counselling older patients should include an emphasis on reducing the total sedentary time, as well as bouts spent engaging in sedentary activities.

On the other extreme end, there has been some observational evidence to suggest early atherosclerotic disease development in those engaged in an excessive volume of high intensity exercise [251]. The exact mechanisms for atherosclerotic development in athletes is unknown, but some potential speculative pathways include altered coronary hemodynamics, increased inflammation, imbalanced diet, performance-enhancing drugs, increased systolic blood pressure and increased mechanical stress [252]. Contrasting these findings, cohorts of elite athletes have been shown to have improved life expectancy and lower CVD mortality [253]. Therefore, while the curvilinear association between exercise and CVD is well established, suggesting diminishing returns in terms of CVD benefit from more excessive exercise practices, whether too much exercise can cause harm is not fully known and the data to date are mixed.

The FITT-VP principle (Frequency, Intensity, Time, Type, Volume and Progression) can be a useful guide when discussing an individualised exercise regime with older adults [254]. Older adults with more complex comorbidities may need health screening prior to engaging in more vigorous exercise programmes. However, it is important to realise that exercise is safe for most people, particularly at lower to moderate intensity levels where benefits far outweigh the risks, and therefore efforts should be made not to over screen or place unnecessary obstacles for patients who are keen to engage in regular physical activity [255].

5.2   Identifying Barriers and Motivators to Exercise in Older Adults

Although the benefits of regular physical activity are well established, most older adults do not maintain the guideline recommended levels. In fact, it is estimated that almost 90% of older adults have at least one perceived barrier to exercise participation [256]. Frequently cited barriers to regular physical activity include presence of co-morbidities (e.g. osteoporosis), lack of time, fear of injury, lack of access to an area for exercising, lack of knowledge and lack of motivation, fear of "slowing others down" or lack of belief in their capabilities [257–259].On the contrary, motivators for regular exercise include physician advice, family influences, health benefits, and psychosocial reasons such as enjoying group activities and meeting friends [257]. It has been suggested that older adults may be more likely to respect physician advice compared to younger patients, and therefore physicians and healthcare providers should make it a priority to regularly counsel older adults about the continued benefits from regular physical activity with aging [260]. To help sustain regular exercise, it is important to encourage patients to find an activity that they enjoy and can include into their daily routine [84]. Increased access to group based physical activity programs may also help in increasing participation in regular exercise [261]. Use of technology, such as step counters or wearable devices and fitness apps can be helpful adjuncts in promoting physical activity, even in older patients [238].

5.3　Cardiac Rehabilitation in Secondary Prevention

Cardiac rehabilitation (CR) remains a critical component in the continuum of care for older patients who have known cardiovascular disease. Using a combination of patient education, health behaviour modification and exercise training, CR has been shown to improve mortality, hospital readmissions, and health related quality of life in secondary prevention patients. Significantly, cardiac rehab has been shown to confer a similar benefit for older patients compared to their younger counterparts [262, 263]. Cardiac rehabilitation is currently recommended for all patients after a myocardial infarction, percutaneous coronary intervention, coronary artery bypass graft surgery or in the setting of chronic coronary syndromes or symptomatic peripheral arterial disease [264–267]. It is also recommended for patients in the setting of heart failure with reduced ejection fraction [268]. Despite the clear indications and benefits, cardiac rehabilitation is often underutilised in older adults, particularly more frail older adults, women or those from minority groups [269–272]. Home based cardiac rehabilitation may be an option for selected older patients in overcoming barriers such as transportation challenges or lack of availability of a programme near a patient's home [273, 274].

6　Conclusion

The prevalence of both cardiovascular risk factors and incident ASVCD increase linearly with advancing age, adding significantly to morbidity, reduced quality of life and early mortality in older adults. With a rapidly ageing population, early and appropriate preventive strategies are therefore a major global health priority. While the risks of CV disease are increased, changing physiology and an increasing prevalence of comorbidities, frailty and polypharmacy, also make this patient cohort more vulnerable to adverse effects of more intensive medical interventions on ASCVD risk factors. Thus, clinicians face unique challenges when considering preventive care strategies for older adults.

The common misperception that it is "too late" to implement changes should be avoided. Assessment of a patient's risk should involve consideration of the potential benefit gained from an intervention, weighed against potential risks. It is particularly important to think outside of chronological age, considering both frailty and potential comorbidities. Undertreatment based on age alone is a common and perilous pitfall. New ASCVD risk prediction tools for older adults, such as the SCORE2 OP, may help overcome age-based therapeutic malaise. Shared clinician-patient decisions are key, both in establishing treatment goals and priorities for all patients.

Going forward, inclusion of older patients with co-morbidities, representative of the everyday older adult, in larger trials is a major research priority. Consideration of outcomes relevant to older adults, such as quality of life, will be key.

Disclosures and Other Relevant Conflicts of Interest　None reported.

References

1. Ference BA, Ginsberg HN, Graham I, et al. Low-density lipoproteins cause atherosclerotic cardiovascular disease. 1. Evidence from genetic, epidemiologic, and clinical studies. A consensus statement from the European Atherosclerosis Society Consensus Panel. Eur Heart J. 2017;38(32):2459–72. https://doi.org/10.1093/eurheartj/ehx144.

2. Lewington S, Whitlock G, Clarke R, et al. Blood cholesterol and vascular mortality by age, sex, and blood pressure: a meta-analysis of individual data from 61 prospective studies with 55,000 vascular deaths. Lancet. 2007;370(9602):1829–39. https://doi.org/10.1016/s0140-6736(07)61778-4.

3. Petersen LK, Christensen K, Kragstrup J. Lipid-lowering treatment to the end? A review of observational studies and RCTs on cholesterol and mortality in 80+−year olds. Age Ageing. 2010;39(6):674–80. https://doi.org/10.1093/ageing/afq129.

4. Gencer B, Marston NA, Im K, et al. Efficacy and safety of lowering LDL cholesterol in older patients: a systematic review and meta-analysis of randomised controlled trials. Lancet. 2020;396(10263):1637–43. https://doi.org/10.1016/s0140-6736(20)32332-1.

5. Mortensen MB, Nordestgaard BG. Elevated LDL cholesterol and increased risk of myocardial infarction and atherosclerotic cardiovascular disease in individuals aged 70-100 years: a contemporary primary prevention cohort. Lancet. 2020;396(10263):1644–52. https://doi.org/10.1016/s0140-6736(20)32233-9.

6. Mortensen MB, Falk E. Primary prevention with statins in the elderly. J Am Coll Cardiol. 2018;71(1):85–94. https://doi.org/10.1016/j.jacc.2017.10.080.

7. Ravnskov U, Diamond DM, Hama R, et al. Lack of an association or an inverse association between low-density-lipoprotein cholesterol and mortality in the elderly: a systematic review. BMJ Open. 2016;6(6):e010401. https://doi.org/10.1136/bmjopen-2015-010401.

8. Takata Y, Ansai T, Soh I, et al. Serum total cholesterol concentration and 10-year mortality in an 85-year-old population. Clin Interv Aging. 2014;9:293–300. https://doi.org/10.2147/CIA.S53754.

9. Johannesen CDL, Langsted A, Mortensen MB, Nordestgaard BG. Association between low density lipoprotein and all cause and cause specific mortality in Denmark: prospective cohort study. BMJ. 2020;371:m4266. https://doi.org/10.1136/bmj.m4266.

10. Yi S-W, Yi J-J, Ohrr H. Total cholesterol and all-cause mortality by sex and age: a prospective cohort study among 12.8 million adults. Sci Rep. 2019;9(1):1596. https://doi.org/10.1038/s41598-018-38461-y.

11. Liang Y, Vetrano DL, Qiu C. Serum total cholesterol and risk of cardiovascular and non-cardiovascular mortality in old age: a population-based study. BMC Geriatr. 2017;17(1):294. https://doi.org/10.1186/s12877-017-0685-z.

12. Brescianini S, Maggi S, Farchi G, et al. Low total cholesterol and increased risk of dying: are low levels clinical warning signs in the elderly? Results from the Italian Longitudinal Study on Aging. J Am Geriatr Soc. 2003;51(7):991–6. https://doi.org/10.1046/j.1365-2389.2003.51313.x.

13. Ranieri P, Rozzini R, Franzoni S, Barbisoni P, Trabucchi M. Serum cholesterol levels as a measure of frailty in elderly patients. Exp Aging Res. 1998;24(2):169–79. https://doi.org/10.1080/036107398244300.

14. Spada RS, Toscano G, Cosentino FII, et al. Low total cholesterol predicts mortality in the nondemented oldest old. Arch Gerontol Geriatr. 2007;44:381–4. https://doi.org/10.1016/j.archger.2007.01.053.

15. Grundy Scott M, Stone Neil J, Bailey Alison L, et al. 2018 AHA/ACC/AACVPR/AAPA/ABC/ACPM/ADA/AGS/APhA/ASPC/NLA/PCNA Guideline on the Management of Blood Cholesterol: A Report of the American College of Cardiology/American Heart Association Task Force on Clinical Practice Guidelines. Circulation. 2019;139(25):e1082–143. https://doi.org/10.1161/CIR.0000000000000625.

16. Mach F, Baigent C, Catapano AL, et al. 2019 ESC/EAS Guidelines for the management of dyslipidaemias: lipid modification to reduce cardiovascular risk: The Task Force for the management of dyslipidaemias of the European Society of Cardiology (ESC) and European Atherosclerosis Society (EAS). Eur Heart J. 2019;41(1):111–88. https://doi.org/10.1093/eurheartj/ehz455.

17. Arps K, Pallazola VA, Cardoso R, et al. Clinician's guide to the updated ABCS of cardiovascular disease prevention: a review part 2. Am J Med. 2019;132(7):e599–609. https://doi.org/10.1016/j.amjmed.2019.01.031.

18. Armitage J, Baigent C, Barnes E, et al. Efficacy and safety of statin therapy in older people: a meta-analysis of individual participant data from 28 randomised controlled trials. Lancet. 2019;393(10170):407–15. https://doi.org/10.1016/S0140-6736(18)31942-1.

19. Pearson GJ, Thanassoulis G, Anderson TJ, et al. Canadian cardiovascular society guidelines for the management of dyslipidemia for the prevention of cardiovascular disease in the adult. Can J Cardiol. 2021;37(8):1129–50. https://doi.org/10.1016/j.cjca.2021.03.016.

20. Cardiovascular disease: risk assessment and reduction, including lipid modification (2014 (updated 2016)).

21. The West of Scotland Coronary Prevention Study Group. A coronary primary prevention study of Scottish men aged 45-64 years: Trial design. J Clin Epidemiol. 1992;45(8):849–60. https://doi.org/10.1016/0895-4356(92)90068-X.

22. Shepherd J, Cobbe SM, Ford I, et al. Prevention of Coronary Heart Disease with Pravastatin in Men with Hypercholesterolemia. N Engl J Med. 1995;333(20):1301–8. https://doi.org/10.1056/NEJM199511163332001.

23. Downs JR, Clearfield M, Weis S, et al. Primary prevention of acute coronary events with lovastatin in men and women with average cholesterol levels: results of AFCAPS/TexCAPS. Air Force/Texas Coronary Atherosclerosis Prevention Study. JAMA. 1998;279(20):1615–22. https://doi.org/10.1001/jama.279.20.1615.

24. Downs JR, Beere PA, Whitney E, et al. Design & rationale of the air force/texas coronary atherosclerosis prevention study (AFCAPS/TexCAPS). Am J Cardiol. 1997;80(3):287–93. https://doi.org/10.1016/s0002-9149(97)00347-0.

25. The ALLHAT Officers Coordinators for the ALLHAT Collaborative Research Group. Major outcomes in moderately hypercholesterolemic, hypertensive patients randomized to pravastatin vs usual carethe antihypertensive and lipid-lowering treatment to prevent heart attack trial (ALLHAT-LLT). JAMA. 2002;288(23):2998–3007. https://doi.org/10.1001/jama.288.23.2998.

26. Han BH, Sutin D, Williamson JD, et al. Effect of statin treatment vs usual care on primary cardiovascular prevention among older adults: the ALLHAT-LLT randomized clinical trial. JAMA Intern Med. 2017;177(7):955–65. https://doi.org/10.1001/jamainternmed.2017.1442.

27. Shepherd J, Blauw GJ, Murphy MB, et al. Pravastatin in elderly individuals at risk of vascular disease (PROSPER): a randomised controlled trial. Lancet. 2002;360(9346):1623–30. https://doi.org/10.1016/S0140-6736(02)11600-X.

28. Sever PS, Dahlöf B, Poulter NR, et al. Prevention of coronary and stroke events with atorvastatin in hypertensive patients who have average or lower-than-average cholesterol concentrations, in the Anglo-Scandinavian Cardiac Outcomes Trial—Lipid Lowering Arm (ASCOT-LLA): a multicentre randomised controlled trial. Lancet. 2003;361(9364):1149–58. https://doi.org/10.1016/s0140-6736(03)12948-0.

29. Sever PS, Dahlöf B, Poulter NR, et al. Rationale, design, methods and baseline demography of participants of the Anglo-Scandinavian Cardiac Outcomes Trial. ASCOT investigators. J Hypertens. 2001;19(6):1139–47. https://doi.org/10.1097/00004872-200106000-00020.

30. Colhoun HM, Thomason MJ, Mackness MI, et al. Design of the collaborative atorvastatin diabetes study (CARDS) in patients with type 2 diabetes. Diabet Med. 2002;19(3):201–11. https://doi.org/10.1046/j.1464-5491.2002.00643.x.

31. Colhoun HM, Betteridge DJ, Durrington PN, et al. Primary prevention of cardiovascular disease with atorvastatin in type 2 diabetes in the Collaborative Atorvastatin Diabetes Study

(CARDS): multicentre randomised placebo-controlled trial. Lancet. 2004;364(9435):685–96. https://doi.org/10.1016/s0140-6736(04)16895-5.

32. Nakamura H, Arakawa K, Itakura H, et al. Primary prevention of cardiovascular disease with pravastatin in Japan (MEGA Study): a prospective randomised controlled trial. Lancet. 2006;368(9542):1155–63. https://doi.org/10.1016/S0140-6736(06)69472-5.

33. Management of Elevated Cholesterol in the Primary Prevention Group of Adult Japanese (MEGA) Study Group. Design and baseline characteristics of a study of primary prevention of coronary events with pravastatin among Japanese with mildly elevated cholesterol levels. Circ J. 2004;68(9):860–7. https://doi.org/10.1253/circj.68.860.

34. Ridker PM, Danielson E, Fonseca FAH, et al. Rosuvastatin to prevent vascular events in men and women with elevated C-reactive protein. N Engl J Med. 2008s;359(21):2195–207. https://doi.org/10.1056/NEJMoa0807646.

35. Yusuf S, Bosch J, Dagenais G, et al. Cholesterol lowering in intermediate-risk persons without cardiovascular disease. N Engl J Med. 2016;374(21):2021–31. https://doi.org/10.1056/NEJMoa1600176.

36. Savarese G, Gotto AM, Paolillo S, et al. Benefits of Statins in Elderly Subjects Without Established Cardiovascular Disease: A Meta-Analysis. J Am Coll Cardiol. 2013;62(22):2090–9. https://doi.org/10.1016/j.jacc.2013.07.069.

37. Neil HA, DeMicco DA, Luo D, et al. Analysis of efficacy and safety in patients aged 65-75 years at randomization: Collaborative Atorvastatin Diabetes Study (CARDS). Diabetes Care. 2006;29(11):2378–84. https://doi.org/10.2337/dc06-0872.

38. Teng M, Lin L, Zhao YJ, et al. Statins for primary prevention of cardiovascular disease in elderly patients: systematic review and meta-analysis. Drugs Aging. 2015;32(8):649–61. https://doi.org/10.1007/s40266-015-0290-9.

39. Glynn RJ, Koenig W, Nordestgaard BG, Shepherd J, Ridker PM. Rosuvastatin for primary prevention in older persons with elevated C-reactive protein and low to average low-density lipoprotein cholesterol levels: exploratory analysis of a randomized trial. Ann Intern Med. 2010;152(8):488–96, w174. https://doi.org/10.7326/0003-4819-152-8-201004200-00005.

40. Ridker PM, Lonn E, Paynter NP, Glynn R, Yusuf S. Primary prevention with statin therapy in the elderly. Circulation. 2017;135(20):1979–81. https://doi.org/10.1161/CIRCULATIONAHA.117.028271.

41. de Lorgeril M, Salen P, Abramson J, et al. Cholesterol lowering, cardiovascular diseases, and the rosuvastatin-JUPITER controversy: a critical reappraisal. Arch Intern Med. 2010;170(12):1032–6. https://doi.org/10.1001/archinternmed.2010.184.

42. Nissen SE. The Jupiter trial: key findings, controversies, and implications. Curr Cardiol Rep. 2009;11(2):81–2. https://doi.org/10.1007/s11886-009-0013-0.

43. Vaccarino V, Bremner JD, Kelley ME. JUPITER: a few words of caution. Circ Cardiovasc Qual Outcomes. 2009;2(3):286–8. https://doi.org/10.1161/CIRCOUTCOMES.109.850404.

44. Kleipool EEF, Dorresteijn JAN, Smulders YM, Visseren FLJ, Peters MJL, Muller M. Treatment of hypercholesterolaemia in older adults calls for a patient-centred approach. Heart. 2020;106(4):261. https://doi.org/10.1136/heartjnl-2019-315600.

45. Ouchi Y, Sasaki J, Arai H, et al. Ezetimibe lipid-lowering trial on prevention of atherosclerotic cardiovascular disease in 75 or older (EWTOPIA 75). Circulation. 2019;140(12):992–1003. https://doi.org/10.1161/CIRCULATIONAHA.118.039415.

46. Orkaby AR, Driver JA, Ho Y-L, et al. Association of statin use with all-cause and cardiovascular mortality in US veterans 75 years and older. JAMA. 2020;324(1):68–78. https://doi.org/10.1001/jama.2020.7848.

47. Kim K, Lee CJ, Shim CY, et al. Statin and clinical outcomes of primary prevention in individuals aged >75 years: The SCOPE-75 study. Atherosclerosis. 2019;284:31–6. https://doi.org/10.1016/j.atherosclerosis.2019.02.026.

48. Jun JE, Cho IJ, Han K, et al. Statins for primary prevention in adults aged 75 years and older: A nationwide population-based case-control study. Atherosclerosis. 2019;283:28–34. https://doi.org/10.1016/j.atherosclerosis.2019.01.030.

49. Bezin J, Moore N, Mansiaux Y, Steg PG, Pariente A. Real-life benefits of statins for cardiovascular prevention in elderly subjects: a population-based cohort study. Am J Med. 2019;132(6):740–748.e7. https://doi.org/10.1016/j.amjmed.2018.12.032.

50. Giral P, Neumann A, Weill A, Coste J. Cardiovascular effect of discontinuing statins for primary prevention at the age of 75 years: a nationwide population-based cohort study in France. Eur Heart J. 2019;40(43):3516–25. https://doi.org/10.1093/eurheartj/ehz458.

51. Gitsels LA, Bakbergenuly I, Steel N, Kulinskaya E. Do statins reduce mortality in older people? Findings from a longitudinal study using primary care records. Fam Med Community Health. 2021;9(2):e000780. https://doi.org/10.1136/fmch-2020-000780.

52. Ramos R, Comas-Cufí M, Martí-Lluch R, et al. Statins for primary prevention of cardiovascular events and mortality in old and very old adults with and without type 2 diabetes: retrospective cohort study. BMJ. 2018;362:k3359. https://doi.org/10.1136/bmj.k3359.

53. Baik SH, McDonald CJ. Independent effects of 15 commonly prescribed drugs on all-cause mortality among US elderly patients with type 2 diabetes mellitus. BMJ Open Diab Res Care. 2020;8(1):e000940. https://doi.org/10.1136/bmjdrc-2019-000940.

54. Orkaby AR, Gaziano JM, Djousse L, Driver JA. Statins for primary prevention of cardiovascular events and mortality in older men. J Am Geriatr Soc. 2017;65(11):2362–8. https://doi.org/10.1111/jgs.14993.

55. Singh S, Zieman S, Go AS, et al. Statins for primary prevention in older adults—moving toward evidence-based decision-making. J Am Geriatr Soc. 2018;66(11):2188–96. https://doi.org/10.1111/jgs.15449.

56. Cannon CP, Blazing MA, Giugliano RP, et al. Ezetimibe added to statin therapy after acute coronary syndromes. N Engl J Med. 2015;372(25):2387–97. https://doi.org/10.1056/NEJMoa1410489.

57. Bach RG, Cannon CP, Giugliano RP, et al. Effect of simvastatin-ezetimibe compared with simvastatin monotherapy after acute coronary syndrome among patients 75 years or older: a secondary analysis of a randomized clinical trial. JAMA Cardiol. 2019;4(9):846–54. https://doi.org/10.1001/jamacardio.2019.2306.

58. Sabatine MS, Giugliano RP, Keech AC, et al. Evolocumab and clinical outcomes in patients with cardiovascular disease. N Engl J Med. 2017;376(18):1713–22. https://doi.org/10.1056/NEJMoa1615664.

59. Sever P, Gouni-Berthold I, Keech A, et al. LDL-cholesterol lowering with evolocumab, and outcomes according to age and sex in patients in the FOURIER trial. Eur J Prev Cardiol. 2021;28(8):805–12. https://doi.org/10.1177/2047487320902750.

60. Sinnaeve PR, Schwartz GG, Wojdyla DM, et al. Effect of alirocumab on cardiovascular outcomes after acute coronary syndromes according to age: an ODYSSEY OUTCOMES trial analysis. Eur Heart J. 2020;41(24):2248–58. https://doi.org/10.1093/eurheartj/ehz809.

61. Thompson PD, Panza G, Zaleski A, Taylor B. Statin-Associated Side Effects. J Am Coll Cardiol. 2016;67(20):2395–410. https://doi.org/10.1016/j.jacc.2016.02.071.

62. Iwere RB, Hewitt J. Myopathy in older people receiving statin therapy: a systematic review and meta-analysis. Br J Clin Pharmacol. 2015;80(3):363–71. https://doi.org/10.1111/bcp.12687.

63. Macedo AF, Taylor FC, Casas JP, Adler A, Prieto-Merino D, Ebrahim S. Unintended effects of statins from observational studies in the general population: systematic review and meta-analysis. BMC Med. 2014;12(1):51. https://doi.org/10.1186/1741-7015-12-51.

64. Newman CB, Preiss D, Tobert JA, et al. Statin safety and associated adverse events: a scientific statement from the american heart association. Arterioscler Thromb Vasc Biol. 2019;39(2):e38–81. https://doi.org/10.1161/ATV.0000000000000073.

65. Jones M, Tett S, Peeters GMEE, Mishra GD, Dobson A. New-onset diabetes after statin exposure in elderly women: the australian longitudinal study on women's health. Drugs Aging. 2017;34(3):203–9. https://doi.org/10.1007/s40266-017-0435-0.

66. Ott BR, Daiello LA, Dahabreh IJ, et al. Do statins impair cognition? A systematic review and meta-analysis of randomized controlled trials. J Gen Intern Med. 2015;30(3):348–58. https://doi.org/10.1007/s11606-014-3115-3.

67. Hale M, Zaman H, Mehdizadeh D, et al. Association between statins prescribed for primary and secondary prevention and major adverse cardiac events among older adults with frailty: a systematic review. Drugs Aging. 2020;37(11):787–99. https://doi.org/10.1007/s40266-020-00798-3.

68. Thompson W, Pottegård A, Nielsen JB, Haastrup P, Jarbøl DE. How common is statin use in the oldest old? Drugs Aging. 2018;35(8):679–86. https://doi.org/10.1007/s40266-018-0567-x.

69. Gulliford M, Ravindrarajah R, Hamada S, Jackson S, Charlton J. Inception and deprescribing of statins in people aged over 80 years: cohort study. Age Ageing. 2017;46(6):1001–5. https://doi.org/10.1093/ageing/afx100.

70. Kutner JS, Blatchford PJ, Taylor DH Jr, et al. Safety and benefit of discontinuing statin therapy in the setting of advanced, life-limiting illness: a randomized clinical trial. JAMA Intern Med. 2015;175(5):691–700. https://doi.org/10.1001/jamainternmed.2015.0289.

71. Ambrose JA, Barua RS. The pathophysiology of cigarette smoking and cardiovascular disease: an update. J Am Coll Cardiol. 2004;43(10):1731–7. https://doi.org/10.1016/j.jacc.2003.12.047.

72. Cornelius M, Wang T, Jamal A, Loretan C, Neff L. Tobacco product use among adults - United States, 2019. MMWR Morb Mortal Wkly Rep. 2020;69:1736–42. https://doi.org/10.15585/mmwr.mm6946a4.

73. Mons U, Müezzinler A, Gellert C, et al. Impact of smoking and smoking cessation on cardiovascular events and mortality among older adults: meta-analysis of individual participant data from prospective cohort studies of the CHANCES consortium. BMJ. 2015;350:h1551. https://doi.org/10.1136/bmj.h1551.

74. Gellert C, Schöttker B, Brenner H. Smoking and all-cause mortality in older people: systematic review and meta-analysis. Arch Intern Med. 2012;172(11):837–44. https://doi.org/10.1001/archinternmed.2012.1397.

75. Müezzinler A, Mons U, Gellert C, et al. Smoking and all-cause mortality in older adults: results from the CHANCES consortium. Am J Prev Med. 2015;49(5):e53–63. https://doi.org/10.1016/j.amepre.2015.04.004.

76. Doll R, Peto R, Boreham J, Sutherland I. Mortality in relation to smoking: 50 years' observations on male British doctors. BMJ. 2004;328(7455):1519. https://doi.org/10.1136/bmj.38142.554479.AE.

77. Taylor DH Jr, Hasselblad V, Henley SJ, Thun MJ, Sloan FA. Benefits of smoking cessation for longevity. Am J Public Health. 2002;92(6):990–6. https://doi.org/10.2105/ajph.92.6.990.

78. Burns DM. Cigarette smoking among the elderly: disease consequences and the benefits of cessation. Am J Health Promot. 2000;14(6):357–61. https://doi.org/10.4278/0890-1171-14.6.357.

79. Qiu D, Chen T, Liu T, Song F. Smoking cessation and related factors in middle-aged and older Chinese adults: evidence from a longitudinal study. PLoS One. 2020;15(10):e0240806. https://doi.org/10.1371/journal.pone.0240806.

80. Doolan DM, Froelicher ES. Smoking cessation interventions and older adults. Prog Cardiovasc Nurs. 2008;23(3):119–27. https://doi.org/10.1111/j.1751-7117.2008.00001.x.

81. Appel DW, Aldrich TK. Smoking cessation in the elderly. Clin Geriatr Med. 2003;19(1):77–100. https://doi.org/10.1016/S0749-0690(02)00053-8.

82. Henley SJ, Asman K, Momin B, et al. Smoking cessation behaviors among older U.S. adults. Prev Med Rep. 2019;16:100978. https://doi.org/10.1016/j.pmedr.2019.100978.

83. Arnett DK, Blumenthal RS, Albert MA, et al. 2019 ACC/AHA Guideline on the Primary Prevention of Cardiovascular Disease: A Report of the American College of Cardiology/American Heart Association Task Force on Clinical Practice Guidelines. Circulation. 2019;140(11):e596–646. https://doi.org/10.1161/CIR.0000000000000678.

84. Piepoli MF, Hoes AW, Agewall S, et al. 2016 European Guidelines on cardiovascular disease prevention in clinical practice: The Sixth Joint Task Force of the European Society of Cardiology and Other Societies on Cardiovascular Disease Prevention in Clinical Practice (constituted by representatives of 10 societies and by invited experts) Developed with the special contribution of the European Association for Cardiovascular Prevention & Rehabilitation (EACPR). Eur Heart J. 2016;37(29):2315–81. https://doi.org/10.1093/eurheartj/ehw106.

85. Stead LF, Perera R, Bullen C, et al. Nicotine replacement therapy for smoking cessation. Cochrane Database Syst Rev. 2012;11:Cd000146. https://doi.org/10.1002/14651858. CD000146.pub4.

86. Roddy E. Bupropion and other non-nicotine pharmacotherapies. BMJ. 2004;328(7438): 509–11. https://doi.org/10.1136/bmj.328.7438.509.

87. Koegelenberg CF, Noor F, Bateman ED, et al. Efficacy of varenicline combined with nicotine replacement therapy vs varenicline alone for smoking cessation: a randomized clinical trial. JAMA. 2014;312(2):155–61. https://doi.org/10.1001/jama.2014.7195.

88. Anthenelli RM, Benowitz NL, West R, et al. Neuropsychiatric safety and efficacy of varenicline, bupropion, and nicotine patch in smokers with and without psychiatric disorders (EAGLES): a double-blind, randomised, placebo-controlled clinical trial. Lancet. 2016;387(10037):2507–20. https://doi.org/10.1016/s0140-6736(16)30272-0.

89. Gonzales D, Rennard SI, Nides M, et al. Varenicline, an α4β2 nicotinic acetylcholine receptor partial agonist, vs sustained-release bupropion and placebo for smoking cessationa randomized controlled trial. JAMA. 2006;296(1):47–55. https://doi.org/10.1001/jama.296.1.47.

90. Qasim H, Karim ZA, Rivera JO, Khasawneh FT, Alshbool FZ. Impact of electronic cigarettes on the cardiovascular system. J Am Heart Assoc. 2017;6(9):e006353. https://doi.org/10.1161/JAHA.117.006353.

91. Alzahrani T, Pena I, Temesgen N, Glantz SA. Association between electronic cigarette use and myocardial infarction. Am J Prev Med. 2018;55(4):455–61. https://doi.org/10.1016/j.amepre.2018.05.004.

92. Pisinger C, Døssing M. A systematic review of health effects of electronic cigarettes. Prev Med. 2014;69:248–60. https://doi.org/10.1016/j.ypmed.2014.10.009.

93. Sarwar N, Gao P, Seshasai SR, et al. Diabetes mellitus, fasting blood glucose concentration, and risk of vascular disease: a collaborative meta-analysis of 102 prospective studies. Lancet. 2010;375(9733):2215–22. https://doi.org/10.1016/s0140-6736(10)60484-9.

94. National Diabetes Statistics Report 2020: Estimates of Diabetes and Its Burden in the United States (2020).

95. American Diabetes A. 2. classification and diagnosis of diabetes: standards of medical care in diabetes—2021. Diabetes Care. 2021;44(Suppl 1):S15. https://doi.org/10.2337/dc21-S002.

96. Meneilly GS, Knip A, Miller DB, Sherifali D, Tessier D, Zahedi A. Diabetes in older people. Can J Diabetes. 2018;42(Suppl 1):S283–s295. https://doi.org/10.1016/j.jcjd.2017.10.021.

97. Sattar N, Rawshani A, Franzén S, et al. Age at diagnosis of type 2 diabetes mellitus and associations with cardiovascular and mortality risks. Circulation. 2019;139(19):2228–37. https://doi.org/10.1161/circulationaha.118.037885.

98. Masuch A, Friedrich N, Roth J, Nauck M, Müller UA, Petersmann A. Preventing misdiagnosis of diabetes in the elderly: age-dependent HbA1c reference intervals derived from two population-based study cohorts. BMC Endocr Disord. 2019;19(1):20. https://doi.org/10.1186/s12902-019-0338-7.

99. Roth J, Müller N, Lehmann T, Heinemann L, Wolf G, Müller UA. HbA1c and age in non-diabetic subjects: an ignored association? Exp Clin Endocrinol Diabetes. 2016;124(10):637–42. https://doi.org/10.1055/s-0042-105440.

100. Pani LN, Korenda L, Meigs JB, et al. Effect of aging on A1C levels in individuals without diabetes: evidence from the Framingham Offspring Study and the National Health and Nutrition Examination Survey 2001-2004. Diabetes Care. 2008;31(10):1991–6. https://doi.org/10.2337/dc08-0577.

101. Lipska KJ, De Rekeneire N, Van Ness PH, et al. Identifying dysglycemic states in older adults: implications of the emerging use of hemoglobin A1c. J Clin Endocrinol Metab. 2010;95(12):5289–95. https://doi.org/10.1210/jc.2010-1171.

102. Cosentino F, Grant PJ, Aboyans V, et al. 2019 ESC Guidelines on diabetes, pre-diabetes, and cardiovascular diseases developed in collaboration with the EASD: The Task Force for diabetes, pre-diabetes, and cardiovascular diseases of the European Society of Cardiology (ESC) and the European Association for the Study of Diabetes (EASD). Eur Heart J. 2019;41(2):255–323. https://doi.org/10.1093/eurheartj/ehz486.

103. American Diabetes A. 11. Microvascular complications and foot care: standards of medical care in diabetes—2021. Diabetes Care. 2021;44(Supplement 1):S151. https://doi.org/10.2337/dc21-S011.

104. Zoungas S, Arima H, Gerstein HC, et al. Effects of intensive glucose control on microvascular outcomes in patients with type 2 diabetes: a meta-analysis of individual participant data from randomised controlled trials. Lancet Diabetes Endocrinol. 2017;5(6):431–7. https://doi.org/10.1016/s2213-8587(17)30104-3.

105. Nathan DM, Genuth S, Lachin J, et al. The effect of intensive treatment of diabetes on the development and progression of long-term complications in insulin-dependent diabetes mellitus. N Engl J Med. 1993;329(14):977–86. https://doi.org/10.1056/nejm199309303291401.

106. The Diabetes Control and Complications Trial/Epidemiology of Diabetes Interventions and Complications (DCCT/EDIC) Study Research Group. Intensive diabetes treatment and cardiovascular disease in patients with type 1 diabetes. N Engl J Med. 2005;353(25):2643–53. https://doi.org/10.1056/NEJMoa052187.

107. Ohkubo Y, Kishikawa H, Araki E, et al. Intensive insulin therapy prevents the progression of diabetic microvascular complications in Japanese patients with non-insulin-dependent diabetes mellitus: a randomized prospective 6-year study. Diabetes Res Clin Pract. 1995;28(2):103–17. https://doi.org/10.1016/0168-8227(95)01064-K.

108. UK Prospective Diabetes Study (UKPDS) Group. Intensive blood-glucose control with sulphonylureas or insulin compared with conventional treatment and risk of complications in patients with type 2 diabetes (UKPDS 33). Lancet. 1998;352(9131):837–53. https://doi.org/10.1016/S0140-6736(98)07019-6.

109. UK Prospective Diabetes Study (UKPDS) Group. Effect of intensive blood-glucose control with metformin on complications in overweight patients with type 2 diabetes (UKPDS 34). Lancet. 1998;352(9131):854–65. https://doi.org/10.1016/S0140-6736(98)07037-8.

110. Azad N, Emanuele NV, Abraira C, et al. The effects of intensive glycemic control on neuropathy in the VA cooperative study on type II diabetes mellitus (VA CSDM). J Diabetes Complications. 1999;13(5–6):307–13. https://doi.org/10.1016/s1056-8727(99)00062-8.

111. Abraira C, Emanuele N, Colwell J, et al. Glycemic control and complications in type II diabetes. Design of a feasibility trial. VA CS Group (CSDM). Diabetes Care. 1992;15(11):1560–71. https://doi.org/10.2337/diacare.15.11.1560.

112. Bagg W, Plank LD, Gamble G, Drury PL, Sharpe N, Braatvedt GD. The effects of intensive glycaemic control on body composition in patients with type 2 diabetes. Diabetes, Obesity and Metabolism. 2001;3(6):410–6. https://doi.org/10.1046/j.1463-1326.2001.00153.x.

113. Becker A, van der Does FE, van Hinsbergh VW, Heine RJ, Bouter LM, Stehouwer CD. Improvement of glycaemic control in type 2 diabetes: favourable changes in blood pressure, total cholesterol and triglycerides, but not in HDL cholesterol, fibrinogen, Von Willebrand factor and (pro)insulin. Neth J Med. 2003;61(4):129–36.

114. van der Does FE, de Neeling JN, Snoek FJ, et al. Randomized study of two different target levels of glycemic control within the acceptable range in type 2 diabetes. Effects on well-being at 1 year. Diabetes Care. 1998;21(12):2085–93. https://doi.org/10.2337/diacare.21.12.2085.

115. Gæde P, Vedel P, Larsen N, Jensen GVH, Parving H-H, Pedersen O. Multifactorial intervention and cardiovascular disease in patients with type 2 diabetes. N Engl J Med. 2003;348(5):383–93. https://doi.org/10.1056/NEJMoa021778.

116. Gæde P, Vedel P, Parving H-H, Pedersen O. Intensified multifactorial intervention in patients with type 2 diabetes mellitus and microalbuminuria: the Steno type 2 randomised study. Lancet. 1999;353(9153):617–22. https://doi.org/10.1016/S0140-6736(98)07368-1.

117. Charbonnel B, Dormandy J, Erdmann E, Massi-Benedetti M, Skene A. The prospective pioglitazone clinical trial in macrovascular events (PROactive): can pioglitazone reduce cardiovascular events in diabetes? Study design and baseline characteristics of 5238 patients. Diabetes Care. 2004;27(7):1647–53. https://doi.org/10.2337/diacare.27.7.1647.

118. Dormandy JA, Charbonnel B, Eckland DJ, et al. Secondary prevention of macrovascular events in patients with type 2 diabetes in the PROactive Study (PROspective pioglitAzone Clinical Trial In macroVascular Events): a randomised controlled trial. Lancet. 2005;366(9493):1279–89. https://doi.org/10.1016/s0140-6736(05)67528-9.

119. Patel A, MacMahon S, Chalmers J, et al. Intensive blood glucose control and vascular outcomes in patients with type 2 diabetes. N Engl J Med. 2008;358(24):2560–72. https://doi.org/10.1056/NEJMoa0802987.

120. The Action to Control Cardiovascular Risk in Diabetes Study Group. Effects of intensive glucose lowering in type 2 diabetes. N Engl J Med. 2008;358(24):2545–59. https://doi.org/10.1056/NEJMoa0802743.

121. Hage C, Norhammar A, Grip L, et al. Glycaemic control and restenosis after percutaneous coronary interventions in patients with diabetes mellitus: a report from the Insulin Diabetes Angioplasty study. Diab Vasc Dis Res. 2009;6(2):71–9. https://doi.org/10.1177/1479164109336042.

122. Duckworth W, Abraira C, Moritz T, et al. Glucose control and vascular complications in veterans with type 2 diabetes. N Engl J Med. 2009;360(2):129–39. https://doi.org/10.1056/NEJMoa0808431.

123. Abraira C, Duckworth W, McCarren M, et al. Design of the cooperative study on glycemic control and complications in diabetes mellitus type 2: veterans affairs diabetes trial. J Diabetes Complications. 2003;17(6):314–22. https://doi.org/10.1016/s1056-8727(02)00277-5.

124. Araki A, Iimuro S, Sakurai T, et al. Long-term multiple risk factor interventions in Japanese elderly diabetic patients: the Japanese Elderly Diabetes Intervention Trial--study design, baseline characteristics and effects of intervention. Geriatr Gerontol Int. 2012;12(Suppl 1):7–17. https://doi.org/10.1111/j.1447-0594.2011.00808.x.

125. Holman RR, Paul SK, Bethel MA, Matthews DR, Neil HAW. 10-year follow-up of intensive glucose control in type 2 diabetes. N Engl J Med. 2008;359(15):1577–89. https://doi.org/10.1056/NEJMoa0806470.

126. Gaede P, Lund-Andersen H, Parving HH, Pedersen O. Effect of a multifactorial intervention on mortality in type 2 diabetes. N Engl J Med. 2008;358(6):580–91. https://doi.org/10.1056/NEJMoa0706245.

127. Zoungas S, Chalmers J, Neal B, et al. Follow-up of blood-pressure lowering and glucose control in type 2 diabetes. N Engl J Med. 2014;371(15):1392–406. https://doi.org/10.1056/NEJMoa1407963.

128. The Accord Study Group. Long-term effects of intensive glucose lowering on cardiovascular outcomes. N Engl J Med. 2011;364(9):818–28. https://doi.org/10.1056/NEJMoa1006524.

129. The Accord Study Group. Nine-year effects of 3.7 years of intensive glycemic control on cardiovascular outcomes. Diabetes Care. 2016;39(5):701. https://doi.org/10.2337/dc15-2283.

130. Hayward RA, Reaven PD, Wiitala WL, et al. Follow-up of glycemic control and cardiovascular outcomes in type 2 diabetes. N Engl J Med. 2015;372(23):2197–206. https://doi.org/10.1056/NEJMoa1414266.

131. Reaven PD, Emanuele NV, Wiitala WL, et al. Intensive glucose control in patients with type 2 diabetes — 15-year follow-up. N Engl J Med. 2019;380(23):2215–24. https://doi.org/10.1056/NEJMoa1806802.

132. Lee AK, Warren B, Lee CJ, et al. The association of severe hypoglycemia with incident cardiovascular events and mortality in adults with type 2 diabetes. Diabetes Care. 2017;41(1):104–11. https://doi.org/10.2337/dc17-1669.

133. Lee AK, McEvoy JW, Hoogeveen RC, Ballantyne CM, Selvin E. Severe hypoglycemia and elevated high-sensitivity cardiac troponin t in older adults with diabetes: the ARIC study. J Am Coll Cardiol. 2016;68(12):1370–1. https://doi.org/10.1016/j.jacc.2016.06.049.

134. Boussageon R, Bejan-Angoulvant T, Saadatian-Elahi M, et al. Effect of intensive glucose lowering treatment on all cause mortality, cardiovascular death, and microvascular events in type 2 diabetes: meta-analysis of randomised controlled trials. BMJ. 2011;343:d4169. https://doi.org/10.1136/bmj.d4169.

135. Ray KK, Seshasai SR, Wijesuriya S, et al. Effect of intensive control of glucose on cardiovascular outcomes and death in patients with diabetes mellitus: a meta-analysis of randomised controlled trials. Lancet. 2009;373(9677):1765–72. https://doi.org/10.1016/s0140-6736(09)60697-8.

136. Turnbull FM, Abraira C, Anderson RJ, et al. Intensive glucose control and macrovascular outcomes in type 2 diabetes. Diabetologia. 2009;52(11):2288–98. https://doi.org/10.1007/s00125-009-1470-0.

137. Hemmingsen B, Lund SS, Gluud C, et al. Intensive glycaemic control for patients with type 2 diabetes: systematic review with meta-analysis and trial sequential analysis of randomised clinical trials. BMJ. 2011;343:d6898. https://doi.org/10.1136/bmj.d6898.

138. Hemmingsen B, Lund SS, Gluud C, et al. Targeting intensive glycaemic control versus targeting conventional glycaemic control for type 2 diabetes mellitus. Cochrane Database Syst Rev. 2013;(11):Cd008143. https://doi.org/10.1002/14651858.CD008143.pub3.

139. Giorgino F, Home PD, Tuomilehto J. Glucose control and vascular outcomes in type 2 diabetes: is the picture clear? Diabetes Care. 2016;39(Supplement 2):S187. https://doi.org/10.2337/dcS15-3023.

140. Huang ES, Liu JY, Moffet HH, John PM, Karter AJ. Glycemic control, complications, and death in older diabetic patients. Diabetes Care. 2011;34(6):1329. https://doi.org/10.2337/dc10-2377.

141. Palta P, Huang ES, Kalyani RR, Golden SH, Yeh H-C. Hemoglobin A 1c and mortality in older adults with and without diabetes: results from the national health and nutrition examination surveys (1988–2011). Diabetes Care. 2017;40(4):453. https://doi.org/10.2337/dci16-0042.

142. Currie CJ, Peters JR, Tynan A, et al. Survival as a function of HbA(1c) in people with type 2 diabetes: a retrospective cohort study. Lancet. 2010;375(9713):481–9. https://doi.org/10.1016/s0140-6736(09)61969-3.

143. Rodriguez-Gutierrez R, Gonzalez-Gonzalez JG, Zuñiga-Hernandez JA, McCoy RG. Benefits and harms of intensive glycemic control in patients with type 2 diabetes. BMJ. 2019;367:l5887. https://doi.org/10.1136/bmj.l5887.

144. Home PD, Pocock SJ, Beck-Nielsen H, et al. Rosiglitazone evaluated for cardiovascular outcomes in oral agent combination therapy for type 2 diabetes (RECORD): a multicentre, randomised, open-label trial. Lancet. 2009;373(9681):2125–35. https://doi.org/10.1016/S0140-6736(09)60953-3.

145. White WB, Cannon CP, Heller SR, et al. Alogliptin after acute coronary syndrome in patients with type 2 diabetes. N Engl J Med. 2013;369(14):1327–35. https://doi.org/10.1056/NEJMoa1305889.

146. Scirica BM, Bhatt DL, Braunwald E, et al. Saxagliptin and cardiovascular outcomes in patients with type 2 diabetes mellitus. N Engl J Med. 2013;369(14):1317–26. https://doi.org/10.1056/NEJMoa1307684.

147. Lincoff AM, Tardif J-C, Schwartz GG, et al. Effect of aleglitazar on cardiovascular outcomes after acute coronary syndrome in patients with type 2 diabetes mellitus: the AleCardio randomized clinical trial. JAMA. 2014;311(15):1515–25. https://doi.org/10.1001/jama.2014.3321.

148. Zinman B, Wanner C, Lachin JM, et al. Empagliflozin, cardiovascular outcomes, and mortality in type 2 diabetes. N Engl J Med. 2015;373(22):2117–28. https://doi.org/10.1056/NEJMoa1504720.

149. Pfeffer MA, Claggett B, Diaz R, et al. Lixisenatide in patients with type 2 diabetes and acute coronary syndrome. N Engl J Med. 2015;373(23):2247–57. https://doi.org/10.1056/NEJMoa1509225.
150. Green JB, Bethel MA, Armstrong PW, et al. Effect of sitagliptin on cardiovascular outcomes in type 2 diabetes. N Engl J Med. 2015;373(3):232–42. https://doi.org/10.1056/NEJMoa1501352.
151. Marso SP, Daniels GH, Brown-Frandsen K, et al. Liraglutide and cardiovascular outcomes in type 2 diabetes. N Engl J Med. 2016;375(4):311–22. https://doi.org/10.1056/NEJMoa1603827.
152. Marso SP, Bain SC, Consoli A, et al. Semaglutide and cardiovascular outcomes in patients with type 2 diabetes. N Engl J Med. 2016;375(19):1834–44. https://doi.org/10.1056/NEJMoa1607141.
153. Neal B, Perkovic V, Mahaffey KW, et al. Canagliflozin and cardiovascular and renal events in type 2 diabetes. N Engl J Med. 2017;377(7):644–57. https://doi.org/10.1056/NEJMoa1611925.
154. Marso SP, McGuire DK, Zinman B, et al. Efficacy and safety of degludec versus glargine in type 2 diabetes. N Engl J Med. 2017;377(8):723–32. https://doi.org/10.1056/NEJMoa1615692.
155. Holman RR, Bethel MA, Mentz RJ, et al. Effects of once-weekly exenatide on cardiovascular outcomes in type 2 diabetes. N Engl J Med. 2017;377(13):1228–39. https://doi.org/10.1056/NEJMoa1612917.
156. Hernandez AF, Green JB, Janmohamed S, et al. Albiglutide and cardiovascular outcomes in patients with type 2 diabetes and cardiovascular disease (Harmony Outcomes): a double-blind, randomised placebo-controlled trial. Lancet. 2018;392(10157):1519–29. https://doi.org/10.1016/S0140-6736(18)32261-X.
157. Rosenstock J, Perkovic V, Johansen OE, et al. Effect of linagliptin vs placebo on major cardiovascular events in adults with type 2 diabetes and high cardiovascular and renal risk: the CARMELINA randomized clinical trial. JAMA. 2019;321(1):69–79. https://doi.org/10.1001/jama.2018.18269.
158. Wiviott SD, Raz I, Bonaca MP, et al. Dapagliflozin and cardiovascular outcomes in type 2 diabetes. N Engl J Med. 2019;380(4):347–57. https://doi.org/10.1056/NEJMoa1812389.
159. Gerstein HC, Colhoun HM, Dagenais GR, et al. Dulaglutide and cardiovascular outcomes in type 2 diabetes (REWIND): a double-blind, randomised placebo-controlled trial. Lancet. 2019;394(10193):121–30. https://doi.org/10.1016/S0140-6736(19)31149-3.
160. Rosenstock J, Kahn SE, Johansen OE, et al. Effect of linagliptin vs glimepiride on major adverse cardiovascular outcomes in patients with type 2 diabetes: the CAROLINA randomized clinical trial. JAMA. 2019;322(12):1155–66. https://doi.org/10.1001/jama.2019.13772.
161. Husain M, Birkenfeld AL, Donsmark M, et al. Oral semaglutide and cardiovascular outcomes in patients with type 2 diabetes. N Engl J Med. 2019;381(9):841–51. https://doi.org/10.1056/NEJMoa1901118.
162. Cannon CP, Pratley R, Dagogo-Jack S, et al. Cardiovascular outcomes with ertugliflozin in type 2 diabetes. N Engl J Med. 2020;383(15):1425–35. https://doi.org/10.1056/NEJMoa2004967.
163. Bhatt DL, Szarek M, Pitt B, et al. Sotagliflozin in patients with diabetes and chronic kidney disease. N Engl J Med. 2021;384(2):129–39. https://doi.org/10.1056/NEJMoa2030186.
164. Strain WD, Hope SV, Green A, Kar P, Valabhji J, Sinclair AJ. Type 2 diabetes mellitus in older people: a brief statement of key principles of modern day management including the assessment of frailty. A national collaborative stakeholder initiative. Diabet Med. 2018;35(7):838–45. https://doi.org/10.1111/dme.13644.
165. Lee SJ, Eng C. Goals of glycemic control in frail older patients with diabetes. JAMA. 2011;305(13):1350–1. https://doi.org/10.1001/jama.2011.404.
166. Visseren FLJ, Mach F, Smulders YM, et al. 2021 ESC Guidelines on cardiovascular disease prevention in clinical practice: Developed by the Task Force for cardiovascular disease prevention in clinical practice with representatives of the European Society of Cardiology and

12 medical societies With the special contribution of the European Association of Preventive Cardiology (EAPC). Eur Heart J. 2021;42(34):3227–337. https://doi.org/10.1093/eurheartj/ehab484.

167. Qaseem A, Wilt TJ, Kansagara D, et al. Hemoglobin A1c targets for glycemic control with pharmacologic therapy for nonpregnant adults with type 2 diabetes mellitus: a guidance statement update from the American College of Physicians. Ann Intern Med. 2018;168(8):569–76. https://doi.org/10.7326/m17-0939.

168. American Diabetes A. 12. Older adults: standards of medical care in diabetes—2021. Diabetes Care. 2021;44(Supplement 1):S168. https://doi.org/10.2337/dc21-S012.

169. Griffith KN, Prentice JC, Mohr DC, Conlin PR. Predicting 5- and 10-year mortality risk in older adults with diabetes. Diabetes Care. 2020;43(8):1724–31. https://doi.org/10.2337/dc19-1870.

170. Pratley RE, Kanapka LG, Rickels MR, et al. Effect of continuous glucose monitoring on hypoglycemia in older adults with type 1 diabetes: a randomized clinical trial. JAMA. 2020;323(23):2397–406. https://doi.org/10.1001/jama.2020.6928.

171. Sinclair A, Morley JE, Rodriguez-Mañas L, et al. Diabetes Mellitus in Older People: Position Statement on behalf of the International Association of Gerontology and Geriatrics (IAGG), the European Diabetes Working Party for Older People (EDWPOP), and the International Task Force of Experts in Diabetes. J Am Med Dir Assoc. 2012;13(6):497–502. https://doi.org/10.1016/j.jamda.2012.04.012.

172. American Geriatrics Society Expert Panel on Care of Older Adults with Diabetes M, Moreno G, Mangione CM, Kimbro L, Vaisberg E. Guidelines abstracted from the American Geriatrics Society Guidelines for Improving the Care of Older Adults with Diabetes Mellitus: 2013 update. J Am Geriatr Soc. 2013;61(11):2020–6. https://doi.org/10.1111/jgs.12514.

173. d'Emden MC, Shaw J, Jones G, Wah CN. Guidance concerning the use of glycated haemoglobin (HbA1c) for the diagnosis of diabetes mellitus. Med J Aust. 2015;203(2):89–90. https://doi.org/10.5694/mja15.00041.

174. Australian Diabetes Society Position Statement: Individualisation of HbA1c Targets for Adults with Diabetes Mellitus. 2009.

175. American Association of Clinical Endocrinologists. Comprehensive Type 2 Diabetes Management Algorithm (2020) - EXECUTIVE SUMMARY. https://pro.aace.com/disease-state-resources/diabetes-diabetes-technology/clinical-practice-guidelines-treatment

176. Handelsman Y, Bloomgarden ZT, Grunberger G, et al. American association of clinical endocrinologists and american college of endocrinology - clinical practice guidelines for developing a diabetes mellitus comprehensive care plan - 2015. Endocr Pract. 2015;21 Suppl 1(Suppl 1):1–87. https://doi.org/10.4158/ep15672.Gl.

177. Type 2 diabetes in adults: management (2015 (last updated 2020)).

178. Type 2 diabetes: prevention in people at high risk (2012 (updated 2017)).

179. Cosentino F, Grant PJ, Aboyans V, et al. 2019 ESC Guidelines on diabetes, pre-diabetes, and cardiovascular diseases developed in collaboration with the EASD: The Task Force for diabetes, pre-diabetes, and cardiovascular diseases of the European Society of Cardiology (ESC) and the European Association for the Study of Diabetes (EASD). Eur Heart J. 2020;41(2):255–323. https://doi.org/10.1093/eurheartj/ehz486.

180. Knowler WC, Barrett-Connor E, Fowler SE, et al. Reduction in the incidence of type 2 diabetes with lifestyle intervention or metformin. N Engl J Med. 2002;346(6):393–403. https://doi.org/10.1056/NEJMoa012512.

181. Diabetes Prevention Program Research G. 10-year follow-up of diabetes incidence and weight loss in the diabetes prevention program outcomes study. Lancet. 2009;374(9702):1677–86. https://doi.org/10.1016/S0140-6736(09)61457-4.

182. Crandall J, Schade D, Ma Y, et al. The influence of age on the effects of lifestyle modification and metformin in prevention of diabetes. J Gerontol A Biol Sci Med Sci. 2006;61(10):1075–81. https://doi.org/10.1093/gerona/61.10.1075.

183. Buse JB, Wexler DJ, Tsapas A, et al. 2019 update to: Management of hyperglycaemia in type 2 diabetes, 2018. A consensus report by the American Diabetes Association (ADA) and the European Association for the Study of Diabetes (EASD). Diabetologia. 2020;63(2):221–8. https://doi.org/10.1007/s00125-019-05039-w.

184. Sherifali D, Bai JW, Kenny M, Warren R, Ali MU. Diabetes self-management programmes in older adults: a systematic review and meta-analysis. Diabet Med. 2015;32(11):1404–14. https://doi.org/10.1111/dme.12780.

185. Murray CM, Shah BR. Diabetes self-management education improves medication utilization and retinopathy screening in the elderly. Prim Care Diabetes. 2016;10(3):179–85. https://doi.org/10.1016/j.pcd.2015.10.007.

186. Schlender L, Martinez YV, Adeniji C, et al. Efficacy and safety of metformin in the management of type 2 diabetes mellitus in older adults: a systematic review for the development of recommendations to reduce potentially inappropriate prescribing. BMC Geriatr. 2017;17(1):227. https://doi.org/10.1186/s12877-017-0574-5.

187. Nissen SE, Wolski K. Effect of Rosiglitazone on the Risk of Myocardial Infarction and Death from Cardiovascular Causes. N Engl J Med. 2007;356(24):2457–71. https://doi.org/10.1056/NEJMoa072761.

188. Gallo LA, Wright EM, Vallon V. Probing SGLT2 as a therapeutic target for diabetes: basic physiology and consequences. Diab Vasc Dis Res. 2015;12(2):78–89. https://doi.org/10.1177/1479164114561992.

189. Karagiannis T, Tsapas A, Athanasiadou E, et al. GLP-1 receptor agonists and SGLT2 inhibitors for older people with type 2 diabetes: A systematic review and meta-analysis. Diabetes Res Clin Pract. 2021;174:108737. https://doi.org/10.1016/j.diabres.2021.108737.

190. Sun F, Wu S, Wang J, et al. Effect of glucagon-like peptide-1 receptor agonists on lipid profiles among type 2 diabetes: a systematic review and network meta-analysis. Clin Ther. 2015;37(1):225–241.e8. https://doi.org/10.1016/j.clinthera.2014.11.008.

191. Onoviran OF, Li D, Toombs Smith S, Raji MA. Effects of glucagon-like peptide 1 receptor agonists on comorbidities in older patients with diabetes mellitus. Ther Adv Chronic Dis. 2019;10:2040622319862691. https://doi.org/10.1177/2040622319862691.

192. Robinson LE, Holt TA, Rees K, Randeva HS, Hare JP. Effects of exenatide and liraglutide on heart rate, blood pressure and body weight: systematic review and meta-analysis. BMJ Open. 2013;3(1):e001986. https://doi.org/10.1136/bmjopen-2012-001986.

193. Umezawa S, Kubota A, Maeda H, et al. Two-year assessment of the efficacy and safety of sitagliptin in elderly patients with type 2 diabetes: post hoc analysis of the ASSET-K study. BMC Endocr Disord. 2015;15:34. https://doi.org/10.1186/s12902-015-0033-2.

194. Schott G, Martinez YV, Ediriweera de Silva RE, et al. Effectiveness and safety of dipeptidyl peptidase 4 inhibitors in the management of type 2 diabetes in older adults: a systematic review and development of recommendations to reduce inappropriate prescribing. BMC Geriatr. 2017;17(Suppl 1):226. https://doi.org/10.1186/s12877-017-0571-8.

195. Karagiannis T, Paschos P, Paletas K, Matthews DR, Tsapas A. Dipeptidyl peptidase-4 inhibitors for treatment of type 2 diabetes mellitus in the clinical setting: systematic review and meta-analysis. BMJ. 2012;344:e1369. https://doi.org/10.1136/bmj.e1369.

196. Kahn SE, Haffner SM, Heise MA, et al. Glycemic durability of rosiglitazone, metformin, or glyburide monotherapy. N Engl J Med. 2006;355(23):2427–43. https://doi.org/10.1056/NEJMoa066224.

197. Graham DJ, Ouellet-Hellstrom R, MaCurdy TE, et al. Risk of acute myocardial infarction, stroke, heart failure, and death in elderly Medicare patients treated with rosiglitazone or pioglitazone. JAMA. 2010;304(4):411–8. https://doi.org/10.1001/jama.2010.920.

198. Winkelmayer WC, Setoguchi S, Levin R, Solomon DH. Comparison of cardiovascular outcomes in elderly patients with diabetes who initiated rosiglitazone vs pioglitazone therapy. Arch Intern Med. 2008;168(21):2368–75. https://doi.org/10.1001/archinte.168.21.2368.

199. Gerstein HC, Bosch J, Dagenais GR, et al. Basal insulin and cardiovascular and other outcomes in dysglycemia. N Engl J Med. 2012;367(4):319–28. https://doi.org/10.1056/NEJMoa1203858.
200. By the American Geriatrics Society Beers Criteria Update Expert P. American Geriatrics Society 2015 Updated Beers Criteria for Potentially Inappropriate Medication Use in Older Adults. J Am Geriatr Soc. 2015;63(11):2227–46. https://doi.org/10.1111/jgs.13702.
201. Whelton PK, Appel LJ, Espeland MA, et al. Sodium reduction and weight loss in the treatment of hypertension in older persons: a randomized controlled trial of nonpharmacologic interventions in the elderly (TONE). JAMA. 1998;279(11):839–46. https://doi.org/10.1001/jama.279.11.839.
202. World Health Organization. Body Mass Index (BMI). 2021. https://www.euro.who.int/en/health-topics/disease-prevention/nutrition/a-healthy-lifestyle/body-mass-index-bmi. Accessed 2nd August.
203. Stevens J, Cai J, Pamuk ER, Williamson DF, Thun MJ, Wood JL. The effect of age on the association between body-mass index and mortality. N Engl J Med. 1998;338(1):1–7. https://doi.org/10.1056/NEJM199801013380101.
204. Prospective Studies Collaboration. Body-mass index and cause-specific mortality in 900,000 adults: collaborative analyses of 57 prospective studies. Lancet. 2009;373(9669):1083–96. https://doi.org/10.1016/S0140-6736(09)60318-4.
205. Flegal KM, Carroll MD, Ogden CL, Curtin LR. Prevalence and trends in obesity among US adults, 1999-2008. JAMA. 2010;303(3):235–41. https://doi.org/10.1001/jama.2009.2014.
206. Peralta M, Ramos M, Lipert A, Martins J, Marques A. Prevalence and trends of overweight and obesity in older adults from 10 European countries from 2005 to 2013. Scand J Public Health. 2018;46(5):522–9. https://doi.org/10.1177/1403494818764810.
207. Sorkin JD. BMI, age, and mortality: the slaying of a beautiful hypothesis by an ugly fact. Am J Clin Nutr. 2014;99(4):759–60. https://doi.org/10.3945/ajcn.114.084780.
208. Janssen I, Mark AE. Elevated body mass index and mortality risk in the elderly. Obes Rev. 2007;8(1):41–59. https://doi.org/10.1111/j.1467-789X.2006.00248.x.
209. Winter JE, MacInnis RJ, Wattanapenpaiboon N, Nowson CA. BMI and all-cause mortality in older adults: a meta-analysis. Am J Clin Nutr. 2014;99(4):875–90. https://doi.org/10.3945/ajcn.113.068122.
210. Batsis JA, Mackenzie TA, Bartels SJ, Sahakyan KR, Somers VK, Lopez-Jimenez F. Diagnostic accuracy of body mass index to identify obesity in older adults: NHANES 1999–2004. Int J Obes. 2016;40(5):761–7. https://doi.org/10.1038/ijo.2015.243.
211. Bouchonville MF, Villareal DT. Sarcopenic obesity: how do we treat it? Curr Opin Endocrinol Diabetes Obes. 2013;20(5):412–9. https://doi.org/10.1097/01.med.0000433071.11466.7f.
212. Stephen WC, Janssen I. Sarcopenic-obesity and cardiovascular disease risk in the elderly. J Nutr Health Aging. 2009;13(5):460–6. https://doi.org/10.1007/s12603-009-0084-z.
213. de Hollander EL, Bemelmans WJ, Boshuizen HC, et al. The association between waist circumference and risk of mortality considering body mass index in 65- to 74-year-olds: a meta-analysis of 29 cohorts involving more than 58 000 elderly persons. Int J Epidemiol. 2012;41(3):805–17. https://doi.org/10.1093/ije/dys008.
214. Powell-Wiley TM, Poirier P, Burke LE, et al. Obesity and cardiovascular disease: a scientific statement from the American Heart Association. Circulation. 2021;143(21):e984–e1010. https://doi.org/10.1161/CIR.0000000000000973.
215. Aune D, Giovannucci E, Boffetta P, et al. Fruit and vegetable intake and the risk of cardiovascular disease, total cancer and all-cause mortality-a systematic review and dose-response meta-analysis of prospective studies. Int J Epidemiol. 2017;46(3):1029–56. https://doi.org/10.1093/ije/dyw319.
216. Appel LJ, Moore TJ, Obarzanek E, et al. A clinical trial of the effects of dietary patterns on blood pressure. N Engl J Med. 1997;336(16):1117–24. https://doi.org/10.1056/NEJM199704173361601.

217. Wang DD, Li Y, Chiuve SE, et al. Association of specific dietary fats with total and cause-specific mortality. JAMA Intern Med. 2016;176(8):1134–45. https://doi.org/10.1001/jamainternmed.2016.2417.
218. Bao Y, Han J, Hu FB, et al. Association of nut consumption with total and cause-specific mortality. N Engl J Med. 2013;369(21):2001–11. https://doi.org/10.1056/NEJMoa1307352.
219. Yang Q, Zhang Z, Gregg EW, Flanders WD, Merritt R, Hu FB. Added sugar intake and cardiovascular diseases mortality among US adults. JAMA Intern Med. 2014;174(4):516–24. https://doi.org/10.1001/jamainternmed.2013.13563.
220. Micha R, Wallace SK, Mozaffarian D. Red and processed meat consumption and risk of incident coronary heart disease, stroke, and diabetes mellitus. Circulation. 2010;121(21):2271–83. https://doi.org/10.1161/CIRCULATIONAHA.109.924977.
221. Song M, Fung TT, Hu FB, et al. Association of animal and plant protein intake with all-cause and cause-specific mortality. JAMA Intern Med. 2016;176(10):1453–63. https://doi.org/10.1001/jamainternmed.2016.4182.
222. Sacks FM, Svetkey LP, Vollmer WM, et al. Effects on blood pressure of reduced dietary sodium and the Dietary Approaches to Stop Hypertension (DASH) diet. DASH-Sodium Collaborative Research Group. N Engl J Med. 2001;344(1):3–10. https://doi.org/10.1056/nejm200101043440101.
223. Cook NR, Cutler JA, Obarzanek E, et al. Long term effects of dietary sodium reduction on cardiovascular disease outcomes: observational follow-up of the trials of hypertension prevention (TOHP). BMJ. 2007;334(7599):885–8. https://doi.org/10.1136/bmj.39147.604896.55.
224. Reedy J, Krebs-Smith SM, Miller PE, et al. Higher diet quality is associated with decreased risk of all-cause, cardiovascular disease, and cancer mortality among older adults. J Nutr. 2014;144(6):881–9. https://doi.org/10.3945/jn.113.189407.
225. Keys A, Menotti A, Karvonen MJ, et al. The diet and 15-year death rate in the seven countries study. Am J Epidemiol. 1986;124(6):903–15. https://doi.org/10.1093/oxfordjournals.aje.a114480.
226. Salas-Salvadó J, Becerra-Tomás N, García-Gavilán JF, Bulló M, Barrubés L. Mediterranean diet and cardiovascular disease prevention: what do we know? Prog Cardiovasc Dis. 2018;61(1):62–7. https://doi.org/10.1016/j.pcad.2018.04.006.
227. Sanches Machado d'Almeida K, Ronchi Spillere S, Zuchinali P, Corrêa Souza G. Mediterranean diet and other dietary patterns in primary prevention of heart failure and changes in cardiac function markers: a systematic review. Nutrients. 2018;10(1) https://doi.org/10.3390/nu10010058.
228. Estruch R, Ros E, Salas-Salvadó J, et al. Primary prevention of cardiovascular disease with a Mediterranean diet. N Engl J Med. 2013;368(14):1279–90. https://doi.org/10.1056/NEJMoa1200303.
229. Trichopoulou A, Kouris-Blazos A, Wahlqvist ML, et al. Diet and overall survival in elderly people. BMJ. 1995;311(7018):1457. https://doi.org/10.1136/bmj.311.7018.1457.
230. Estruch R, Ros E, Salas-Salvadó J, et al. Primary prevention of cardiovascular disease with a mediterranean diet supplemented with extra-virgin olive oil or nuts. N Engl J Med. 2018;378(25):e34. https://doi.org/10.1056/NEJMoa1800389.
231. Karanja NM, Obarzanek E, Lin PH, et al. Descriptive characteristics of the dietary patterns used in the Dietary Approaches to Stop Hypertension Trial. DASH Collaborative Research Group. J Am Diet Assoc. Aug 1999;99(8 Suppl):S19–27. https://doi.org/10.1016/s0002-8223(99)00412-5.
232. Seidelmann SB, Claggett B, Cheng S, et al. Dietary carbohydrate intake and mortality: a prospective cohort study and meta-analysis. Lancet Public Health. 2018;3(9):e419–28. https://doi.org/10.1016/S2468-2667(18)30135-X.
233. Kalla A, Figueredo VM. Alcohol and cardiovascular disease in the geriatric population. Clin Cardiol. 2017;40(7):444–9. https://doi.org/10.1002/clc.22681.
234. Guthold R, Stevens GA, Riley LM, Bull FC. Worldwide trends in insufficient physical activity from 2001 to 2016: a pooled analysis of 358 population-based surveys with 1.9

million participants. Lancet Glob Health. 2018;6(10):e1077–86. https://doi.org/10.1016/S2214-109X(18)30357-7.

235. Kyu HH, Bachman VF, Alexander LT, et al. Physical activity and risk of breast cancer, colon cancer, diabetes, ischemic heart disease, and ischemic stroke events: systematic review and dose-response meta-analysis for the Global Burden of Disease Study 2013. BMJ. 2016;354:i3857. https://doi.org/10.1136/bmj.i3857.

236. Sattelmair J, Pertman J, Ding EL, Kohl HW 3rd, Haskell W, Lee IM. Dose response between physical activity and risk of coronary heart disease: a meta-analysis. Circulation. 2011;124(7):789–95. https://doi.org/10.1161/circulationaha.110.010710.

237. Physical activity strategy for the WHO European Region 2016–2025; 2016.

238. Piercy KL, Troiano RP, Ballard RM, et al. The physical activity guidelines for Americans. JAMA. 2018;320(19):2020–8. https://doi.org/10.1001/jama.2018.14854.

239. Ferraro RA, Pallazola VA, Michos ED. Physical activity, CVD, and older adults. Aging (Albany NY). 2019;11(9):2545–6. https://doi.org/10.18632/aging.101942.

240. van der Ploeg HP, Chey T, Ding D, Chau JY, Stamatakis E, Bauman AE. Standing time and all-cause mortality in a large cohort of Australian adults. Prev Med. 2014;69:187–91. https://doi.org/10.1016/j.ypmed.2014.10.004.

241. Zheng H, Orsini N, Amin J, Wolk A, Nguyen VT, Ehrlich F. Quantifying the dose-response of walking in reducing coronary heart disease risk: meta-analysis. Eur J Epidemiol. 2009;24(4):181–92. https://doi.org/10.1007/s10654-009-9328-9.

242. O'Donovan G, Lee IM, Hamer M, Stamatakis E. Association of "weekend warrior" and other leisure time physical activity patterns with risks for all-cause, cardiovascular disease, and cancer mortality. JAMA Intern Med. 2017;177(3):335–42. https://doi.org/10.1001/jamainternmed.2016.8014.

243. Chomistek AK, Manson JE, Stefanick ML, et al. Relationship of sedentary behavior and physical activity to incident cardiovascular disease: results from the Women's Health Initiative. J Am Coll Cardiol. 2013;61(23):2346–54. https://doi.org/10.1016/j.jacc.2013.03.031.

244. Patterson R, McNamara E, Tainio M, et al. Sedentary behaviour and risk of all-cause, cardiovascular and cancer mortality, and incident type 2 diabetes: a systematic review and dose response meta-analysis. Eur J Epidemiol. 2018;33(9):811–29. https://doi.org/10.1007/s10654-018-0380-1.

245. Rezende LFM, Rey-López JP, Matsudo VKR, Luiz OC. Sedentary behavior and health outcomes among older adults: a systematic review. BMC Public Health. 2014;14(1):333. https://doi.org/10.1186/1471-2458-14-333.

246. Matthews CE, George SM, Moore SC, et al. Amount of time spent in sedentary behaviors and cause-specific mortality in US adults. Am J Clin Nutr. 2012;95(2):437–45. https://doi.org/10.3945/ajcn.111.019620.

247. Du Y, Liu B, Sun Y, Snetselaar LG, Wallace RB, Bao W. Trends in adherence to the physical activity guidelines for americans for aerobic activity and time spent on sedentary behavior among US adults, 2007 to 2016. JAMA Netw Open. 2019;2(7):–e197597. https://doi.org/10.1001/jamanetworkopen.2019.7597.

248. Prince SA, Melvin A, Roberts KC, Butler GP, Thompson W. Sedentary behaviour surveillance in Canada: trends, challenges and lessons learned. Int J Behav Nutr Phys Act. 2020;17(1):34. https://doi.org/10.1186/s12966-020-00925-8.

249. Bellettiere J, LaMonte MJ, Evenson KR, et al. Sedentary behavior and cardiovascular disease in older women. Circulation. 2019;139(8):1036–46. https://doi.org/10.1161/CIRCULATIONAHA.118.035312.

250. Katzmarzyk PT, Church TS, Craig CL, Bouchard C. Sitting time and mortality from all causes, cardiovascular disease, and cancer. Med Sci Sports Exerc. 2009;41(5):998–1005. https://doi.org/10.1249/MSS.0b013e3181930355.

251. Eijsvogels TMH, Molossi S, Lee D-c, Emery MS, Thompson PD. Exercise at the extremes: the amount of exercise to reduce cardiovascular events. J Am Coll Cardiol. 2016;67(3):316–29. https://doi.org/10.1016/j.jacc.2015.11.034.

252. Aengevaeren VL, Mosterd A, Sharma S, et al. Exercise and coronary atherosclerosis. Circulation. 2020;141(16):1338–50. https://doi.org/10.1161/CIRCULATIONAHA.119.044467.
253. Kettunen JA, Kujala UM, Kaprio J, et al. All-cause and disease-specific mortality among male, former elite athletes: an average 50-year follow-up. Br J Sports Med. 2015;49(13):893–7. https://doi.org/10.1136/bjsports-2013-093347.
254. Zaleski AL, Taylor BA, Panza GA, et al. Coming of age: considerations in the prescription of exercise for older adults. Methodist Debakey Cardiovasc J. 2016;12(2):98–104. https://doi.org/10.14797/mdcj-12-2-98.
255. Riebe D, Franklin BA, Thompson PD, et al. Updating ACSM's recommendations for exercise preparticipation health screening. Med Sci Sports Exerc. 2015;47(11):2473–9.
256. O'Neill K, Reid G. Perceived barriers to physical activity by older adults. Can J Public Health. 1991;82(6):392–6.
257. Costello E, Kafchinski M, Vrazel J, Sullivan P. Motivators, barriers, and beliefs regarding physical activity in an older adult population. J Geriatr Phys Ther. 2011;34(3):138–47.
258. Spiteri K, Broom D, Bekhet AH, de Caro JX, Laventure B, Grafton K. Barriers and motivators of physical activity participation in middle-aged and older-adults - a systematic review. J Aging Phys Act. 2019;27(4):929–44. https://doi.org/10.1123/japa.2018-0343.
259. Franco MR, Tong A, Howard K, et al. Older people's perspectives on participation in physical activity: a systematic review and thematic synthesis of qualitative literature. Br J Sports Med. 2015;49(19):1268–76. https://doi.org/10.1136/bjsports-2014-094015.
260. Schutzer KA, Graves BS. Barriers and motivations to exercise in older adults. Prev Med. 2004;39(5):1056–61. https://doi.org/10.1016/j.ypmed.2004.04.003.
261. Beauchamp MR, Ruissen GR, Dunlop WL, et al. Group-based physical activity for older adults (GOAL) randomized controlled trial: Exercise adherence outcomes. Health Psychol. 2018;37(5):451–61. https://doi.org/10.1037/hea0000615.
262. Suaya JA, Stason WB, Ades PA, Normand SL, Shepard DS. Cardiac rehabilitation and survival in older coronary patients. J Am Coll Cardiol. 2009;54(1):25–33. https://doi.org/10.1016/j.jacc.2009.01.078.
263. Jepma P, Jorstad HT, Snaterse M, et al. Lifestyle modification in older versus younger patients with coronary artery disease. Heart. 2020;106(14):1066–72. https://doi.org/10.1136/heartjnl-2019-316056.
264. Collet J-P, Thiele H, Barbato E, et al. 2020 ESC Guidelines for the management of acute coronary syndromes in patients presenting without persistent ST-segment elevation: The Task Force for the management of acute coronary syndromes in patients presenting without persistent ST-segment elevation of the European Society of Cardiology (ESC). Eur Heart J. 2021;42(14):1289–367. https://doi.org/10.1093/eurheartj/ehaa575.
265. Knuuti J, Wijns W, Saraste A, et al. 2019 ESC guidelines for the diagnosis and management of chronic coronary syndromes: The Task Force for the diagnosis and management of chronic coronary syndromes of the European Society of Cardiology (ESC). Eur Heart J. 2019;41(3):407–77. https://doi.org/10.1093/eurheartj/ehz425.
266. Ibanez B, James S, Agewall S, et al. 2017 ESC Guidelines for the management of acute myocardial infarction in patients presenting with ST-segment elevation: The Task Force for the management of acute myocardial infarction in patients presenting with ST-segment elevation of the European Society of Cardiology (ESC). Eur Heart J. 2017;39(2):119–77. https://doi.org/10.1093/eurheartj/ehx393.
267. O'Gara PT, Kushner FG, Ascheim DD, et al. 2013 ACCF/AHA guideline for the management of ST-elevation myocardial infarction. Circulation. 2013;127(4):e362–425. https://doi.org/10.1161/CIR.0b013e3182742cf6.
268. McDonagh TA, Metra M, Adamo M, et al. 2021 ESC Guidelines for the diagnosis and treatment of acute and chronic heart failure: Developed by the Task Force for the diagnosis and treatment of acute and chronic heart failure of the European Society of Cardiology (ESC) With the special contribution of the Heart Failure Association (HFA) of the ESC. Eur Heart J. 2021;42(36):3599–726. https://doi.org/10.1093/eurheartj/ehab368.

269. Vigorito C, Abreu A, Ambrosetti M, et al. Frailty and cardiac rehabilitation: a call to action from the EAPC cardiac rehabilitation section. Eur J Prev Cardiol. 2017;24(6):577–90. https://doi.org/10.1177/2047487316682579.
270. Norekvål TM, Allore HG. Cardiac rehabilitation in older adults: is it just lifestyle? Heart. 2020;106(14):1035. https://doi.org/10.1136/heartjnl-2019-316497.
271. Suaya JA, Shepard DS, Normand SL, Ades PA, Prottas J, Stason WB. Use of cardiac rehabilitation by Medicare beneficiaries after myocardial infarction or coronary bypass surgery. Circulation. 2007;116(15):1653–62. https://doi.org/10.1161/circulationaha.107.701466.
272. Doll JA, Hellkamp A, Ho PM, et al. Participation in cardiac rehabilitation programs among older patients after acute myocardial infarction. JAMA Intern Med. 2015;175(10):1700–2. https://doi.org/10.1001/jamainternmed.2015.3819.
273. Thomas RJ, Beatty AL, Beckie TM, et al. Home-based cardiac rehabilitation: a scientific statement from the American Association of Cardiovascular and Pulmonary Rehabilitation, the American Heart Association, and the American College of Cardiology. Circulation. 2019;140(1):e69–89. https://doi.org/10.1161/CIR.0000000000000663.
274. Snoek JA, Prescott EI, van der Velde AE, et al. Effectiveness of home-based mobile guided cardiac rehabilitation as alternative strategy for nonparticipation in clinic-based cardiac rehabilitation among elderly patients in Europe: a randomized clinical trial. JAMA Cardiol. 2021;6(4):463–8. https://doi.org/10.1001/jamacardio.2020.5218.

Cardiovascular Pharmacology of the Older Patient

Brent G. Petty

1 Concentration of Medication in Our Bodies: Pharmacokinetics

Pharmacokinetics has been described as "what our bodies do to medications." The factors that influence the concentrations of medications in our bodies include absorption, distribution, metabolism, and elimination. Absorption usually depends on the gastrointestinal tract, but alternative routes are sometimes effective for adequate absorption (e.g., sublingual, buccal, rectal, or transdermal). The most important organs involved with metabolism are the liver and the gastrointestinal mucosa, which both contain metabolizing enzymes. Elimination of medications and their metabolites may involve the liver, gastrointestinal mucosa, biliary tract, and kidneys.

2 Physiology of Aging

Our bodies are fantastic machines, but they tend to wear over time. All organ systems are affected in the physiology of aging [1], but the ones that are most important concerning medications are the renal and hepatic systems, and to a small degree, the gastrointestinal system.

B. G. Petty (✉)
Pharmacy & Therapeutics Committee, Johns Hopkins University School of Medicine, Baltimore, MD, USA
e-mail: bgp@jhmi.edu, bpetty1@jh.edu

© The Author(s), under exclusive license to Springer Nature Switzerland AG 2023
T. M. Leucker, G. Gerstenblith (eds.), *Cardiovascular Disease in the Elderly*, Contemporary Cardiology, https://doi.org/10.1007/978-3-031-16594-8_3

2.1 Reduction of Kidney Function

With the passage of time, there is a reduction in the number and size of nephrons. There is also glomerular sclerosis, glomerular basement membrane thickening, and reduction of renal blood flow [1]. All of these factors contribute to the progressive reduction of renal function. This impairs the body's ability to eliminate certain medications and/or metabolites, consequently exposing the elderly patient to higher medication concentrations and longer persistence of increased concentrations compared to younger patients.

2.2 Reduction of Liver Function

As humans age, both liver mass and hepatic blood flow fall [1]. The ability of hepatic enzymes to metabolize medications is reduced in advancing age. This slows the conversion of medications to metabolites and slows the conversion of active metabolites to inactive molecules. It may also delay the change of an inactive "prodrug" (e.g., codeine) to its active form (morphine).

2.3 Gastrointestinal Absorption

There is little influence of aging on gastrointestinal absorption. The bioavailability of medications, or the fraction of medication absorbed, is not substantially altered with advancing age. For compounds that are better absorbed in an acidic gastric environment, such as iron or calcium, the reduction of gastric acid production sometimes seen in elderly patients affects absorption [1, 2].

Figure 1 shows a representative example of the blood concentrations of verapamil in a young patient compared to an elderly patient. The peak level with the first dose does not differ much between young and elderly patients, but the idifference in the peaks will increase between them over time with continued dosing. The lowest (trough) concentration will also be higher and will progressively increase in the elderly patient compared to the younger patient.

The overall conclusion regarding pharmacokinetics in elderly patients is that both medication concentrations and half-lives will be increased compared to younger patients [3]. This means that lower doses, perhaps given less frequently, may be sufficient for the desired effect and/or to avoid concentration-related toxicities. Upward titration of doses for greater effect should be done more conservatively in older patients because they will have a greater rise in concentrations.

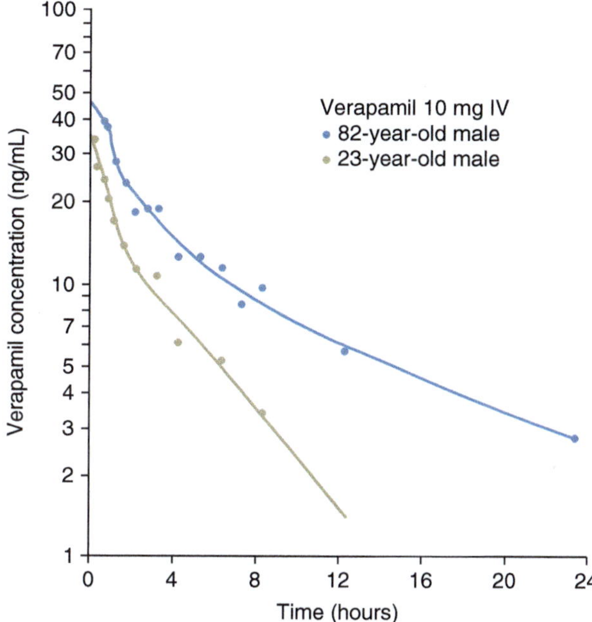

Fig. 1 A representative example of the blood concentrations of verapamil in a young patient compared to an elderly patient

3   Effects of Medication on Our Bodies: Pharmacodynamics

The influence of aging on medication effect is variable. A variety of medications and their pharmacodynamic responses are outlined in Table 1. The effect of age on medication responses varies not only among medications but varies with the particular response measured [3]. In many cases, elderly patients can be more sensitive than younger people to the effect of a given dose or blood concentration of a medication [4]. Yet in other cases, including the sensitivity of the same individual and to the same medication, the nature of the response can be different. For example, the effect of diltiazem at equal concentrations on reducing blood pressure is greater with elderly patients compared to young patients, yet the effect of diltiazem on prolongation of the PR interval is less with elderly compared to young patients. And while the effects of verapamil on blood pressure and heart rate are greater in older than younger patients, elderly patients are less sensitive to the effects on cardiac conduction.

Table 1 Selected pharmacodynamic changes with age[a]

Medication	Measured effect	Response to equal blood concentrations in elderly compared to younger patients
Adenosine	Heart-rate response	↔
Amlodipine [24]	Blood pressure response	↔
Diazepam	Sedation, postural sway	↑
Diltiazem	Acute and chronic antihypertensive effect	↑
	Acute PR interval prolongation	↓
Diphenhydramine	Postural sway	↔
Enalapril	ACE inhibition	↔
Furosemide	Peak diuretic response	↓
Heparin	Anticoagulant effect	↔
Isoproterenol	Chronotropic effect	↓
Phenylephrine	$Alpha_1$-adrenergic responsiveness	↔
Propranolol	Antagonism of chronotropic effects of isoproterenol	↓
Verapamil	Acute antihypertensive effect	↑
	Cardiac conduction	↓
Warfarin	Anticoagulant effect	↑

↑ = increase; ↓ = decrease; ↔ = no significant change; ACE = angiotensin-converting enzyme
[a]Adapted from Mangoni and Jackson [3]

4 Polypharmacy

As patients age, they tend to develop more medical problems, they consult more medical providers, and they are treated with more and more medications. Over 90% of patients in long-term care take five or more medications daily [5]. As the number of medications taken increases, the patient is more likely to have adverse effects and/or clinically significant drug interactions [6]. The principle should always be to use the lowest doses of the fewest number of medications to adequately (not perfectly) control the patient's problems.

The conscious effort to reduce the number of medications that patients take is called "deprescribing." This has become more and more popular in recent years [5–7]. There have even been calls for investigating the deprescribing of medications as part of the process of new drug development in order to reduce the risk of withdrawal-associated harms and to include this information in product labels [8]. Epidemiologic data suggest that statins used for primary prevention of cardiovascular events might best be continued after age 75 and not be deprescribed [9].

In summary, the cautious and reasonable approach to take with regard to dosing most medications in the elderly is to "start low and go slow" [10]. This will help avoid excessively high concentrations of medications in the elderly and takes into account the potential synergistic effect of multiple, simultaneous pharmacodynamic responses in these patients. Consideration of age is incorporated into recommended dose reduction for some drugs, such as apixaban [11].

5   Drug Interactions

As mentioned above, drug interactions are common and increase with the number of medications a patient is taking. Access to drug interaction data is widely available on medication databases such as Lexicomp and Micromedex, or on the internet through sites such as the FDA [12] or Indiana University [13]. It is important to remember that drug interactions are influenced not only by the addition of medications to a patient's regimen but also by removals. For example, in a patient taking both simvastatin and diltiazem, stopping the diltiazem can lead to a reduction in the simvastatin concentration because the diltiazem no longer slows the elimination of simvastatin.

6   Interventions

6.1   Avoidance

One strategy to avoid toxicity due to medications in the elderly is simply to avoid using all medications that may contribute to problems in elderly patients. That was the approach proposed in the original Beers list [14], which called for certain medications not to be used in elderly patients. In recent years, as the American Geriatric Society has been revising and rewording the list, their approach has become more realistic and reasonable [15]. Now there is a recognition that the plurality of medications are just relatively contraindicated, and with appropriate dose adjustment these drugs can be used safely and effectively in most elderly patients.

6.2   Therapeutic Drug Monitoring

Treatment of any patient should follow the "ideal therapeutic algorithm" (Table 2). First, the prescriber should have a therapeutic goal in mind, whether it is to lower the blood pressure to a certain point, reduce the hemoglobin A1c below a certain threshold, or drive the LDL cholesterol down under some concentration. With the goal in mind, an appropriate agent is selected, and then an appropriate starting dose of the agent is chosen. When relevant patient characteristics or concomitant medications are known, the dose may be individualized somewhat. After allowing a

Table 2 Ideal therapeutic algorithm[a]

1. Determine the therapeutic goal.
2. Choose an appropriate agent.
3. Choose the appropriate dose, individualizing for each patient when possible.
4. Know when/how to monitor for effectiveness and safety, including the essential criteria for appropriate therapeutic drug monitoring.
5. Properly adjust the therapy (e.g., increase the dose, add another medication, switch to another agent, etc.) to attain the therapeutic goal and avoid toxicity.

[a] From "Rational Therapeutics" course, the Johns Hopkins University School of Medicine

Table 3 Criteria for appropriate therapeutic drug monitoring

1. Medication concentration or effects can be measured reliably and accurately
AND
2. The efficacy of medication treatment can be enhanced by achieving a certain concentration or effect range
AND/OR
3. The toxicity of medication treatment can be reduced by maintaining a certain concentration or effect range

sufficient period of time for the intervention to reach a substantial or peak effect, which may be days or weeks, a repeat measurement is performed and is compared to the pre-treatment reading and the therapeutic goal. Then, whatever the starting dose may have been, adjustments in the dose may well be needed to achieve the therapeutic goal. After the response to the new dose is observed, another adjustment in dose, or adding or substituting another medication, can be considered. All the while there is monitoring for evidence of adverse effects.

Therapeutic drug monitoring is a term that usually implies the measurement in some body fluid of a substance that is either the medication that is being monitored or a related substance. Therapeutic drug monitoring is best employed when certain criteria can be met (Table 3). If measuring a drug concentration or a physiological result [e.g., activated partial thromboplastin time (aPTT)] is part of the monitoring, one must be confident that the laboratory to be used can measure the item accurately and in a timely fashion. Then, it must be known that the efficacy of the drug is enhanced or the toxicity of the drug is reduced by adjusting the dose of the medication. If the efficacy or toxicity of a medication cannot reliably be improved by adjusting the dose to achieve a result in the "therapeutic range," then therapeutic drug monitoring is without value. We should avoid the temptation to measure drug concentrations just because we can. Achieving and maintaining results in the "therapeutic range" should reduce the risk of toxicity or improve efficacy, or both. It should be emphasized that measuring drug concentrations in plasma or serum establishes individual patient pharmacokinetics. One well-done drug concentration is more valuable than any algorithm that seeks to predict concentration or effect using patient characteristics, co-morbidities, or other factors.

6.3 Proper Medication Use [16]

The choice of initiating medication treatment or not should always be carefully weighed. Before a medication is ordered for a hospitalized patient or prescribed for an outpatient, the prescriber needs to consider the (1) efficacy, (2) safety, and (3) cost of the medication, in that order of importance. Without efficacy for the condition being treated, no medication should be given. "It's not likely to be harmful" is no justification for giving a medication without demonstrated efficacy for the patient's problem.

It is always an option in medicine to do nothing (offer no treatment), and sometimes no treatment is the best option. For example, in a patient with an acute inferior wall myocardial infarction who develops Mobitz I block (Wenkebach), the occasional missed beat is often of no clinical consequence, creates no risk for the patient, and almost always resolves without intervention. Treating such a problem with atropine or a pacemaker would be a mistake, introducing some risk of toxicity or complication for no clinical benefit, so no treatment is the best approach for the transient conduction defect in such patients.

Additionally, there are often "non-pharmacologic approaches" that may be alternatives or adjuncts to medications for certain medical conditions. These non-pharmacologic approaches include lifestyle modification and behavioral therapies. Weight loss, dietary changes, smoking cessation, stopping alcohol, and prudent exercise are among the options.

6.3.1 Evidence for Efficacy

The quality of medical studies supporting the use of medications varies widely. The strongest studies that direct medical practice are clinical trials that are well designed, randomized, controlled, "blinded" or "masked," and prospective. Each of these elements is important to increase the likelihood that the results of the study can be accepted as accurate rather than be the result of chance. The study question is framed as a "null hypothesis," which is often not what the investigators actually expect to find. In fact, most investigators begin with the expectation of showing a difference between the test compound and either standard treatment or inactive (placebo) treatment. So for example, if one were comparing the effect of two HMG-CoA reductase inhibitors ("statins") on serum cholesterol, a null hypothesis could be, "There is no difference between atorvastatin and rosuvastatin in patients with hypercholesterolemia and symptomatic coronary artery disease." Then the study is conducted with a sufficient sample size to attempt to disprove the null hypothesis with a certainty of at least 95% that the degree of difference between the two drugs is greater than zero and not just the result of chance (alpha or type I error = 0.05). More frequently now than in the past, the investigators may propose that there will not be a significant difference between the two arms, or what is called a "non-inferiority" study. The confidence of saying that two medications are "equivalent" or "non-inferior" often requires a larger sample size because (1) the difference for a treatment to be considered inferior (the margin of clinical equivalence) is often smaller than the treatment effect hypothesized in a superiority study, and (2) the beta, or probability of type II, error is normally set at 0.2, but when investigators want more certainty that they are not missing a treatment difference that truly exists, the beta may be reduced to 0.1.

Once the study is completed, having achieved the intended sample size, the results are analyzed. The most balanced approach is to assume that either of the two groups could be superior to the other, which leads to a "two-tailed" statistical test. It is especially interesting to see how close each group actually performed compared to the predicted response when the study hypothesis was developed and the sample size was calculated. The analysis can determine whether one group had a more favorable outcome than the other, and by how much they differed. The difference is "statistically significant" if it is less likely than 5% to have reached that difference through chance alone. The 5% threshold is, of course, arbitrary as a level to embrace an observation with absolute conviction vs. 6% to discount as nothing very meaningful. In fact, when the difference reaches a 6% degree of certainty for being beyond a chance finding, it seems inappropriate to say that the outcomes of the groups were "not different." The truth is that the groups' outcomes *were* different, but there was not sufficient evidence to reject the null hypothesis. Regrettably, in such cases, one often hears the term "trend" used to describe the difference, with the assumption that the difference would have reached statistical significance if only the sample size were larger *and* the proportional responses held the same levels with additional subjects. What is important to emphasize is that the difference may be clinically meaningful and that further research should be done to assess the difference.

Too often readers ignore the Methods sections of published papers, giving their limited time instead to the Abstract, a few figures or tables in the Results, and the highlights of the Discussion section. This approach may save time, but it ignores the critical information about characteristics of the study population recruited, what kinds of patients were excluded, how other medications were managed, and many other aspects that ultimately determine whether the results of the study are valid and whether they can be applied to any other population/patient group besides those enrolled into the study. The paper rises or falls on its Methods, so results or conclusions are not valid if the procedures involved in conducting the study are seriously flawed.

Among the difficult issues with clinical trials is whether the results can be extrapolated to all drugs in the same class. Extrapolation across a class is somewhat common but also hazardous, as drug formulation, absorption, duration of effect, and frequency and severity of drug interactions differ among drugs in the same class. Even with HMG-CoA reductase inhibitors, whose effects on LDL cholesterol are mostly affected by drug potency and can often be equated through adjustment of dose, the efficacy related to clinical outcomes and frequency of adverse effects may vary. Thus, what is true for one drug in a certain class may not always be true for other drugs in the same class.

Another issue regarding the validity of clinical trials is the use of "surrogate markers" in place of "hard clinical endpoints." An example is a reduction of HIV RNA levels as a surrogate for medication efficacy instead of prolonged survival in patients with AIDS. Some surrogate markers have been demonstrated through rigorous clinical studies to be closely associated with hard clinical endpoints, providing assurance that they can be trusted as substitutes. Other surrogate markers have less data to justify their use as substitutes. A published study points out the hazard of surrogate markers: a study of interleukin-2 therapy in patients with HIV infection showed a substantial and sustained elevation of CD4+ cell count over a period of 7–8 years average follow-up, but no improvement in survival or in the incidence of opportunistic infections [17]. In this case, the positive effect of the medication on the surrogate marker was not accompanied by improvement in the clinical endpoints. And recent emphasis has been focused on a questionable surrogate marker related to a controversial medication for treatment of Alzheimer's Disease [18].

Another common outcome strategy in clinical trials is "composite endpoints," combining as an "event" any one of several conditions, such as cardiac death, nonfatal myocardial infarction, and admission to a hospital for unstable angina. Obviously, all of these conditions are defensible as outcomes in patients with coronary artery disease, but they are decreasingly reliable as "hard clinical endpoints" for an intervention intended to influence the course of coronary artery disease. Especially when the most frequent of the three conditions contributing to the composite endpoint is the result of variable clinician judgment (e.g., the threshold for when to admit a patient for unstable angina), the reliability of the composite endpoint decreases. In the words of one author, "…inconsistent or even inappropriate construction of composite endpoints is a common and completely avoidable threat to appropriate understanding and interpretation of trial results" [19].

6.3.2 Safety

Throughout all phases of drug development before drug approval (Phases I, II, and III), safety is assessed, but at best these studies involve only a few thousand study subjects for the vast majority of drugs. With this number of patients, only side effects of moderate frequency (around 1–10 per thousand) will be identified. More rare (and often more serious) side effects may only become recognized with much more extensive use, involving tens of thousands of people. The experience with drugs such as troglitazone [20] emphasizes the importance of post-marketing reporting of toxicities associated with newly-approved medications to MedWatch and/or to the manufacturer.

There is a risk of toxicity with virtually all medications, so there must be a consideration of risk and benefit before starting or continuing medications. In many cases, the toxicity emerges without warning ("idiosyncratic"), such as rashes in response to penicillin. These "adverse drug events" are usually unpredictable and are not considered "medication errors." In other cases, the possible toxicities of medications can be identified and treated before they become clinically dangerous (e.g., hypokalemia with loop diuretics or hyperkalemia with ACE inhibitors). These adverse drug events are not medication errors either unless the patient is not monitored appropriately with occasional serum potassium measures.

6.3.3 Cost

The cost of medical care seems to steadily rise. Spending on healthcare in the U.S. in 2019 rose 4.6%, to a total of $3.8 trillion. This represented 17.7% of our overall economy [21]. Interestingly, while the spending on drugs continues to go up each year, the rates of increase have varied [22]. Data for the annual increases in total U.S. drug expenditures for the past 10 years are shown in Table 4.

Retail prescription drug expenditures rose by 2.2%, 3.8%, and 5.7% in calendar years 2017, 2018, and 2019, respectively [22]. No wonder patients sometimes find that they are unable to afford their medications, and as a result they go without them. This "economic non-compliance" increases during difficult economic periods or when people have fixed incomes and must choose between paying for these medications or their food or housing. Additionally, if hospitals and health systems could pay less for their medications, they would have more funds available for capital improvements or expanded personnel services.

The drug that contributed the most to overall drug expenditures in 2020 was adalimumab [22]. In second place, with about half the total expenditure, was apixaban (Table 5). Other cardiovascular drugs in the top 25 for 2020 included rivaroxiban and epinephrine, and their costs for 2020 are also shown.

Clinical trials have increasingly been including assessment of quality of life, not just the survival rate. The measure of quality-adjusted life year (QALY) is a standard and internationally-recognized method to assess the relative benefit of medical interventions [23]. It combines the duration of survival and the quality of life during

Table 4 Increase of U.S. drug costs year-to-year[a]

Year	% increase over previous year
2011	4.0
2012	0.02
2013	0.03
2014	13.3
2015	11.7
2016	5.8
2017	1.7
2018	5.5
2019	5.4
2020	4.9
Mean	5.24
Median	5.15

[a]Adapted from Tichy et al. [22]

Table 5 Selected drugs from among the top 25 according to overall U.S. drug expenditures in 2020[a]

Rank	Drug	2020 Expenditures ($ Thousands)	Percentage change (from 2019)
1.	Adalimumab	24,856,877	11.5
2.	Apixaban	12,805,307	29.9
3.	Insulin glargine	9,702,808	2.1
8.	Etanercept	7,768,483	−3.5
9.	Rivaroxaban	6,628,084	10.2
24.	Epinephrine	3,848,533	−1.4

[a]Adapted from Tichy et al. [22]

each year of life. Although one treatment might help someone live longer, it might also have serious side effects (for example, it might make them feel sick or put them at risk of other illnesses). Another treatment might not extend survival but it may improve quality of life (for example, by reducing pain). The quality of life rating can range from 0 (worst possible health) to 1 (best possible health). Having the QALY measurement allows one to consider, how much the treatment costs per QALY gained. This is the cost of providing a year of the best quality of life available, which could be one person receiving one QALY, but is more likely to be a number of people receiving a portion of a QALY—for example, 4 people receiving 0.25 QALY.

The combination of cost and effectiveness merge into cost-effectiveness analysis. This is another increasingly popular approach to assessing the impact of interventions that may have financial benefits. For example, aspirin's cost is much less than the cost of caring for the heart attacks or strokes it prevents. Sometimes a medication's benefit is secondary or indirect. For example, acetycholinesterase inhibitors are reported to cause a temporary delay in the cognitive decline of patients with dementia. If this delay in cognitive decline can postpone a patient from requiring institutionalization in a nursing home or full-time care at their home for a period of months or years, the costs of such medication may be much less than the cost of the care that must otherwise be provided.

Policymakers, including governmental bodies, payers, and influential foundations are interested in maximizing cost-effectiveness. They are convinced, with some justification, that many practices and interventions might well be replaced with less costly approaches, without diminishing the quality of health care and the benefit our patients derive.

6.3.4 Patient Preferences and Values

With rare exceptions, prescribers have a number of possible medications for managing diseases, and each may cause likely responses (good or bad) in addition to the intended response. In all cases, the patient's inclination to accept the proposed therapy should be considered.

The prescriber should also consider co-existing medical conditions that might likewise benefit from the same therapy, as this may magnify the benefit of the medication without adding the additional risk of toxicity. For example, in a patient with hypertension who also suffers from frequent migraine headaches, a beta blocker or verapamil might be favored by the patient over other medications because they may reduce the frequency and/or severity of the migraine episodes at the same time the blood pressure is being reduced. On the other hand, a patient with hypertension who also suffers from asthma may have increased bronchospasm if a beta blocker is given as part of the hypertension regimen.

Patients with potentially life-threatening conditions (e.g., metastatic cancer) are often treated with potent medications with the potential of side effects that are not only miserable but may be life-threatening themselves. When treatments are similar in efficacy but differ in types of toxicities, the patients' preferences are important, since hair loss may be more adverse for some patients than risk of infection or incidence of diarrhea. Tailoring the medications used in such cases preserves the patient's autonomy and properly respects their right to choose among reasonable options.

6.3.5 Medication Reconciliation

During hospitalization, patients may receive a different drug than when they were home. This may be the result of provider preference or formulary restriction. Hospital formularies are either "open" or "closed," and may have additional restrictions. "Open" formularies mean that prescribers can order any marketed product and the patient will get whatever specific product was ordered. "Closed" formularies limit the selection of medications to a smaller number of products within either a chemical class or indication class. For example, rather than having all H2-receptor blockers and all proton pump inhibitors on the hospital's formulary, the hospital may restrict the choice to famotidine and/or omeprazole. These determinations are generally made based on the assumptions of (1) equal, or at least adequate, efficacy, (2) no worse toxicity profile for the selected product, and (3) substantial cost savings.

Medication treatment may be either specific (based on the establishment of a definite diagnosis) or empiric (based on the best guess of a diagnosis using the available evidence and considering the usual etiology responsible for the condition, such as the most likely bacterial pathogens for a community-acquired pneumonia). Oftentimes it is hazardous to withhold treatment until a specific diagnosis is confirmed, so empiric treatment is well accepted in many situations.

The initiation of a new medication in the hospital or in the outpatient setting must be framed on the background of the medications that the patient previously had taken. The process of considering the immediate previous medications (the patient's "home medications") when ordering new treatment is called medication reconciliation. "Home medications" may not always have been taken at a patient's house, as the patient may have come to the hospital from a nursing home or may have been transferred from another hospital. Medication reconciliation is not simply copying the "home medications" into the hospital's order system, but rather it is a thoughtful consideration of the value of continuing each medication in light of the patient's new medical condition. There should be a conscious decision, for each and every medication, whether to stop, continue, or modify the administration of the drug.

At the time of transfer to a new service or level of care, and at the end of the patient's hospitalization, another medication reconciliation should occur. This one differs from the one at admission because the consideration of medications to prescribe upon transfer or at discharge should take into account not only the medications the patient was taking in the hospital just before transfer or discharge but the "home medications." The purpose of this dual consideration is to avoid costly and potentially hazardous duplication of medications. As explained above, patients may receive one proton pump inhibitor while in the hospital (e.g., pantoprazole), which is different than the one they took at home (e.g., omeprazole) or the one they might be prescribed at discharge (e.g., lansoprazole). Patients have been known to be taking supplies of both "warfarin" and "Coumadin" following hospital discharge because one had been provided by prescription from their family doctor while the other came from their hospital doctors. Since generic and brand products may look different, it is easy to understand how patients may not recognize the hazardous duplication. Conscientious medication reconciliation can reduce the risk of adverse drug events, save unnecessary drug costs, and minimize drug interactions.

References

1. Preston J, Biddell B. The physiology of ageing and how these changes affect older people. Medicine. 2020;49:1–5.
2. Bhutti A, Morley J. The clinical significance of gastrointestinal changes with aging. Curr Opin Clin Nutr Metab Care. 2008;11:651–60.
3. Mangoni AA, Jackson SHD. Age-related changes in pharmacokinetics and pharmacodynamics: basic principles and practical applications. Br J Clin Pharmacol. 2004;57:6–14.
4. Bowie MW, Slattum PW. Pharmacodynamics in older adults: a review. Am J Geriatr Pharmacother. 2007;5:263–303.
5. Halli-Tierney AD, Scarborough C, Carroll D. Polypharmacy: evaluating risks and deprescribing. Am Fam Physician. 2019;100:32–8.
6. Hoel RWS, Giddings Connolly RM, Takahashi PY. Polypharmacy management in older patients. Mayo Clin Proc. 2021;96:242–56.
7. Scott IA, Hilmer SN, Le Couteur DG. Going beyond the guidelines in individualising the use of antihypertensive drugs in older patients. Drugs Aging. 2019;36:675–85.
8. Lau SWJ, Schlender J-F, Slattum PW, et al. Geriatrics 2030: developing drugs to care for older persons—a neglected and growing population. Clin Pharmacol Ther. 2020;107:53–6.
9. Giral P, Neumann A, Weill A, Coste J. Cardiovascular effect of discontinuing statins for primary prevention at the age of 75 years: a nationwide population-based cohort study in France. Eur Heart J. 2019;40:3516–25.
10. ElDesoky ES. Pharmacokinetic-pharmacodynamic crisis in the elderly. Am J Ther. 2007;14:488–98.

11. Bristol-Myers Squibb. Eliquis® (apixaban tablets). Prescribing information. https://packagein-serts.bms.com/pi/pi_eliquis.pdf. Accessed 31 Aug 2021.
12. https://www.fda.gov/drugs/drug-interactions-labeling/drug-development-and-drug-interactions-table-substrates-inhibitors-and-inducers. Accessed 30 Aug 2021.
13. https://drug-interactions.medicine.iu.edu/MainTable.aspx. Accessed 30 Aug 2021.
14. Beers MH, Ouslander JG, Rollinger I, et al. Explicit criteria for determining inappropriate medication use in nursing home residents. Arch Intern Med. 1991;151:1825–32.
15. American Geriatrics Society Beers Criteria® Update Expert Panel. American Geriatrics Society 2019 updated AGS Beers Criteria® for potentially inappropriate medication use in older adults. J Am Geriatr Soc. 2019;67:674–94.
16. Petty BG. Principles of evidence-based prescribing. In: McKean SC, Ross JJ, Dressler DD, Scheurer DB, editors. Principles and practice of hospital medicine. 2nd ed. New York: McGraw Hill; 2017. p. 56–61.
17. The INSIGHT-ESPRIT Study Group and SILCAAT Scientific Committee. Interleukin-2 therapy in patients with HIV infection. N Engl J Med. 2009;361:1548–59.
18. Alexander GC, Knopman DS, Emerson SS, et al. Revisiting FDA approval of aducanumab. N Engl J Med. 2021;385:769–71.
19. West CP. Outcomes, outcomes everywhere, nor any stop to think? J Gen Intern Med. 2011;26:1239–40.
20. Gale EAM. Troglitazone: the lesson that nobody learned? Diabetologia. 2006;49:1–6.
21. Martin AB, Hartman M, Lassman D, Catlin A. National health care spending in 2019: steady growth for the fourth consecutive year. Health Aff (Milwood). 2021;40:1–14.
22. Tichy EM, Hoffman JM, Suda KJ, et al. National trends in prescription drug expenditures and projections for 2021. Am J Health-Syst Pharm. 2021;78:1294–308.
23. www.nice.org.uk/Glossary?letter=Q#QALY. Accessed 30 Aug 2021.
24. Abernethy DR. An overview of the pharmacokinetics and pharmacodynamics of amlodipine in elderly persons with systemic hypertension. Am J Cardiol. 1994;73:10A–7A.

Aging of the Vasculature

Thorsten M. Leucker, Joseph Goldenberg, and Gary Gerstenblith

1 Introduction

Longevity is a vascular question, which has been well expressed in the axiom that man is only as old as his arteries. To a majority of men death comes primarily or secondarily through this portal. The onset of what may be called physiological arterio-sclerosis depends, in the first place, on the quality of arterial tissue which the individual has inherited, and secondarily on the amount of wear and tear to which he has subjected it.—Sir William Osler, 1891 [1].

Sir William Osler's famous quotation is as relevant today as it was in the late nineteenth century. Vascular disease and its consequences remain the most common causes of mortality and significant lifelong disability in developed, and most developing, countries. Age is the most potent risk factor for the responsible vascular changes and although these are in part dependent on the "quality of the arterial tissue" we inherit, their trajectory can be impacted by the environment our vessels are exposed to. This chapter will review the molecular, cellular, structural, and functional changes associated with aging, the impact of these changes on cardiovascular outcomes, and lifestyle and pharmacologic interventions designed to modify them.

T. M. Leucker (✉) · G. Gerstenblith
Division of Cardiology, Department of Medicine, Johns Hopkins University School of Medicine, Baltimore, MD, USA
e-mail: tleucke1@jhmi.edu; gblith@jhmi.edu

J. Goldenberg
Divison of Cardiology, School of Medicine, Johns Hopkins University, Baltimore, MD, USA
e-mail: jgolde17@jhu.edu

T. M. Leucker, G. Gerstenblith (eds.), *Cardiovascular Disease in the Elderly*, Contemporary Cardiology, https://doi.org/10.1007/978-3-031-16594-8_4

2   Molecular and Cellular Mechanisms of Vascular Aging

The vasculature consists of two primary cell types: endothelial cells and vascular smooth muscle cells. The endothelium is the innermost, lumen-facing layer of the vasculature [2]. Endothelial cells communicate with vascular smooth muscle cells via a variety of mechanisms including paracrine mediators such as endothelial nitric oxide synthase-derived nitric oxide, extracellular vesicles, and microRNAs, as well as interactions via the extracellular matrix and direct cell-cell pathways [3, 4]. Endothelial cell function is considered a "barometer" of vascular health because it is a driver of the development, progression, and clinical manifestations of cardio-vascular and cerebrovascular diseases. Endothelial dysfunction is considered a major risk factor for cardiovascular disease, the leading cause of mortality and loss of independence in older Americans [5]. The number of older individuals in the USA is rapidly growing with a projected increase in those >65 years of age from 56.2 million in 2021 to 80.8 million in 2040 [6]. Thus, there is an unmet need to understand responsible mechanisms, which can inform the development and testing of novel treatments for the amelioration of the age-associated increased cardiovas-cular risk.

Several mechanisms are involved in vascular aging. Among them are reduced nitric oxide bioavailability, increased oxidative stress, mitochondrial dysfunction, sterile inflammation or "inflammaging", genomic/epigenetic alterations, telomere shortening, and stem cell depletion.

The following sections highlight aging-associated vascular cell changes, and their contribution to the pathogenesis of both microvascular and macrovascular dis-eases (Fig. 1).

Fig. 1 Conceptual model for the role of cell-autonomous and noncell-autonomous mechanisms in vascular aging. The model predicts that circulating progeronic (e.g., inflammatory cytokines, renin-angiotensin system [RAS], and aldosterone) and antigeronic factors (e.g., IGF-1 [insulin-like growth factor 1], mediators of caloric restriction, estrogen) derived from the brain, the endo-crine system, cells of the immune system, and the adipose tissue orchestrate aging processes simultaneously in the endothelial and smooth muscle cells within the large vessels and microcir-culation. The hierarchical regulatory cascade for vascular aging involves modulation of cell-autonomous cellular and molecular aging processes. The resulting functional dysregulation of vascular cells (i.e., impaired vasomotor, barrier, secretory, and transport functions of the vascula-ture, as well as adverse structural remodeling) promotes the development of a wide range of age-related vascular pathologies. *AMI* acute myocardial infarction, *GDF11* growth differentiation factor 11, *PAD* peripheral artery disease. (From: Circulation Research. 2018;123:849–867)

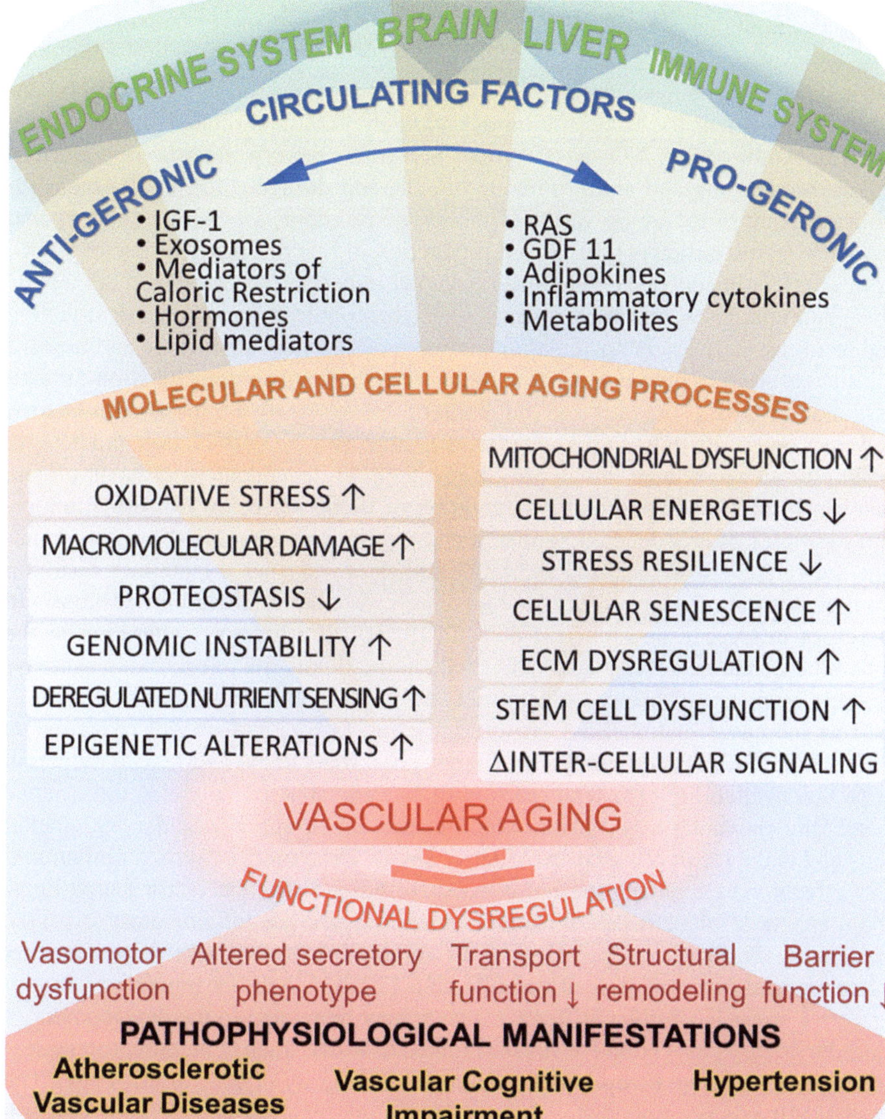
ENDOCRINE SYSTEM BRAIN LIVER IMMUNE SYSTEM
CIRCULATING FACTORS
ANTI-GERONIC
PRO-GERONIC
• IGF-1
• Exosomes
• Mediators of Caloric Restriction
• Hormones
• Lipid mediators
• RAS
• GDF 11
• Adipokines
• Inflammatory cytokines
• Metabolites
MOLECULAR AND CELLULAR AGING PROCESSES
OXIDATIVE STRESS ↑
MACROMOLECULAR DAMAGE ↑
PROTEOSTASIS ↓
GENOMIC INSTABILITY ↑
DEREGULATED NUTRIENT SENSING ↑
EPIGENETIC ALTERATIONS ↑
MITOCHONDRIAL DYSFUNCTION ↑
CELLULAR ENERGETICS ↓
STRESS RESILIENCE ↓
CELLULAR SENESCENCE ↑
ECM DYSREGULATION ↑
STEM CELL DYSFUNCTION ↑
ΔINTER-CELLULAR SIGNALING
VASCULAR AGING
FUNCTIONAL DYSREGULATION
Vasomotor dysfunction
Altered secretory phenotype
Transport function ↓
Structural remodeling
Barrier function ↓
PATHOPHYSIOLOGICAL MANIFESTATIONS
Atherosclerotic Vascular Diseases (AMI, stroke, PAD)
Vascular Cognitive Impairment
Hypertension
Macular Degeneration
Intracerebral Hemorrhages
Alzheimer's Disease
Aneurysms

2.1 Role of Oxidative and Nitrative Stress

Nitric oxide (NO) bioavailability and its endocrine and paracrine effects are fundamentally important for orchestration of endothelial cell and related vascular function [3]. Additionally, NO exerts potent anti-inflammatory actions, i.e., reduced leukocyte adhesion and antithrombotic effects, and the reduction in NO bioavailability present in the aging vascular phenotype promotes a pro-inflammatory and pro-atherogenic milieu [4]. Increased production of reactive oxygen species (ROS) from a variety of sources, e.g. reduced NADPH (nicotinamide adenine dinucleotide phosphate) oxidases, and mitochondria likely contribute to endothelial dysfunction and resulting large artery stiffening in animal models of advancing age and humans [7]. Increased ROS production has a variety of effects on vascular function through oxidation of critical proteins and induction of redox-sensitive transcription factors; however, one of its most important effects is impairing NO production and activity leading to an age-related imbalance of endothelium-dependent vasorelaxation and vasoconstriction and resulting dysregulation of tissue perfusion [8]. Some important examples of NO-deficiency-related end-organ dysfunction in the aging organism are related to myocardial ischemia and neurovascular uncoupling resulting from impaired coronary artery and cerebral vascular dilatation in response to increases in oxygen and nutrient demand [9, 10]. Furthermore, alteration in the activation of the key enzyme for NO production, endothelial nitric oxide synthase (eNOS), by means of reduced substrate (L-arginine) and co-factor (BH4) activity, as well as increased endothelin-1 (vasoconstricting factor) and overall reduction in eNOS protein expression likely play fundamental roles in the age-related reduction in NO bioavailability [11]. The reaction of NO and superoxide yields the reactive metabolite oxidant peroxynitrite, which is present in aging vascular endothelial cells and is the result of vascular oxidative stress. Peroxinitrite exerts proinflammatory effects via enhancing the redox-sensitive NF-κB (nuclear factor kappa-light-chain-enhancer of activated B cells), which triggers pro-inflammatory cytokine expression. Furthermore, peroxinitrite exerts direct cytotoxic effects and impairs mitochondrial function of aged vascular cells [12, 13]. Another impact of vascular oxidative stress is vascular stiffening, which may be related to the development of vascular aneurysms. Oxidative stress is linked to MMP (matrix metalloproteinases) activation leading to disruption of the structural integrity of aged arteries [14]. The ROS-MMP axis is associated with a variety of age-related changes in the cerebral micro- and macro-circulation, e.g., development of cerebral microhemorrhages leading to cognitive decline [15]. Finally, anti-oxidant interventions decrease vascular stiffness in preclinical models [16].

2.2 Mitochondrial Function

Similar to NO-bioavailability, orchestrated mitochondrial activity plays a fundamental role in normal vascular function and impaired mitochondrial function related to aging leads to diminished respiratory chain function and electron leakage associated with increased ROS-production and resulting reduced energy production, e.g. reduced ATP [17]. Further, mitochondria-derived H_2O_2 is associated with low-grade vascular inflammation via inducing NF-κB activation [18]. Increases in mitochondrial ROS (mtROS) and the associated impaired electron transport mechanism, can be further exaggerated by peroxynitrite-mediated nitration and inhibition of MnSOD (manganese-dependent superoxide dismutase), reduced cellular glutathione content, and impaired Nrf2 (nuclear factor [erythroid-derived 2]-like 2)-mediated antioxidant defense responses [19]. Additionally, models of hypertension-induced mtROS production in aged vascular smooth muscle cells (VSMCs) increased MMP activation in the vascular wall, resulted in disruption of the structural integrity of aged arteries and led to formation of cerebral microhemorrhages [20]. Targeted mitochondrial antioxidant interventions with the mitochondrial antioxidant MitoQ, resveratrol, and the tetrapeptide SS-31, were demonstrated to attenuate ROS production and improve endothelial function in arteries from rodent models of aging and specifically treatment with SS-31 improved neurovascular coupling and improved cognitive function in these models [21, 22].

Normal aging increases mutations and deletions in mitochondrial DNA (mtDNA) leading to decreased mitochondrial energy production. Furthermore, mitochondrial oxidative stress results in mtDNA damage. MtDNA is subject to an accelerated mutation rate due to a variety of factors, including proximity to sites of ROS production in the mitochondria, a lack of protective histone coverage in the mtDNA, and limited efficiency of mtDNA repair mechanisms [23, 24]. The impact of such changes in aging was explored in a limited body of literature to date. Mitochondrial mutations likely play a causal role in atherogenesis in rodent models of atherosclerosis. For example, apolipoprotein E knock-out mice have an mtDNA polymerase (polG [DNA polymerase subunit gamma]) deficient in proof-reading activity, leading to accumulating mutations in mtDNA and demonstrate dysfunctional proliferation and apoptosis of vascular smooth muscle cells and accelerated atherosclerosis [25].

Vascular mitochondrial function depends on the NAD+ (nicotinamide adenine dinucleotide)-dependent pro-survival enzyme SIRT1 (sirtuin1) for mitochondrial biogenesis and cellular energy metabolism, as well as on controlling mtROS production and sequestration of damaged mitochondria by autophagy. Studies have demonstrated that treatment with the NAD+ intermediate nicotinamide mononucleotide through activation of sirtuin-mediated pathways can improve age-related functional alterations in the rodent aorta and reverse the age-related decline in mitochondrial function. Additional, and potential related mechanisms contributing to impaired bioenergetics in aged vascular cells include oxidation or nitration of mitochondrial proteins, impairment of the different electron transport chain complexes, and impaired mitochondrial autophagy (mitophagy) [26].

2.3 Vascular Inflammation

Age-associated inflammation, or "inflammaging", is associated with macrovascular and microvascular pathologies, ranging from atherogenesis and aneurysm formation to microvascular dysfunction, blood-brain barrier disruption, and Alzheimer pathologies. The sterile, low-grade inflammation in aging individuals impacts the microenvironment in the vascular wall and promotes vascular dysfunction. Several mechanisms have been proposed including a pro-inflammatory shift in the gene expression profile of vascular endothelial and smooth muscle cells leading to the production of a variety of inflammatory cytokines and mediators [27]. Additional mechanisms contributing to vascular inflammation in aging will be discussed in the following paragraph.

Aged endothelial and smooth muscle cells exhibit significant activation of the inflammatory "gatekeeper" NF-κB [12, 13]. Additional mediators of pro-inflammatory pathways described in aging or senescent endothelium and leading to the production and release of a wide range of inflammatory cytokines and chemokines are p38MAPK, the DNA damage response pathway, and GATA4 (transcription factor GATA-4) [28, 29]. As previously discussed, increases in ROS mediate proinflammatory signaling pathways, including NF-κB activation leading to vascular endothelial activation and expression of proinflammatory paracrine mediators and ultimately promote atherogenesis. Impaired resilience to oxidative stress in aging also exacerbates vascular inflammation induced by cardiovascular risk factors, e.g. hypertension, obesity, and metabolic syndrome [30, 31]. NF-κB inhibition decreases systemic inflammation and extends health span [32]. Additionally, NF-κB-mediated cytokine production is a potent activator of cellular oxidative stress (e.g., TNF-α activates NADPH oxidases). Pharmacological activators of SIRT1 have anti-inflammatory effects in aging rodents [33].

Activation of the innate immune system by TLRs (toll-like receptors) and the NLRP3 (NACHT, LRR, and PYD domains-containing protein 3) inflammasome complex is associated with the sterile inflammation in the vascular wall [34]. Activation of TLR4-mediated, MyD88-dependent signaling pathways in aging VSMCs is associated with the production of several proinflammatory paracrine mediators (e.g., IL-1, IL-6, IL-8, and TNF-α). Furthermore, the canonical Nlrp3 inflammasome contributes to systemic inflammation in aged rodent models [35].

Finally, the interaction between aging and environmental inflammatory factors (e.g., particulate exposure) has been proposed to exacerbate vascular inflammation. For example, bacterial breakdown products entering the circulation through a leaky intestinal barrier or by chronic infection with viruses that exhibit endothelial tropism likely play a role in vascular inflammation. Some viruses, such as the cytomegalovirus, replicate in vascular endothelial cells and long-term exposure and chronic infection are shown to predict increased incidences of frailty and mortality [36].

2.4   Genomic Instability

Experimental evidence indicates that a variety of genetic lesions accumulate within aged cells, including somatic mutations, chromosomal aneuploidies, copy number variations, and telomere shortening. Age-related oxidative stress-induced DNA damage is often proposed as an interconnecting mechanism between the oxidative stress hypothesis of aging and the genomic instability associated with vascular aging [37]. Endothelial cells have impaired DNA repair pathways compared to other cell types and interventions that cause DNA damage (e.g. radiation) result in phenotypic and functional changes in endothelial cells, decrease microvascular density, impair vasodilation, and promote proinflammatory changes, mimicking several aspects of the aging phenotype. Several rodent models have been developed to further investigate the impact of genetic stability changes in aging. For example, one model with defective nucleotide excision repair genes (ERCC1 and XPD) results in an aging-like vascular phenotypes, including endothelial cell dysfunction, increased vascular stiffness and senescence cell count, as well as hypertension [38]. Further, a second model of genetic deficiency in the spindle assembly checkpoint protein BubR1 (budding uninhibited by benzimidazole-related 1), also shows aging-like vascular phenotypes, with a phenotype similar to those outlined above [39]. However, both models also exhibit a short life span associated with severe functional deficits in multiple organ systems and the relevance of this model to normal aging has been questioned. Finally, telomere shortening and associated cellular senescence (see following paragraph below for more details) have been proposed as an important mechanism in vascular aging [40].

2.5   Epigenetic Alterations

Vascular aging is associated with a variety of cellular epigenetic alterations such as DNA methylation changes, posttranslational modification of histones, and dysregulation of microRNAs (miRNAs). Among these, modification in DNA methylation is the central regulator of genomic function and aging is associated with adverse changes in vascular cell methylation patterns [41]. Furthermore, interventions such as caloric restriction can partially reverse alterations in the aging-associated methylation pattern of several organ systems and altered methylation of genes important for vascular function have been observed in a rodent model [42]. Next, posttranslational histone modifications are regulated by histone acetyltransferases and histone deacetylases. Changes in expression and reduced activity of class III histone deacetylases, which are the NAD+ utilizing sirtuin family, contribute to vascular endothelial cell aging [43]. Most human protein coding genes are controlled via posttranscriptional repression by noncoding micro RNAs. Vascular cell micro RNAs contribute to the regulation of important biological processes, such as angiogenesis, atherogenesis, aging related impairment of the angiogenic processes, decreased cellular stress resilience, and atherosclerotic plaque formation and desta-bilization and are all associated with dysregulation of miRNA expression in vascu-lar endothelial and VSMCs [44]. More specifically insulin-like growth factor 1 (IGF-1) deficiency early in life can lead to adverse changes in posttranscriptional miRNA-mediated control of vascular function associated genes and may contribute to the known adverse cardiovascular late-life effects observed in IGF-deficiency [45]. Finally, several of these epigenetic changes are reversible and epigenome-influencing interventions may prove to be successful in limiting, preventing, or even reversing aging related vascular dysfunction [46].

2.6 Vascular Cell Senescence

As part of the aging process, vascular endothelial and smooth muscle cells, similar to other cell types, can permanently withdraw from the cell cycle in response to endogenous and exogenous stressors such as oxidative stress, dysfunctional telo-meres, DNA damage, and a variety of paracrine signals, and undergo distinctive phenotypic alterations, including changes to the proinflammatory secretome. This process is called cellular senescence and particular endothelial cell senescence con-tributes to endothelial dysfunction in aging and pathophysiological conditions asso-ciated with accelerated vascular aging [47, 48]. Additionally, studies have demonstrated that elimination of senescent cells can extend the life span in rodents, suggesting that cellular senescence plays a fundamental role in the physiological decline associated with aging [49]. Accelerating this process in a model of irradiation-induced, DNA damage-mediated senescence in a neurovascular rodent model was associated with significant cerebral-microvascular dysfunction, simulat-ing the vascular aging phenotype [50]. Furthermore, genetic and pharmacologic interference to eliminate senescent cells in an LDL receptor knockout mouse model of atherosclerosis resulted in marked changes in atherosclerotic plaque morphology and suggested a role of senescent cells in facilitating plaque instability, e.g., promot-ing inflammation, and upregulation of MMPs [49]. Different pharmacologic seno-lytic interventions to clear senescent cells have been shown to improve endothelial cell function and are proposed to exhibit an atheroprotective effect. Finally, vascular senescence-associated secretory pathways can induce paracrine senescence, and alter the function of neighboring endothelial cells and VSMCs, adversely impacting vascular function [51].

2.7 The Renin–Angiotensin–Aldosterone System (RAAS)

Alterations of the RAAS via the angiotensin converting enzyme (ACE) homologue acn-1 in a model organism, genetic or pharmacological interference with the RAAS in a rodent model, and pharmacological ACE inhibition were shown to have a regulatory effect on the life span and may reverse age-related phenotypic and functional changes in the aged vasculature, such as reducing arterial stiffness [52]. Further, human data in elderly subjects suggest that upregulation of tissue RAAS can lead to intimal thickening and remodeling in large conduit arteries associated with an aging vascular phenotype [53]. Additionally, infusion of angiotensin II in young rats accelerates vascular aging, e.g., carotid media thickening and intima infiltration by VSMCs [54]. A variety of other aging-related changes have been observed in experimental models of RAAS upregulation in the vascular wall, e.g. inducing low-grade inflammatory and oxidative stress responses, development of cerebral microhemorrhages, and disruption of the blood-brain barrier [53, 55]. More specifically, local expression of mineralocorticoids and their receptors in the vasculature, e.g., aldosterone, promotes vascular inflammatory changes and leads to adverse vascular remodeling of VSMCs [56]. Overall, the overwhelming data of RAAS involvement in aging emphasizes the importance of the enzyme system and associated peptide hormones in regulating fundamental aging processes.

2.8 Extracellular Matrix (ECM) Remodeling in Vascular Aging

Aging of the vasculature is associated with a variety of changes to the ECM of the subendothelial basement membrane, intima, media, adventitia, and interstitial matrix. Some examples of these changes are decreases in ECM biosynthesis, post-translational modifications of ECM components, and alterations in cell-matrix interactions [57]. ECM integrity is fundamentally important for vascular integrity as it provides mechanical scaffolding as well as mediates the signal transduction required for vascular homeostasis, morphogenesis, and cell differentiation. Aging is associated with changes in the expression of growth factors that regulate ECM biosynthesis and decreased synthesis of several elasticity and resilience-associated components such as elastin, which renders the vasculature more susceptible to wall tension changes related to pulsatile pressure waves and can result in structural vascular damage [58]. Furthermore, collagen synthesis is impacted by aging-associated increased transforming growth factor-β (TGF-β) leading to vascular fibrosis and arterial stiffening [59]. Next, changes in the secretory phenotype of vascular cells, e.g. endothelial and smooth muscle cells, are observed with aging. An increase in MMP secretion and increased MMP activation related to oxidative stress further impair structural integrity and promote pathological remodeling, which can lead to stiffening, hypertension, and aneurysm formation [60]. Several lines of evidence suggest that age-associated activation of the RAAS as well as a decline in IGF-1 are also involved and impact the ECM changes observed in aging [61]. Finally, the described alterations in the biomechanical properties of large arteries associated with age-related ECM remodeling likely also affect microvascular transport mechanism, barrier function, and vein function.

2.9 Progenitor Cell Exhaustion

Exhaustion of the vascular progenitor cell pool and an inability to replenish the pool with functional and differentiated endothelial cells and VSMCs compromise the biological functions and impair neovasculariztion of the aged vasculature. Additionally, age-associated sterile inflammation, oxidative stress, and activation of the RAAS alter the function of circulating EPCs by decreasing differentiation, migration, and survival factors [62, 63]. Animal studies highlighted the importance of circulating factors, e.g., serum from young rats improved function in EPCs previously isolated from old rats [64]. Additionally, studies in ApoE knockout mice demonstrated that bone marrow derived EPCs from young rats slowed atherosclerosis progression whereas EPCs from older rats was ineffective [63]. However, to date, human data are conflicting, and additional data are needed to more clearly define the contribution of changes in EPC number and functionality to the aging vasculature phenotype.

3 Structural Changes Accompanying Age-Associated Increased Stiffness

One of the most important age-associated vascular changes is an increase in central vascular, primarily aortic, stiffness, which alters the pressure and flow characteristics of the wave as it travels through the central, to the peripheral, vessels (Fig. 2) [65]. With the contraction of the left ventricle, ejection of blood from the heart creates a pressure wave that travels along the aorta at a velocity dependent on the stiffness and thickness of the artery. As the pressure wave moves forward, it encounters resistance due to the branching of the arterial tree. This creates a reflected pressure wave that returns at a velocity-dependent, as well, on the stiffness and other properties of the arterial wall. In healthy young individuals, the reflected pressure wave returns to the central aorta during diastole. The expansion of the aorta during systole dampens the pressure at that time and forward stroke volume is reduced by the volume within the expanded aorta. Recoil during diastole increases diastolic pressure and forward stroke volume at that time. The elastic aorta in young individuals thus dampens central pressure during systole, increases it during diastole, and converts the pulsatile flow generated by the heart during systole to a more continuous flow throughout the cycle. However, with advancing age the large elastic arteries stiffen, and therefore expand less, and the left ventricle must generate more systolic pressure for any given stroke volume. In addition, the lower recoil during diastole results in lower central pressure and less forward flow during diastole. The increased "pulsatility" causes microvascular damage, particularly in high flow dependent organs such as the brain, heart, and kidneys.

The major components of the aorta are elastin and collagen and the significant changes both undergo with advancing age are responsible for the increase in

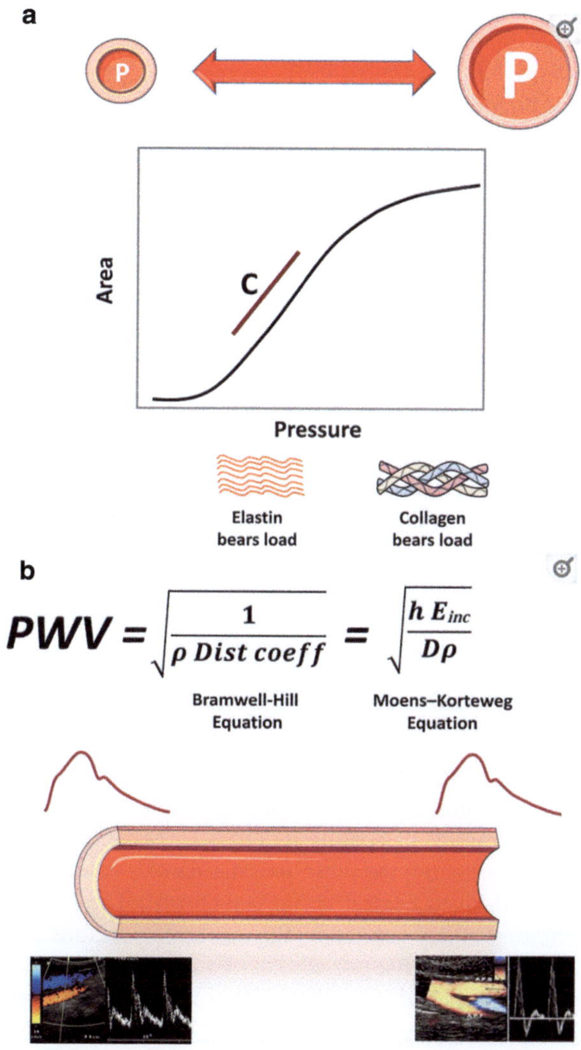

$$PWV = \sqrt{\frac{1}{\rho \, Dist \, coeff}} = \sqrt{\frac{h \, E_{inc}}{D\rho}}$$

Fig. 2 Compliance, distensibility and PWV. (**a**) Typical relationship between intra-arterial pressure and lumen area when varying the pressure over a sufficiently large range. The area compliance (red line) is the slope to the pressure-area relationship, which can be calculated at any pressure level. At low pressure, the load is mainly taken by elastin, and the artery has a high compliance. As pressure increases, the load is progressively shifted to stiffer collagen fibers, leading to a functionally lower compliance. Vascular smooth muscle tone also affects compliance, particularly in distal aortic segments and intermediate-sized arteries. Normalizing area compliance to the local radius yields the distensibility coefficient (see Table 1). (**b**) For a homogenous tube, the distensibility coefficient (Dist coeff) is theoretically linked to the PWV via the Bramwell-Hill equation (where ρ is the density of the blood) in an inverse, non-linear fashion; an increase in PWV by a factor 2 (which is about the change observed in humans from the age of 20 to the age of 70) implies a decrease in distensibility by a factor 4. An alternative formulation is the Moens-Korteweg equation, linking PWV to the stiffness of the wall material (incremental elastic modulus, Einc), the wall thickness (h) and lumen diameter (D). (From: J Am Coll Cardiol. 2019 Sep 3;74(9):1237–1263)

stiffness [65–68]. There is a decrease and fraying of elastin that results from increased activity of matrix metallo proteinases and other enzymes regulated, in part, by pro-inflammatory cytokines [68]. Increased activity of the RAAS also increases elastin loss and decreases elastin synthesis. Accumulation of collagen, also stimulated by the RAAS, is accompanied by cross-links between collagen molecules and condensates of glucose produced by nonenzymatic reactions. These advanced glycation end-products form cross-links between collagen molecules that increase stiffness and are resistant to enzymatic degradation [69]. Increased stiffness decreases stretch-induced increases in nitric oxide (NO) bioavailability and by interacting with receptors on immune and other cells increases oxidant stress and upregulates cytokines, stimulating vascular inflammation. There is, as well, proliferation and migration of vascular smooth muscle cells to the intima and osteogenic transdifferentiation of the cells, which increases the mineralization of the extracellular matrix [70, 71]. These changes are not passive, but rather dynamic processes triggered by cellular senescence, autophagy, and mediated, at least in part, by oxidative stress, inflammation, RAAS, and angiotensin II signaling [72]. Furthermore, the consequent higher systolic and pulse pressures due to stiffening may stimulate the production of these factors, resulting in further stiffening and a repeating cycle.

3.1 Measures of Aortic Stiffness

Aortic stiffness is best defined by the change in intra-aortic distending pressure relative to the change in volume. The invasive nature of this assessment, however, precludes its use in large studies of healthy individuals. More easily assessed indices include brachial pulse pressure, the pulse pressure/stroke volume ratio, and carotid and radial tonometry-derived central aortic waveforms. The latter can be used to assess the augmentation index, defined by the increased pressure accompanying the reflected wave divided by the pulse pressure, with higher values indicating increased stiffness. One of the first, and remarkably prescient, studies were reported by Bramwell and Hill in The Lancet 100 years ago [73]. They studied healthy individuals and measured pulse wave velocity using the time between the arrival of the pulse in the carotid and radial arteries and the estimated distance the pulse traveled through the aorta by subtracting the distance between the sternoclavicular joint and the carotid artery from the distance between the sternoclavicular joint and the radial artery. A similar non-invasive technique is still used with the exception that the femoral, rather than the radial, pulse is recorded, and the distance is obtained by subtracting the distance between the carotid measurement site and the sternal notch from the distance between the sternal notch and the femoral measurement site. Reference values for pulse wave velocity in 11,092 individuals without known cardiovascular disease and diabetes and who were not receiving anti-hypertensive or lipid lowering therapies are presented in Table 1 [74]. Optimal blood pressure was defined as <120/80, normal as ≥120/80 and <130/85; high normal as ≥130/85 and

Table 1 Distribution of pulse wave velocity (PWV) values (m/s) in the reference value population (11,092 subjects) according to age and blood pressure category

Age category (years)	Blood pressure category				
	Optimal	Normal	High normal	Grade I HT	Grade II/III HT
PWV as mean (±2 SD)					
<30	6.1 (4.6–7.5)	6.6 (4.9–8.2)	6.8 (5.1–8.5)	7.4 (4.6–10.1)	7.7 (4.4–11.0)
30–39	6.6 (4.4–8.9)	6.8 (4.2–9.4)	7.1 (4.5–9.7)	7.3 (4.0–10.7)	8.2 (3.3–13.0)
40–49	7.0 (4.5–9.6)	7.5 (5.1–10.0)	7.9 (5.2–10.7)	8.6 (5.1–12.0)	9.8 (3.8–15.7)
50–59	7.6 (4.8–10.5)	8.4 (5.1–11.7)	8.8 (4.8–12.8)	9.6 (4.9–14.3)	10.5 (4.1–16.8)
60–69	9.1 (5.2–12.9)	9.7 (5.7–13.6)	10.3 (5.5–15.1)	11.1 (6.1–16.2)	12.2 (5.7–18.6)
≥70	10.4 (5.2–15.6)	11.7 (6.0–17.5)	11.8 (5.7–17.9)	12.9 (6.9–18.9)	14.0 (7.4–20.6)
PWV as median (10–90 pc)					
<30	6.0 (5.2–7.0)	6.4 (5.7–7.5)	6.7 (5.8–7.9)	7.2 (5.7–9.3)	7.6 (5.9–9.9)
30–39	6.5 (5.4–7.9)	6.7 (5.3–8.2)	7.0 (5.5–8.8)	7.2 (5.5–9.3)	7.6 (5.8–11.2)
40–49	6.8 (5.8–8.5)	7.4 (6.2–9.0)	7.7 (6.5–9.5)	8.1 (6.8–10.8)	9.2 (7.1–13.2)
50–59	7.5 (6.2–9.2)	8.1 (6.7–10.4)	8.4 (7.0–11.3)	9.2 (7.2–12.5)	9.7 (7.4–14.9)
60–69	8.7 (7.0–11.4)	9.3 (7.6–12.2)	9.8 (7.9–13.2)	10.7 (8.4–14.1)	12.0 (8.5–16.5)
≥70	10.1 (7.6–13.8)	11.1 (8.6–15.5)	11.2 (8.6–15.8)	12.7 (9.3–16.7)	13.5 (10.3–18.2)

SD standard deviation, *10 pc* the upper limit of the 10th percentile, *90 pc* the lower limit of the 90th percentile, *HT* hypertension. From ref. [74]

<140/90, grade 1 hypertension as ≥140/90 and <160/100, and Grade II/III hypertension as ≥160/100 mmHg.

3.2 *Consequences of Increased Stiffness*

3.2.1 Cardiovascular Performance

The relationship between central vascular stiffness and left ventricular contractility is termed arterial-ventricular coupling. It can be quantified using the ratio of effective arterial elastance (Ea) to end-systolic left ventricular elastance (Elv) [75, 76] and estimated non-invasively. A ratio close to 0.5 is associated with optimal cardiovascular efficiency [77, 78]. The Baltimore Longitudinal Study of Aging reported longitudinal changes in left ventricular volumes as assessed by repeated multigated blood pool scans and blood pressures over an average follow-up period of 12.2 years in 129 individuals without evidence of coronary or other cardiac disease [79]. The projected trajectories of Ea, Elv, and the ratio Ea/Elv in different age groups are presented in Fig. 3a, b. Ea increases with age and the rate of increase increases with advancing age. Elv also increases with aging; however, the increase

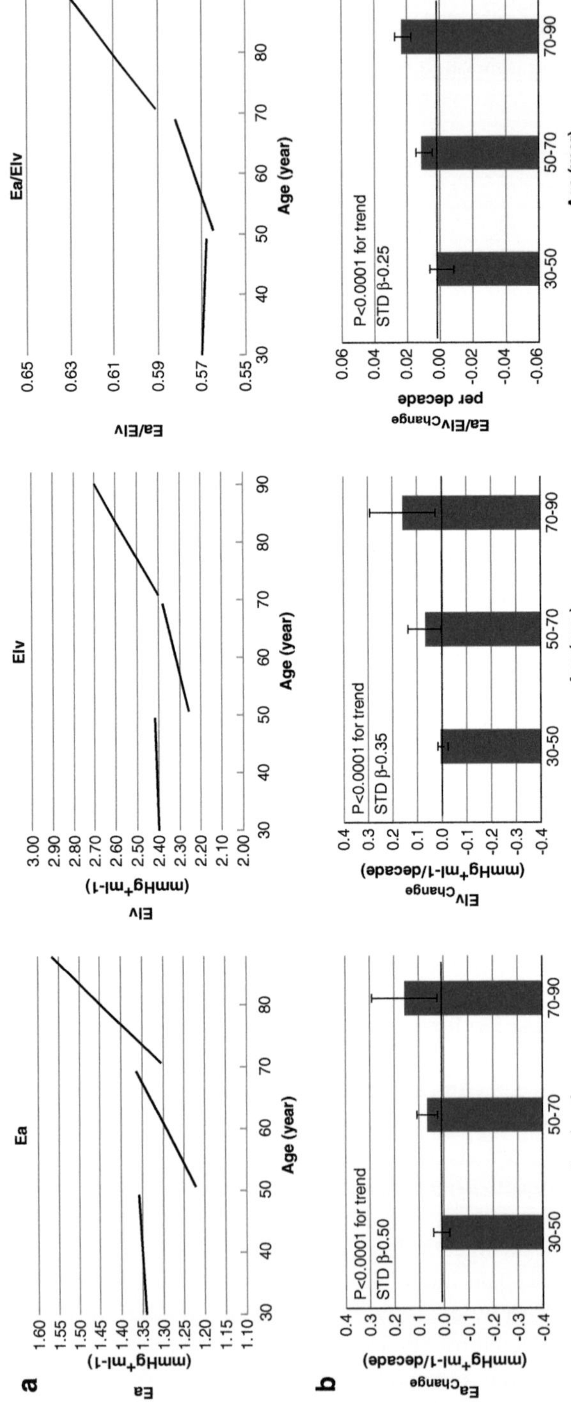

Fig. 3 (**a**) Age-group trajectories generated from averaged individual, model-predicted longitudinal trajectories in Ea, Elv, and Ea/Elv, projected over 20 years follow-up. (**b**) Age-group average rates of changes. (From: Geroscience. 2021 Apr;43(2):551–561)

in Elv is less than that of Ea, which results in an age-associated increase in Ea/Elv indicating progressive AV uncoupling, due primarily to an increase in vascular stiffness. This was associated with left ventricular remodeling characterized by increased end-systolic volume and reduced stroke and end-diastolic volumes, a pattern consistent with that present in individuals with heart failure with a preserved ejection fraction.

In addition to these left ventricular structural changes, increased central vascular stiffness impacts left ventricular performance, primarily by increasing afterload during left ventricular ejection as the pressure required to eject a given volume increases with a progressively stiffer aorta. Due to the increase in pulse wave velocity associated with the stiffer aorta, the reflected wave returns earlier, in systole rather than diastole, further increasing systolic pressure and left ventricular afterload. In addition, the lower diastolic pressure due to both lower "recoil" during diastole, and the absence of the reflected wave at that time, decreases coronary perfusion pressure, which, when combined with the increased myocardial oxygen demand due to the higher afterload, may impact left ventricular performance in the setting of obstructive disease.

3.2.2   Clinical Outcomes

In clinical outcome studies, central vascular stiffness is usually assessed as pulse pressure, pulse wave velocity, or by using radial or carotid tonometry. Although these measures do not precisely define relative changes in aortic volume with aortic pressure, they are non-invasive, safe, predictive of outcomes, and, in many clinical centers, readily available. The Framingham investigators reported the association between stiffness as indexed by carotid-femoral pulse wave velocity on cardiovascular and other events in 7283 Framingham Study participants over a median follow-up period of 15 years [80]. In adjusted analysis, each standard deviation increase in the carotid-femoral pulse wave velocity was associated with an increased risk of hypertension (HR 1.32), diabetes (HR 1.32), chronic kidney disease (HR 1.19), dementia (HR 1.27) coronary heart disease (HR 1.37), transient ischemic attack or stroke (HR 1.24), and death (HR 1.29) (see Fig. 4). In a pooled analysis from 16 studies examining the impact of aortic pulse wave velocity on cardiac outcomes in 17,635 participants [81], for every one standard deviation increase in loge aortic pulse wave velocity, there was a significant 54% increased 5 year stroke risk for those 61–70 years of age and a 37% increase for those over 70 years of age. Similarly, there was a 31% increase in coronary heart disease events for those 61–70 years and a 14% increase for those over 70 years of age. In a community of adults over 70 years of age, the Health ABC Study investigators reported that over a 4.6 year follow-up aortic pulse wave velocity quartiles were significantly associated with cardiovascular mortality, with a relative risk 2.1, 3.0, and 2.3 for quartiles 2, 3, and 4 versus the first quartile 1 [82].

Hypertension is the most common risk factor in the older population and is strongly related to stroke and heart failure risk (see Chap. 1). In the Atherosclerosis

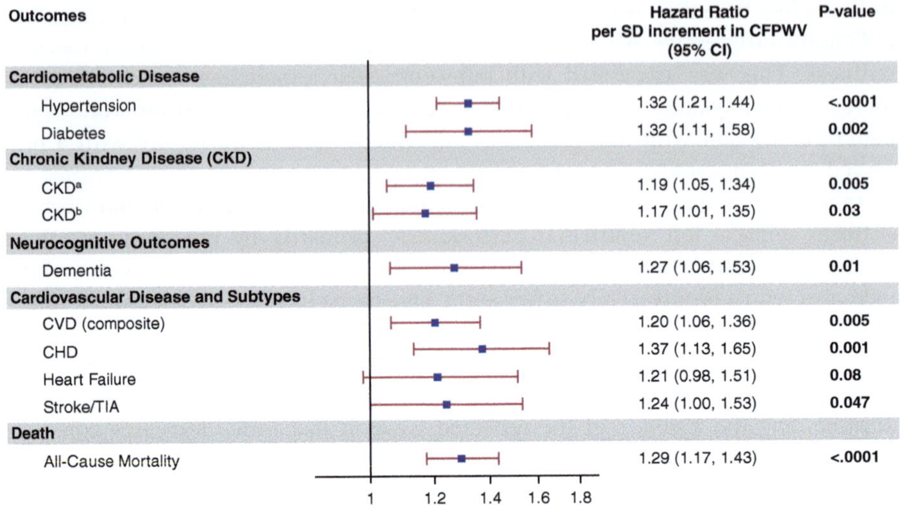

Fig. 4 Relations of carotid-femoral pulse wave velocity (CFPWV) and incidence of outcome events dichotomized by median age (50 years for analyses combining FOS [Framingham Offspring Study] and Gen 3 [Third Generation; incidence of hypertension, diabetes, chronic kidney disease (CKD)b, cardiovascular disease (CVD), CVD subtypes, and death]; 60 years for analyses limited to FOS [incidence of CKDa and dementia]). Hazards ratios are per SD increment in CFPWV from age-stratified models adjusting for model 3 covariates (sex, current smoking status, total cholesterol concentration in blood/HDL (high-density lipoprotein) cholesterol, diabetes [or fasting blood glucose, for incident diabetes], systolic blood pressure, and antihypertensive treatment). Interaction *p* values are from models pooling age groups. CKDa and CKDb refer to definitions of incident disease based on reduced estimated glomerular filtration rate (eGFR) and increased urine albumin to creatinine ratio vs reduced eGFR alone, respectively. *CHD* coronary heart disease, *TIA* transient ischemic attack. (From: Hypertension. 2022;79:1045–1056)

Risk in Communities study, pulse wave velocity was an independent predictor of incident hypertension [83]. Arterial stiffness was assessed by ultrasound detected change in carotid arterial diameter, adjusted for the diastolic and pulse pressures. After adjustment for traditional risk factors, there was a significant increase in the incidence of hypertension over a mean follow-up of 3 years with rates of 9.6% in the least elastic and 6.7% in the most elastic quartiles. For every one standard deviation decrease in elasticity there was a 15% greater risk of hypertension. Najjar et al. reported the impact of pulse wave velocity measured using carotid and femoral tonometry in 306 Baltimore Longitudinal Study of Aging participants who were normotensive at baseline on the development of hypertension over 4 years [84]. Thirty-four percent developed hypertension and for every 1 m/s increase in PWV, the hazard of developing hypertension was 1.10 (CI 1.00–1.30).

Age also impacts the association between different blood pressure indices and coronary heart disease risk. The Framingham Heart Study compared the importance of systolic, diastolic, and pulse pressure blood pressures to the risk for coronary artery disease over a mean follow-up period of 17 years (Table 2) [85]. Diastolic pressure was the strongest predictor for those under 50 years of age and the components were equally predictive for those 50–59 years. However, for those 60 years of age and older, while systolic blood pressure remained significant (hazard ratio 1.17

Table 2 Proportional-hazard regression coefficients relating incidence of CHD to single BP components of SBP, DBP, and PP by age groups

Single BP components[a]	β[b]	SE[b]	Wald χ[c]	HR (95% CI)[b]
Age < 50 years				
SBP	0.13	0.04	10.8	1.14 (1.06–1.24)[d]
DBP	0.29	0.06	21.8	1.34 (1.18–1.51)[e]
PP	0.02	0.07	0.1	1.02 (0.89–1.17)
Age 50–59 years				
SBP	0.08	0.03	6.3	1.08 (1.02–1.15)[f]
DBP	0.10	0.06	2.9	1.11 (0.99–1.24)
PP	0.11	0.05	5.4	1.11 (1.02–1.22)[f]
Age ≥ 60 years				
SBP	0.16	0.03	30.0	1.17 (1.11–1.24)[d]
DBP	0.11	0.06	3.2	1.12 (0.99–1.27)
PP	0.21	0.04	36.9	1.24 (1.16–1.33)[d]

From: Circulation. 2001;103:1245–1249
[a]SBP, DBP, and PP were entered in separate models, adjusted for age, sex, body mass index, cigarette smoking, diabetes mellitus, and ratio of total to HDL cholesterol
[b]HR was associated with a 10 mmHg increase in BP
[c]Wald χ
[d]$p < 0.01$
[e]$p < 0.00$
[f]$p < 0.05$

(1.11–1.24, $p < 0.001$)), the strongest predictor was pulse pressure, with a hazard ratio of 1.24 (1.16–1.33, $p < 0.001$) for every 10 mmHg increase after adjustment for diabetes and other cardiovascular risk factors.

Stiffness, as indexed by pulse pressure, is also related to the development of congestive heart failure (CHF). In a study of 1621 participants 65 years or older, with a mean age of 77.9 years, there was a 14% increase in the risk of CHF for every 10-mmHg increase in pulse pressure over a mean follow-up period of 3.8 years and for those in the highest quartile, the risk was 55% higher than for those in the lowest quartile [86]. In Framingham Heart Study participants 50–79 years of age, there was a 55% increased risk for the development of heart failure over a 17.4 year mean follow-up period for every 16 mmHg increase in pulse pressure [87]. Increased central vascular stiffness is also believed to play an important pathophysiologic role in patients with heart failure and a preserved ejection fraction, a common form of heart failure in older patients [88]. Abnormal central vascular hemodynamics are particularly evident during exercise [89]. In a study comparing measures of cardiac function and arterial parameters, at rest and during exercise in 98 patients with heart failure and a preserved ejection fraction (mean age 68 years) and 22 control patients with hypertension but without heart failure (mean age 62 years), parameters of central stiffness did not differ at rest. At a common 20-W supine cycle exercise workload and adjusted for age and body mass index, stiffness assessed by end-systolic central blood pressure divided by the stroke volume index was significantly higher in the heart failure with preserved ejection fraction group (3.26 ± 0.92) than in the control group (2.64 ± 0.71, $p < 0.004$). The higher arterial stiffness correlated with higher pulmonary capillary wedge pressures and lower cardiac outputs during the exercise period. Peak exercise capacity was about 40% lower, and stiffness about 30% higher in the heart failure with preserved ejection fraction group. Thus, there is a significant association between central vascular stiffness and cardiac function indices of exercise performance in patients with heart failure and a preserved ejection fraction, which is independent of hypertension.

Measures of vascular stiffness are also associated with incident atrial fibrillation, cognitive decline, and renal failure. In Framingham Heart Study offspring and third-generation cohorts all older than 45 years and with a mean age of 61 years, each standard deviation of augmentation index and of central pulse pressure assessed with tonometry wave forms, adjusted for age, sex, and hypertension, was associated with atrial fibrillation hazard ratios of 1.16 (95% CI 1.02–1.32, $p = 0.02$) and 1.14 (95% CI 1.02–1.28 $p = 0.02$) for augmentation index and central pulse pressure respectively [90]. Cognitive changes and central vascular stiffness were assessed in 1101 Framingham Offspring participants, all of whom were 60 years of age or older, over a 10-year follow-up period. Stiffness, defined by the carotid-femoral pulse wave velocity was significantly associated with an increased risk of mild cognitive impairment (HR 1.40, CI 1.13–1.73), all cause dementia (HR 1.45, CI 1.13–1.87) and Alzheimer's Disease (1.41, CI 1.06–1.67) [91]. In a 356 participant subset of the Cardiovascular Health Study, with a mean age of 77.8 years, for whom carotid femoral pulse wave velocity was measured and incident dementia assessed over a 15-year follow-up period, the risk of incident dementia for those in the highest quartile was 57% higher than for those in the lowest quartile, adjusted for conventional risk factors and anti-hypertensive medications [92]. Longitudinal changes in brain MRI scans over a mean 4.9-year follow-up period were analyzed in 278 individuals with normal or mild cognitive impairments from the Vanderbilt Memory and Aging Project. Increased pulse wave velocity was associated with an increase in white matter intensity, likely related to ischemia, and a decrease in gray matter [93]. Measures of arterial stiffness are also associated with decline in kidney function and renal failure in studies of older individuals [94, 95]. The MESA study examined the association of vascular stiffness indexed by pulse pressure and radial artery tonometry and changes in renal function in 4853 persons, all of whom had an initial estimated GFR of >60 mL/min/1.73 m^2 [95]. Higher pulse pressure and vascular stiffness were associated with faster rates of kidney decline. Compared to those with a pulse pressure of 40–50 mmHg the decline in eGFR was 0.29, 0.56 and 0.91 mL/min/1.73 m^2/year faster among those with pulse pressures of 50–60, 60–70, and >71 mmHg respectively, all $p < 0.01$.

3.3 Intervention Strategies

The above studies indicating an association between increased central vascular stiffness and adverse cardiovascular outcomes prompted studies of non-pharmacologic and pharmacologic interventions designed to decrease stiffness. Although the underlying mechanisms cannot be directly assessed, the consequences in terms of stiffness indices can be. The primary non-pharmacologic approaches are changes in dietary pattern and exercise. The benefits of the Dietary Approaches to Stop Hypertension (DASH) and Mediterranean diets on cardiovascular health are well established [96, 97]. The principal components of many of these diets include increased cocoa, coffee, extra virgin olive oil, fermented foods, fiber, fish, fruits, nuts, vegetables, and whole grains along with decreased intake of high glycemic carbohydrates, processed foods, and sugar, and are associated with deceased vascular stiffness [98, 99]. The responsible mechanisms are multifactorial and include impacts on secreted cytokines, function of immune cells, adipose tissue, skeletal muscle, pancreas, and liver. These are believed to be associated with activation of SIRT-1 and AMPK pathways, depression of mTOR, protein catabolism, fatty acid oxidation, autophagy, mitochondrial homeostasis, and protection against oxidative stress and inflammation. In pre-clinical models, caloric restriction is associated with decreased central vascular stiffness, [100] thought to be related to activation of anti-oxidant/and anti-inflammatory pathway systems and of endogenous cellular stress resistance pathways, SIRT-1, AMPK, and mTOR [100]. In addition to the types of foods, the intake of certain elements is also associated with vascular function. Thus, calcium, potassium, and magnesium may be beneficial, while sodium intake is associated with injury to the vessel wall [99]. Gates et al. conducted a double-blind cross-over study demonstrating that decreasing sodium chloride intake improved large artery elastic compliance in older adults [101]. They assessed the impact of two weeks of decreased sodium intake, to about 60 mmol/day, consistent with the DASH diet, on carotid artery compliance in 12 individuals with stage 1 hypertension. In addition to a significant decrease in systolic pressure, carotid artery compliance increased by 46%, % augmentation index decreased from 40 ± 2 to 29 ± 2 ($p < 0.05$) and carotid artery pulse pressure decreased from 50 ± 6 to 40 ± 6 ($p < 0.05$). Potential mechanisms for sodium's detrimental effects include direct injury to the vessel wall, vascular smooth muscle cell hypertrophy, and increased reactive oxygen species, inflammation and resultant fibrosis.

Weight loss reduces arterial stiffness in obese and overweight adults [102, 103]. Following a 12-week 1200–1500 kcal/day diet, 25 individuals with an average body mass index of 30.0 ± 0.6 kg/m^2, lost 7.1 ± 0.7 kg. Carotid-femoral pulse wave velocity decreased by 187 ± 29 cm/s and the decrease was correlated with reduced total body and abdominal obesity [103]. The long-term success of caloric restriction, per se, is low because of difficult adherence. In addition, there are concerns regarding caloric restriction including loss of skeletal muscle mass, decreased bone mineral density, and decreased intake of important nutrients. Potential alternatives include caloric restriction for a few days each week and limiting feeding to a limited number of hours (e.g. 8 h) each day.

Physical activity decreases central vascular stiffness and age-related increases in stiffness can be mitigated by exercise in both men and women [104, 105]. The Baltimore Longitudinal Study of Aging measured VO$_2$ max in rigorously phenotyped adults aged 21–96 years of age [106]. With increasing age, in the entire cohort, augmentation index and aortic PWV increased out of proportion to the blood pressure increase. However, these measures of aortic stiffness were lower in endurance-trained male athletes (defined by a VO$_2$ max 1 standard deviation above their age-matched non-trained controls), compared with sedentary individuals (defined as less than 20 min of aerobic exercise three times weekly) of similar age. Similarly, while augmentation index and pulse wave velocity were higher in sedentary post-menopausal women than comparable pre-menopausal women, these measures were similar in physically active pre- and post-menopausal active women defined by performing endurance training, or actively competing in running races, an average of 6 ± 1 h of activity per week [106].

3.3.1 Drug Effects on Vascular Stiffness

Some pharmacologic agents also decrease measures of vascular stiffness. The majority of the studies are with anti-hypertensive agents. Those which decrease stroke volume will decrease expansion required of the rigid aortic elements during ejection and therefore pressure. Thus, pulse wave velocity may change but there is no change in the pressure/volume relationship per se. Vascular smooth muscle vasodilation induced by ACE-inhibitors and angiotensin receptor II receptor blockers decrease stiffness measures. The benefit of these may extend beyond an impact related to an acute effect on blood pressure due to a decrease in vascular smooth muscle cell proliferation and vascular calcification. The impact of drugs on pressure and stiffness may also differ. Thus, lisinopril and metoprolol reduced blood pressure similarly but the angiotensin converting enzyme inhibitor improved compliance while the beta blocker did not [107]. In general, and in the few studies which have been performed, ACE-inhibitors, angiotensin II receptor blockers, and calcium antagonists improve compliance relative to beta blockers (with the possible exception of those with vasodilating properties), despite similar blood pressure reductions [108]. It should be emphasized, however, that no randomized study has determined whether decreasing compliance independent of blood pressure decreases adverse cardiovascular events.

3.3.2 The Impact of Urban Environments on Age-Associated Vascular Properties

The importance of the environment to which our vasculature is exposed in mediating the age associated vascular changes is also illustrated in studies comparing these properties in rural and urban dwellers. When compared with urban societies, those in isolated rural communities that have been slow to assimilate into urban societies have very low rates of prevalent hypertension and lower age-associated increases in pressure with increasing age.

The prevalence of hypertension and longitudinal changes in blood pressure were studied in 2248 adults aged 20–90 years among the Tsimane, forager-horticulturalists in the Bolivian Amazon [109]. In the entire group the prevalence of hypertension was only 3.9% in women and 5.2% in men. The increases in systolic, diastolic, and pulse pressure per decade, respectively, were 2.86, 0.95, and 1.95 mmHg for women and 0.91, 0.93, and −0.02 mmHg for men, all of which are significantly lower than the same profiles in the United States [110]. In a study comparing pulse wave velocity (PWV), matched for age and blood pressure, PWV in the arm was significantly lower in rural Guangzhou (PWV = 0.61 (age) + 817) than in Beijing (PWV = 4.8 (age) + 998) [111]. One of the most salient studies examining this question was the Yi migrant study, which examined blood pressures in 8241 Yi farmers, 2675 Yi who had migrated from the rural to an urban environment, and 3689 urban residents [112]. The prevalence of borderline or definite hypertension in the farmer population was only 2.69% in men and 2.42% in women 65 years of age or older, and rose to 30.77% in men and 55.55% in women migrants and to 57.57% in men and 70.0% women urban dwellers. For men 65 years of age or older, the mean systolic pressures expressed as mean ± SD were 110.8 ± 12.3 in the farmers, 130.4 ± 14.0 in the migrants, and 136.9 ± 23.6 mmHg in the urban dwellers. For women, the respective numbers were 111.2 ± 12.6, 135.0 ± 17.2 and 146.5 ± 25.6 mmHg. Furthermore, the change in systolic pressure with age, expressed as the mean ± SE mmHg/year was also significantly lower in the farmers (0.13 ± 0.01) than in the migrants (0.33 ± 0.03) and the urban dwellers (0.36 ± 0.02). Migration was associated with decreased physical activity and increased intake of animal products, sugar, salt, fat, and total calories. Furthermore, adjusting for BMI reduced much of the hypertension risk. Although these studies suggest that a significant component of the age-associated increase in measures of central vascular stiffness can be mitigated by lifestyle factors, it is not practical for most currently living in an urban/suburban environment to reproduce the lifestyle practiced in these remote rural areas.

4 Vascular Endothelial Cell Function Testing

The previous sections describe in detail the molecular and cellular mechanisms of vascular aging with an emphasis on vascular endothelial cell function as well as the structural changes accompanying age associated increased stiffness and interventions to improve vascular stiffness. The following paragraphs focus on vascular function testing and the clinical implications of age associated impairments in vascular endothelial cell function.

Endothelial dysfunction is associated with a plethora of cardiovascular diseases and can be observed in larger conduit arteries (macrovascular dysfunction) as well as smaller resistance vessels (microvascular dysfunction). Furthermore, the presence of endothelial dysfunction is a clinical prognosticator for cardiovascular events and associated mortality. Vascular endothelial function testing is a useful tool in selecting therapies and assessing the response to interventions. For this purpose, several invasive as well as non-invasive modalities have emerged for clinical and research purposes and strengths and limitations of these techniques will be discussed in the following sections.

4.1 Invasive Coronary Endothelial Function Assessment

Coronary endothelial dysfunction is a reliable predictor of cardiovascular events and associated mortality and an important vascular bed in studies of vasoreactivity [113]. Endothelial dysfunction diagnosed by invasive methods is prevalent in a variety of cardiometabolic diseases and is associated with future atherosclerotic cardiovascular events [114, 115]. Furthermore, responses to risk factor modifying therapies targeting endothelial cell dysfunction improve vascular function [116].

The gold standard for coronary endothelial functional assessment uses invasive quantitative angiography [117]. Blood flow velocity, measured using a Doppler wire, and epicardial diameter are used to calculate coronary blood flow [118]. To assess endothelial cell-dependent function an endothelial-dependent vasodilator, e.g. acetylcholine, is infused and the response to the acetylcholine-induced increased production of nitric oxide is recorded [119]. The normal, functional, coronary vasculature response to low dose acetylcholine infusion is coronary arterial vasodilation and increased blood flow (by >50%). In the setting of vascular endothelial cell dysfunction, the increases in coronary flow and dimension are less and, at times, even paradoxical vasoconstriction occurs [120]. Other, less commonly used agents for invasive endothelial-dependent coronary vascular function testing are bradykinin, papaverine, Substance P and adenosine [121, 122]. Non-pharmacologic endothelial-dependent stressors to assess coronary vascular function include cold pressor testing [123] and exercise testing using an ergometer [124].

Advantages of the invasive, catheter-based, coronary endothelial assessment include the precision and accuracy of direct rather than surrogate measures of coronary arterial function assessment. These are, however, balanced by the potential risks of vascular access, coronary vessel engagement with the catheter, exposure to radiation and contrast agents, and potential systemic, hemodynamic effects of the pharmacologic intervention. These concerns limit repeated assessments of invasive coronary endothelial function testing outside of clinically indicated procedures.

4.2 Non-invasive Coronary Artery and Peripheral Arterial Endothelial Function Assessment

There are a variety of non-invasive, imaging, modalities to assess endothelial-dependent coronary- and peripheral vascular function including magnetic resonance imaging (MRI) [125], positron emission tomography (PET)/computed tomography (CT) [126, 127], computed tomography angiography (CTA) [128] and ultrasound to assess brachial artery flow - mediated dilatation (FMD) [129]. The following section will focus on the two most used techniques at our institution: MRI for coronary artery endothelial function testing and FMD for peripheral vascular function testing.

4.2.1 Non-invasive Evaluation of Epicardial Coronary Endothelial Function and Microvascular Function Testing: MRI

MRI in combination with isometric handgrip exercise (IHE), a known endothelial-dependent stressor, is a non-invasive, and reproducible method to assess coronary endothelial function (CEF). [3, 125] CEF reflects coronary endothelial NO release and, as such, can be used to test pathophysiologic contributors to cardiovascular diseases [130]. The normal response to IHE is an increase in NO bioavailability with subsequent coronary vascular dilation and increases in coronary flow velocity and flow. Furthermore, our studies showed impaired CEF in patients with CAD [131] and separately in people living with HIV compared to otherwise risk-factor-matched control participants [125]. The coronary artery area and flow responses to stressors as assessed by MRI have been validated when compared to invasive measures using quantitative coronary angiography with Doppler techniques [132]. This MRI technique therefore provides an opportunity to monitor the impact of interventions to improve CEF and therefore decrease the development and progression of atherosclerosis during the early stages of coronary disease [133]. MRI techniques can also be used to interrogate microvascular function. Stress perfusion cardiovascular magnetic resonance (CMR), distinct from the coronary vasoreactivity approaches outlined above, typically use vasodilator stress (e.g., adenosine) to detect changes in myocardial blood flow in response to stress. Several studies support the use of stress perfusion CMR to investigate myocardial perfusion reserve, which reflects microvascular function in the absence of significant CAD [134, 135]. Like MRI for CEF testing, the prognostic value of stress CMR was similar to that of invasive strategies [136].

4.2.2 Peripheral Endothelial Function Assessment: Brachial Artery Flow Mediated Dilatation and Peripheral Artery Tonometry

Flow-mediated vasodilatation (FMD) of the brachial artery measures the response of a focal segment of the vessel to endothelial-dependent NO release induced by a hyperemic stimulus, usually at the time of increased blood flow following a 5 min blood pressure cuff occlusion of flow. FMD is defined as the change in arterial diameter post-stimulus compared to the baseline diameter, measured manually or with edge-detection software [129, 137]. Furthermore, baseline and hyperemic (maximal) blood flows are calculated from the onset of one arterial waveform to the beginning of the next waveform using the time-averaged pulsed Doppler spectral trace time-velocity integral. FMD assessed vascular endothelial cell function is a validated method to detect endothelial dysfunction, which predicts future cardiovascular events [138].

Peripheral artery tonometry (PAT) is also used to assess endothelial function. PAT uses a pneumatic finger probe to measure the arterial pulse wave amplitude at baseline and with reactive hyperemia. There is a poor correlation between the FMD and PAT techniques [139], and it was proposed that PAT is a more accurate assessment of micro- rather than macrovascular, function [140].

4.3 Endothelial Function in the Coronary and Peripheral Vasculature

As outlined in the prior sections, endothelial function assessed by invasive and noninvasive modalities is an important predictor of vascular health and cardiovascular outcomes. However, some studies show only a modest association between systemic and coronary endothelial function assessments [141]. Furthermore, there may be significant variability of the endothelial cell function measures within a vascular territory or even within the coronary vasculature of the same person [131]. A variety of mechanisms may explain these differences, including differences in local shear stress, the resistance of downstream vessels, and neurohormonal regulation. Finally, endothelial function assessment in the coronary and systemic vasculatures, with individual strengths and limitations, may provide complementary insights into vascular endothelial cell function [142].

References

1. Martin CF. Osler as clinician and teacher. Can Med Assoc J. 1920;10(Spec Issue):82–6.
2. Gimbrone MA Jr, Garcia-Cardena G. Endothelial cell dysfunction and the pathobiology of atherosclerosis. Circ Res. 2016;118(4):620–36.
3. Hays AG, et al. Coronary vasomotor responses to isometric handgrip exercise are primarily mediated by nitric oxide: a noninvasive MRI test of coronary endothelial function. Am J Physiol Heart Circ Physiol. 2015;308(11):H1343–50.
4. Jones SP, Bolli R. The ubiquitous role of nitric oxide in cardioprotection. J Mol Cell Cardiol. 2006;40(1):16–23.
5. Virani SS, et al. Heart disease and stroke statistics-2020 update: a report from the American Heart Association. Circulation. 2020;141(9):e139–596.
6. Vespa J, Medina L, Armstrong DM. Demographic turning points for the United States: population projections for 2020 to 2060. Current Population Reports. Washington, DC: Census Bureau; 2020. p. P25–1144.
7. Rizvi F, et al. Effects of aging on cardiac oxidative stress and transcriptional changes in pathways of reactive oxygen species generation and clearance. J Am Heart Assoc. 2021;10(16):e019948.
8. Finkel T, Holbrook NJ. Oxidants, oxidative stress and the biology of ageing. Nature. 2000;408(6809):239–47.
9. Csiszar A, et al. Aging-induced phenotypic changes and oxidative stress impair coronary arteriolar function. Circ Res. 2002;90(11):1159–66.
10. Toth P, et al. Resveratrol treatment rescues neurovascular coupling in aged mice: role of improved cerebromicrovascular endothelial function and downregulation of NADPH oxidase. Am J Physiol Heart Circ Physiol. 2014;306(3):H299–308.
11. Yang YM, et al. eNOS uncoupling and endothelial dysfunction in aged vessels. Am J Physiol Heart Circ Physiol. 2009;297(5):H1829–36.

12. Donato AJ, et al. Direct evidence of endothelial oxidative stress with aging in humans: relation to impaired endothelium-dependent dilation and upregulation of nuclear factor-kappaB. Circ Res. 2007;100(11):1659–66.
13. Csiszar A, et al. Inflammation and endothelial dysfunction during aging: role of NF-kappaB. J Appl Physiol (1985). 2008;105(4):1333–41.
14. Wang M, et al. Matrix metalloproteinases promote arterial remodeling in aging, hypertension, and atherosclerosis. Hypertension. 2015;65(4):698–703.
15. Ungvari Z, et al. Cerebral microhemorrhages: mechanisms, consequences, and prevention. Am J Physiol Heart Circ Physiol. 2017;312(6):H1128–43.
16. Fleenor BS, et al. Superoxide signaling in perivascular adipose tissue promotes age-related artery stiffness. Aging Cell. 2014;13(3):576–8.
17. Ungvari Z, Sonntag WE, Csiszar A. Mitochondria and aging in the vascular system. J Mol Med (Berl). 2010;88(10):1021–7.
18. Ungvari Z, et al. Increased mitochondrial H_2O_2 production promotes endothelial NF-kappaB activation in aged rat arteries. Am J Physiol Heart Circ Physiol. 2007;293(1):H37–47.
19. Ungvari Z, et al. Age-associated vascular oxidative stress, Nrf2 dysfunction, and NF-{kappa} B activation in the nonhuman primate Macaca mulatta. J Gerontol A Biol Sci Med Sci. 2011;66(8):866–75.
20. Springo Z, et al. Aging exacerbates pressure-induced mitochondrial oxidative stress in mouse cerebral arteries. J Gerontol A Biol Sci Med Sci. 2015;70(11):1355–9.
21. Gioscia-Ryan RA, et al. Mitochondria-targeted antioxidant (MitoQ) ameliorates age-related arterial endothelial dysfunction in mice. J Physiol. 2014;592(12):2549–61.
22. Pearson KJ, et al. Resveratrol delays age-related deterioration and mimics transcriptional aspects of dietary restriction without extending life span. Cell Metab. 2008;8(2):157–68.
23. Nissanka N, Moraes CT. Mitochondrial DNA damage and reactive oxygen species in neurodegenerative disease. FEBS Lett. 2018;592(5):728–42.
24. Bratic A, Larsson NG. The role of mitochondria in aging. J Clin Invest. 2013;123(3):951–7.
25. Yu E, et al. Mitochondrial DNA damage can promote atherosclerosis independently of reactive oxygen species through effects on smooth muscle cells and monocytes and correlates with higher-risk plaques in humans. Circulation. 2013;128(7):702–12.
26. Sack MN, Finkel T. Mitochondrial metabolism, sirtuins, and aging. Cold Spring Harb Perspect Biol. 2012;4(12):a013102.
27. Wang M, et al. Proinflammation: the key to arterial aging. Trends Endocrinol Metab. 2014;25(2):72–9.
28. Kang C, et al. The DNA damage response induces inflammation and senescence by inhibiting autophagy of GATA4. Science. 2015;349(6255):aaa5612.
29. Freund A, Patil CK, Campisi J. p38MAPK is a novel DNA damage response-independent regulator of the senescence-associated secretory phenotype. EMBO J. 2011;30(8):1536–48.
30. Bailey-Downs LC, et al. Aging exacerbates obesity-induced oxidative stress and inflammation in perivascular adipose tissue in mice: a paracrine mechanism contributing to vascular redox dysregulation and inflammation. J Gerontol A Biol Sci Med Sci. 2013;68(7):780–92.
31. Tucsek Z, et al. Aging exacerbates obesity-induced cerebromicrovascular rarefaction, neurovascular uncoupling, and cognitive decline in mice. J Gerontol A Biol Sci Med Sci. 2014;69(11):1339–52.
32. Hasegawa Y, et al. Blockade of the nuclear factor-kappaB pathway in the endothelium prevents insulin resistance and prolongs life spans. Circulation. 2012;125(9):1122–33.
33. Gano LB, et al. The SIRT1 activator SRT1720 reverses vascular endothelial dysfunction, excessive superoxide production, and inflammation with aging in mice. Am J Physiol Heart Circ Physiol. 2014;307(12):H1754–63.
34. Karasawa T, Takahashi M. Role of NLRP3 inflammasomes in atherosclerosis. J Atheroscler Thromb. 2017;24(5):443–51.
35. Song Y, et al. Aging enhances the basal production of IL-6 and CCL2 in vascular smooth muscle cells. Arterioscler Thromb Vasc Biol. 2012;32(1):103–9.
36. Wang GC, et al. Cytomegalovirus infection and the risk of mortality and frailty in older women: a prospective observational cohort study. Am J Epidemiol. 2010;171(10):1144–52.

37. Shah AV, Bennett MR. DNA damage-dependent mechanisms of ageing and disease in the macro- and microvasculature. Eur J Pharmacol. 2017;816:116–28.

38. Durik M, et al. Nucleotide excision DNA repair is associated with age-related vascular dysfunction. Circulation. 2012;126(4):468–78.

39. Matsumoto T, et al. Aging-associated vascular phenotype in mutant mice with low levels of BubR1. Stroke. 2007;38(3):1050–6.

40. Liu J, et al. Roles of telomere biology in cell senescence, replicative and chronological ageing. Cells. 2019;8(1):54.

41. Zhang W, et al. Epigenetic modifications in cardiovascular aging and diseases. Circ Res. 2018;123(7):773–86.

42. Gensous N, et al. The impact of caloric restriction on the epigenetic signatures of aging. Int J Mol Sci. 2019;20(8):2022.

43. Kida Y, Goligorsky MS. Sirtuins, cell senescence, and vascular aging. Can J Cardiol. 2016;32(5):634–41.

44. de Lucia C, et al. microRNA in cardiovascular aging and age-related cardiovascular diseases. Front Med (Lausanne). 2017;4:74.

45. Tarantini S, et al. IGF-1 deficiency in a critical period early in life influences the vascular aging phenotype in mice by altering miRNA-mediated post-transcriptional gene regulation: implications for the developmental origins of health and disease hypothesis. Age (Dordr). 2016;38(4):239–58.

46. Lopez-Otin C, et al. The hallmarks of aging. Cell. 2013;153(6):1194–217.

47. Campisi J, d'Adda di Fagagna F. Cellular senescence: when bad things happen to good cells. Nat Rev Mol Cell Biol. 2007;8(9):729–40.

48. Erusalimsky JD. Vascular endothelial senescence: from mechanisms to pathophysiology. J Appl Physiol (1985). 2009;106(1):326–32.

49. Childs BG, et al. Senescent intimal foam cells are deleterious at all stages of atherosclerosis. Science. 2016;354(6311):472–7.

50. Ungvari Z, et al. Ionizing radiation promotes the acquisition of a senescence-associated secretory phenotype and impairs angiogenic capacity in cerebromicrovascular endothelial cells: role of increased DNA damage and decreased DNA repair capacity in microvascular radiosensitivity. J Gerontol A Biol Sci Med Sci. 2013;68(12):1443–57.

51. Roos CM, et al. Chronic senolytic treatment alleviates established vasomotor dysfunction in aged or atherosclerotic mice. Aging Cell. 2016;15(5):973–7.

52. Kumar S, Dietrich N, Kornfeld K. Angiotensin converting enzyme (ACE) inhibitor extends Caenorhabditis elegans life span. PLoS Genet. 2016;12(2):e1005866.

53. Wang M, et al. Proinflammatory profile within the grossly normal aged human aortic wall. Hypertension. 2007;50(1):219–27.

54. Wang M, et al. Angiotensin II activates matrix metalloproteinase type II and mimics age-associated carotid arterial remodeling in young rats. Am J Pathol. 2005;167(5):1429–42.

55. Wang M, et al. Aging increases aortic MMP-2 activity and angiotensin II in nonhuman primates. Hypertension. 2003;41(6):1308–16.

56. McCurley A, Jaffe IZ. Mineralocorticoid receptors in vascular function and disease. Mol Cell Endocrinol. 2012;350(2):256–65.

57. Bonnans C, Chou J, Werb Z. Remodelling the extracellular matrix in development and disease. Nat Rev Mol Cell Biol. 2014;15(12):786–801.

58. Toth P, et al. Aging exacerbates hypertension-induced cerebral microhemorrhages in mice: role of resveratrol treatment in vasoprotection. Aging Cell. 2015;14(3):400–8.

59. Fleenor BS, et al. Arterial stiffening with ageing is associated with transforming growth factor-beta1-related changes in adventitial collagen: reversal by aerobic exercise. J Physiol. 2010;588(Pt 20):3971–82.

60. Jacob MP. Extracellular matrix remodeling and matrix metalloproteinases in the vascular wall during aging and in pathological conditions. Biomed Pharmacother. 2003;57(5–6):195–202.

61. Tarantini S, et al. Insulin-like growth factor 1 deficiency exacerbates hypertension-induced cerebral microhemorrhages in mice, mimicking the aging phenotype. Aging Cell. 2017;16(3):469–79.
62. Keymel S, et al. Impaired endothelial progenitor cell function predicts age-dependent carotid intimal thickening. Basic Res Cardiol. 2008;103(6):582–6.
63. Rauscher FM, et al. Aging, progenitor cell exhaustion, and atherosclerosis. Circulation. 2003;108(4):457–63.
64. Zhu G, et al. Young environment reverses the declined activity of aged rat-derived endothelial progenitor cells: involvement of the phosphatidylinositol 3-kinase/Akt signaling pathway. Ann Vasc Surg. 2009;23(4):519–34.
65. Chirinos JA, et al. Large-artery stiffness in health and disease: JACC state-of-the-art review. J Am Coll Cardiol. 2019;74(9):1237–63.
66. Paneni F, et al. The aging cardiovascular system: understanding it at the cellular and clinical levels. J Am Coll Cardiol. 2017;69(15):1952–67.
67. Angoff R, Mosarla RC, Tsao CW. Aortic stiffness: epidemiology, risk factors, and relevant biomarkers. Front Cardiovasc Med. 2021;8:709396.
68. Fritze O, et al. Age-related changes in the elastic tissue of the human aorta. J Vasc Res. 2012;49(1):77–86.
69. Zieman SJ, Melenovsky V, Kass DA. Mechanisms, pathophysiology, and therapy of arterial stiffness. Arterioscler Thromb Vasc Biol. 2005;25(5):932–43.
70. Monk BA, George SJ. The effect of ageing on vascular smooth muscle cell behaviour—a mini-review. Gerontology. 2015;61(5):416–26.
71. Pescatore LA, Gamarra LF, Liberman M. Multifaceted mechanisms of vascular calcification in aging. Arterioscler Thromb Vasc Biol. 2019;39(7):1307–16.
72. Ungvari Z, et al. Mechanisms of vascular aging. Circ Res. 2018;123(7):849–67.
73. Bramwell JC, Hill AV. The velocity of pulse wave in man. Proc R Soc Lond Ser B Biol Sci. 1922;93(652):298–306.
74. Reference Values for Arterial Stiffness Collaboration. Determinants of pulse wave velocity in healthy people and in the presence of cardiovascular risk factors: 'establishing normal and reference values'. Eur Heart J. 2010;31(19):2338–50.
75. Najjar SS, et al. Age and gender affect ventricular-vascular coupling during aerobic exercise. J Am Coll Cardiol. 2004;44(3):611–7.
76. Redfield MM, et al. Age- and gender-related ventricular-vascular stiffening: a community-based study. Circulation. 2005;112(15):2254–62.
77. De Tombe PP, et al. Ventricular stroke work and efficiency both remain nearly optimal despite altered vascular loading. Am J Phys. 1993;264(6 Pt 2):H1817–24.
78. Segers P, Stergiopulos N, Westerhof N. Relation of effective arterial elastance to arterial system properties. Am J Physiol Heart Circ Physiol. 2002;282(3):H1041–6.
79. AlGhatrif M, et al. Longitudinal uncoupling of the heart and arteries with aging in a community-dwelling population. Geroscience. 2021;43(2):551–61.
80. Vasan RS, et al. Arterial stiffness and long-term risk of health outcomes: the Framingham Heart Study. Hypertension. 2022;79(5):1045–56.
81. Ben-Shlomo Y, et al. Aortic pulse wave velocity improves cardiovascular event prediction: an individual participant meta-analysis of prospective observational data from 17,635 subjects. J Am Coll Cardiol. 2014;63(7):636–46.
82. Sutton-Tyrrell K, et al. Elevated aortic pulse wave velocity, a marker of arterial stiffness, predicts cardiovascular events in well-functioning older adults. Circulation. 2005;111(25):3384–90.
83. Liao D, et al. Arterial stiffness and the development of hypertension. The ARIC study. Hypertension. 1999;34(2):201–6.
84. Najjar SS, et al. Pulse wave velocity is an independent predictor of the longitudinal increase in systolic blood pressure and of incident hypertension in the Baltimore Longitudinal Study of Aging. J Am Coll Cardiol. 2008;51(14):1377–83.

85. Franklin SS, et al. Does the relation of blood pressure to coronary heart disease risk change with aging? The Framingham Heart Study. Circulation. 2001;103(9):1245–9.
86. Chae CU, et al. Increased pulse pressure and risk of heart failure in the elderly. JAMA. 1999;281(7):634–9.
87. Haider AW, et al. Systolic blood pressure, diastolic blood pressure, and pulse pressure as predictors of risk for congestive heart failure in the Framingham Heart Study. Ann Intern Med. 2003;138(1):10–6.
88. Omote K, Verbrugge FH, Borlaug BA. Heart failure with preserved ejection fraction: mechanisms and treatment strategies. Annu Rev Med. 2022;73:321–37.
89. Reddy YNV, et al. Arterial stiffening with exercise in patients with heart failure and preserved ejection fraction. J Am Coll Cardiol. 2017;70(2):136–48.
90. Shaikh AY, et al. Relations of arterial stiffness and brachial flow-mediated dilation with new-onset atrial fibrillation: the Framingham Heart Study. Hypertension. 2016;68(3):590–6.
91. Pase MP, et al. Aortic stiffness and the risk of incident mild cognitive impairment and dementia. Stroke. 2016;47(9):2256–61.
92. Cui C, et al. Aortic stiffness is associated with increased risk of incident dementia in older adults. J Alzheimers Dis. 2018;66(1):297–306.
93. Bown CW, et al. Elevated aortic pulse wave velocity relates to longitudinal gray and white matter changes. Arterioscler Thromb Vasc Biol. 2021;41(12):3015–24.
94. Yannoutsos A, et al. Clinical relevance of aortic stiffness in end-stage renal disease and diabetes: implication for hypertension management. J Hypertens. 2018;36(6):1237–46.
95. Peralta CA, et al. Association of pulse pressure, arterial elasticity, and endothelial function with kidney function decline among adults with estimated GFR >60 mL/min/1.73 m(2): the Multi-Ethnic Study of Atherosclerosis (MESA). Am J Kidney Dis. 2012;59(1):41–9.
96. Appel LJ, et al. A clinical trial of the effects of dietary patterns on blood pressure. DASH Collaborative Research Group. N Engl J Med. 1997;336(16):1117–24.
97. Menotti A, Puddu PE. How the Seven Countries Study contributed to the definition and development of the Mediterranean diet concept: a 50-year journey. Nutr Metab Cardiovasc Dis. 2015;25(3):245–52.
98. LaRocca TJ, Martens CR, Seals DR. Nutrition and other lifestyle influences on arterial aging. Ageing Res Rev. 2017;39:106–19.
99. Mozaffarian D, Wu JHY. Flavonoids, dairy foods, and cardiovascular and metabolic health: a review of emerging biologic pathways. Circ Res. 2018;122(2):369–84.
100. Wang M, et al. Calorie restriction curbs proinflammation that accompanies arterial aging, preserving a youthful phenotype. J Am Heart Assoc. 2018;7(18):e009112.
101. Gates PE, et al. Dietary sodium restriction rapidly improves large elastic artery compliance in older adults with systolic hypertension. Hypertension. 2004;44(1):35–41.
102. Figueroa A, et al. Effects of diet and/or low-intensity resistance exercise training on arterial stiffness, adiposity, and lean mass in obese postmenopausal women. Am J Hypertens. 2013;26(3):416–23.
103. Dengo AL, et al. Arterial destiffening with weight loss in overweight and obese middle-aged and older adults. Hypertension. 2010;55(4):855–61.
104. Santos-Parker JR, LaRocca TJ, Seals DR. Aerobic exercise and other healthy lifestyle factors that influence vascular aging. Adv Physiol Educ. 2014;38(4):296–307.
105. Lopes S, et al. Exercise training reduces arterial stiffness in adults with hypertension: a systematic review and meta-analysis. J Hypertens. 2021;39(2):214–22.
106. Vaitkevicius PV, et al. Effects of age and aerobic capacity on arterial stiffness in healthy adults. Circulation. 1993;88(4 Pt 1):1456–62.
107. De Cesaris R, et al. Forearm arterial distensibility in patients with hypertension: comparative effects of long-term ACE inhibition and beta-blocking. Clin Pharmacol Ther. 1993;53(3):360–7.
108. Dudenbostel T, Glasser SP. Effects of antihypertensive drugs on arterial stiffness. Cardiol Rev. 2012;20(5):259–63.

109. Gurven M, Blackwell AD, Rodríguez DE, Stieglitz J, Kaplan H. Does blood pressure inevitably rise with age?: Longitudinal evidence among forager-horticulturalists. Hypertension. 2012 Jul;60(1):25-33. doi: https://doi.org/10.1161/HYPERTENSIONAHA.111.189100.. Epub 2012 May 21. PMID: 22700319; PMCID: PMC3392307.

110. Tsao CW, Aday AW, Almarzooq ZI, Alonso A, Beaton AZ, Bittencourt MS, Boehme AK, Buxton AE, Carson AP, Commodore-Mensah Y, MSV E, Evenson KR, Eze-Nliam C, Ferguson JF, Generoso G, Ho JE, Kalani R, Khan SS, Kissela BM, Knutson KL, Levine DA, Lewis TT, Liu J, Loop MS, Ma J, Mussolino ME, Navaneethan SD, Perak AM, Poudel R, Rezk-Hanna M, Roth GA, Schroeder EB, Shah SH, Thacker EL, LB VW, Virani SS, Voecks JH, Wang NY, Yaffe K, Martin SS. Heart Disease and Stroke Statistics-2022 Update: A Report From the American Heart Association. Circulation. 2022;145(8):e153–639. https://doi.org/10.1161/CIR.0000000000001052. Epub 2022 Jan 26. Erratum in: Circulation. 2022 Sep 6;146(10):e141

111. Avolio AP, Deng FQ, Li WQ, Luo YF, Huang ZD, Xing LF, O'Rourke MF. Effects of aging on arterial distensibility in populations with high and low prevalence of hypertension: comparison between urban and rural communities in China. Circulation. 1985 Feb;71(2):202-210. doi: https://doi.org/10.1161/01.cir.71.2.202.

112. He J, Klag MJ, Whelton PK, Chen JY, Mo JP, Qian MC, Mo PS, He GQ. Migration, blood pressure pattern, and hypertension: the Yi Migrant Study. Am J Epidemiol. 1991;134(10):1085–101. https://doi.org/10.1093/oxfordjournals.aje.a116012.

113. Halcox JP, et al. Prognostic value of coronary vascular endothelial dysfunction. Circulation. 2002;106(6):653–8.

114. Houghton JL, et al. Effect of African-American race and hypertensive left ventricular hypertrophy on coronary vascular reactivity and endothelial function. Hypertension. 1997;29(3):706–14.

115. Cosson E, et al. Impaired coronary endothelium-dependent vasodilation is associated with microalbuminuria in patients with type 2 diabetes and angiographically normal coronary arteries. Diabetes Care. 2006;29(1):107–12.

116. Treasure CB, et al. Beneficial effects of cholesterol-lowering therapy on the coronary endothelium in patients with coronary artery disease. N Engl J Med. 1995;332(8):481–7.

117. Schachinger V, Britten MB, Zeiher AM. Prognostic impact of coronary vasodilator dysfunction on adverse long-term outcome of coronary heart disease. Circulation. 2000;101(16):1899–906.

118. Doucette JW, et al. Validation of a Doppler guide wire for intravascular measurement of coronary artery flow velocity. Circulation. 1992;85(5):1899–911.

119. Zeiher AM, et al. Modulation of coronary vasomotor tone in humans. Progressive endothelial dysfunction with different early stages of coronary atherosclerosis. Circulation. 1991;83(2):391–401.

120. Ludmer PL, et al. Paradoxical vasoconstriction induced by acetylcholine in atherosclerotic coronary arteries. N Engl J Med. 1986;315(17):1046–51.

121. Niccoli G, Scalone G, Crea F. Coronary functional tests in the catheterization laboratory - pathophysiological and clinical relevance. Circ J. 2015;79(4):676–84.

122. Randaccio P. A program for optimizing radiation beam parameters in radiotherapy (author's transl). Radiol Med. 1979;65(10):741–6.

123. Nabel EG, et al. Dilation of normal and constriction of atherosclerotic coronary arteries caused by the cold pressor test. Circulation. 1988;77(1):43–52.

124. Gordon JB, et al. Atherosclerosis influences the vasomotor response of epicardial coronary arteries to exercise. J Clin Invest. 1989;83(6):1946–52.

125. Leucker TM, et al. Coronary endothelial dysfunction is associated with elevated serum PCSK9 levels in people with HIV independent of low-density lipoprotein cholesterol. J Am Heart Assoc. 2018;7(19):e009996.

126. Beanlands RS, et al. Noninvasive quantification of regional myocardial flow reserve in patients with coronary atherosclerosis using nitrogen-13 ammonia positron emission tomography. Determination of extent of altered vascular reactivity. J Am Coll Cardiol. 1995;26(6):1465–75.

127. Taqueti VR, Di Carli MF. Coronary microvascular disease pathogenic mechanisms and therapeutic options: JACC state-of-the-art review. J Am Coll Cardiol. 2018;72(21):2625–41.
128. George RT, et al. Quantification of myocardial perfusion using dynamic 64-detector computed tomography. Investig Radiol. 2007;42(12):815–22.
129. Corretti MC, et al. Guidelines for the ultrasound assessment of endothelial-dependent flow-mediated vasodilation of the brachial artery: a report of the International Brachial Artery Reactivity Task Force. J Am Coll Cardiol. 2002;39(2):257–65.
130. Sara JD, et al. Prevalence of coronary microvascular dysfunction among patients with chest pain and nonobstructive coronary artery disease. JACC Cardiovasc Interv. 2015;8(11):1445–53.
131. Hays AG, et al. Noninvasive visualization of coronary artery endothelial function in healthy subjects and in patients with coronary artery disease. J Am Coll Cardiol. 2010;56(20):1657–65.
132. Hundley WG, et al. Assessment of coronary arterial flow and flow reserve in humans with magnetic resonance imaging. Circulation. 1996;93(8):1502–8.
133. Leucker TM, et al. Evolocumab, a PCSK9-monoclonal antibody, rapidly reverses coronary artery endothelial dysfunction in people living with HIV and people with dyslipidemia. J Am Heart Assoc. 2020;9(14):e016263.
134. Shufelt CL, et al. Cardiac magnetic resonance imaging myocardial perfusion reserve index assessment in women with microvascular coronary dysfunction and reference controls. Cardiovasc Diagn Ther. 2013;3(3):153–60.
135. Dorbala S, et al. Coronary microvascular dysfunction is related to abnormalities in myocardial structure and function in cardiac amyloidosis. JACC Heart Fail. 2014;2(4):358–67.
136. Kelle S, et al. A bi-center cardiovascular magnetic resonance prognosis study focusing on dobutamine wall motion and late gadolinium enhancement in 3,138 consecutive patients. J Am Coll Cardiol. 2013;61(22):2310–2.
137. Haluska B, et al. Automated edge-detection technique for measurement of brachial artery reactivity: a comparison of concordance with manual measurements. Ultrasound Med Biol. 2001;27(9):1285–9.
138. Matsuzawa Y, et al. Prognostic value of flow-mediated vasodilation in brachial artery and fingertip artery for cardiovascular events: a systematic review and meta-analysis. J Am Heart Assoc. 2015;4(11):e002270.
139. Allan RB, et al. A comparison of flow-mediated dilatation and peripheral artery tonometry for measurement of endothelial function in healthy individuals and patients with peripheral arterial disease. Eur J Vasc Endovasc Surg. 2013;45(3):263–9.
140. Bonetti PO, et al. Noninvasive identification of patients with early coronary atherosclerosis by assessment of digital reactive hyperemia. J Am Coll Cardiol. 2004;44(11):2137–41.
141. Iantorno M, et al. Simultaneous noninvasive assessment of systemic and coronary endothelial function. Circ Cardiovasc Imaging. 2016;9(3):e003954.
142. Minhas AS, et al. Imaging assessment of endothelial function: an index of cardiovascular health. Front Cardiovasc Med. 2022;9:778762.

Peripheral Artery Disease (PAD)

Andrew Cluckey, Cherie N. Dahm, and Matthews Chacko

1   Introduction

Peripheral artery disease (PAD) is a circulatory disease that involves narrowed arteries that reduce blood flow to the limbs, typically due to atherosclerosis or plaque build-up within the arterial wall. In this chapter, we will discuss the clinical manifestations, diagnosis, and management of lower extremity PAD.

PAD generally develops due to fatty or atherosclerotic plaque deposition in the intimal layer of the arterial wall. As the plaque begins to accrue, it can obstruct flow in one of two ways, both of which can be life- or limb-threatening: (1) chronically, as the intimal layer continues to grow and obstruct into the lumen of the vessel or (2) acutely as the plaque ruptures, causing platelet adhesion and aggregation, resulting in thrombosis of the vessel.

PAD is common and is associated with significant cardiovascular morbidity and mortality, even if one is asymptomatic. It is estimated to occur in over 8 million Americans and more than 200 million individuals worldwide. In those older than 70 years of age, the prevalence is ~10% and increases to ~17% in those older than 80 years of age [1].

Key risk factors for atherosclerosis and PAD include diabetes mellitus, hypertension, hypercholesterolemia, older age, and cigarette smoking with cigarette smoking being a very potent risk factor for developing and accelerating atherosclerosis [2]. Other risk factors include coronary artery disease, cerebrovascular disease, chronic kidney disease, obesity, and systemic inflammatory disease.

A. Cluckey · C. N. Dahm · M. Chacko (✉)
Division of Cardiovascular Medicine, Vanderbilt University Medical Center,
Nashville, TN, USA
e-mail: matthews.chacko@vumc.org

© The Author(s), under exclusive license to Springer Nature
Switzerland AG 2023
T. M. Leucker, G. Gerstenblith (eds.), *Cardiovascular Disease in the Elderly*,
Contemporary Cardiology, https://doi.org/10.1007/978-3-031-16594-8_5

2 Clinical Manifestations

Most patients with PAD are asymptomatic, however symptomatic PAD can manifest as a spectrum of symptoms, ranging from exertional crampy or achy leg pain called intermittent claudication to debilitating pain at rest, and even gangrene leading to limb amputation in extreme cases. During rest, there is decreased vascular resistance to maintain muscle perfusion, however, with exercise, there is a supply-demand mismatch leading to limb ischemia. Over time with repeated episodes of ischemia and reperfusion, the release of oxygen free radicals leads to abnormal myocyte metabolism and impaired contractile reserve [3]. For hemodynamically significant stenosis at rest, the vessel diameter is generally reduced by 90% or more. With exertion, there is an increase in distal limb metabolic requirements and therefore even a 50% luminal reduction can have a hemodynamically significant impact in some instances [2], particularly if the vascular bed distal to the stenosis is large.

A careful history and physical examination is important, as several non-vascular diseases can mimic the symptoms of PAD, or vice versa, including lumbosacral spinal stenosis, peripheral neuropathy, and degenerative arthritis. Loss of hair or skin changes such as dependent rubor, poor capillary refill, or ulcerations can signify severe advanced PAD. A detailed pulse examination, including the radial, brachial, femoral, popliteal, posterior tibialis and dorsalis pedis pulses, can clue the examiner to the presence of significant obstructive PAD. Discrepant, diminished, or absent pulses warrants further investigation, however absent dorsalis pedis or posterior tibial pulses can be seen in the general population without PAD. Auscultation of the femoral arteries can suggest the presence of PAD if a bruit is noted. A meta-analysis looking into the most useful history and exam findings include symptoms of intermittent claudication with a likelihood ratio (LR) for PAD of 3.3, skin discoloration (LR 2.8), digital wounds (LR 5.9), arterial bruit (LR 5.6) and abnormal pulse exam (LR 4.7) [4].

3 Diagnosis

The diagnostic test of choice for PAD is an ankle-brachial index (ABI), or a toe-brachial index (TBI) when significant vessel calcification and stiff non-compressible vessels are present as may be the case in the elderly, diabetic, or chronic kidney disease populations. An ABI is obtained by measuring ankle (dorsalis pedis and posterior tibialis) and bilateral brachial systolic pressures while the patient is supine, with the greater of the two ankle pressures being the numerator and the greater of the two brachial pressures being the denominator. An ABI of ≤0.90 is diagnostic for PAD with an index of >1.0 and ≤1.4 considered normal [5]. With exertional symptoms and normal or borderline resting, ABIs present, an exercise ABI may increase the sensitivity of the test [6]. An initial ABI of 0.5 is a significant predictor of disease severity likely to require revascularization [2]. Though varying cut-offs have been used in clinical trials, a TBI cut-off of ≤ 0.7 has been recommended in the AHA PAD guidelines [7]. Segmental blood pressures in the lower extremities may allow for anatomic localization of obstructive PAD with a positive finding defined as a drop of >20 mmHg between levels [7].

Duplex ultrasound, CT angiography, or magnetic resonance angiography (MRA) can further help to localize disease as well as allow for pre-procedural or pre-operative planning with test selection often dependent upon patient factors such as chronic kidney disease or claustrophobia. Catheter-based angiography with digital subtraction angiography (DSA) is considered the gold standard for PAD imaging, however, due to its invasive nature and attendant risks of complications such as bleeding, vascular injury, and contrast nephropathy, it is reserved for instances when intervention may be necessary or when there are divergent findings on diagnostic testing or clinical assessment. When compared with catheter-based angiography, duplex ultrasound has been shown to have a good concordance in diagnosing and localizing lesions, particularly in the femoro-popliteal region [8]. CTA and MRA have also been shown to have high sensitivity and specificity in diagnosing PAD when compared with catheter-based angiography [9, 10].

4   Management

4.1   Lifestyle Modifications

Multiple risk factors contribute and play a significant role in the progression of PAD. As with coronary artery disease, management of risk factors such as diabetes, lipids, hypertension, and smoking cessation are class I recommendations [7]. Smoking is a significant risk factor for PAD, with a dose-response relationship [11]. Smokers are not only at increased risk for developing PAD compared to non-smokers, they also have higher complication rates from PAD, including requiring limb salvage therapies and amputation [12, 13]. Several studies have shown that smoking cessation limits the risk of developing PAD, however, compared with CAD and stroke, the risk never returns to baseline [14, 15]. The Framingham study showed that smokers are twice as likely to develop PAD as they are to develop CAD [2]. Smoking cessation programs and smoking cessation adjunctive therapies should be considered for all patients with PAD. In a randomized control trial of PAD patients, those that underwent intensive counseling and pharmacologic therapy were more likely to have abstained from smoking at 6 months than those in the standard therapy arm (21.3% vs. 6.8%) with 87% of patients in the intensive arm reporting pharmacotherapy use compared with only 67% in the standard arm [13].

While medical therapy and risk factor modification may help to reduce major adverse cardiac events (MACE) and limb events (MALE), few medications have proven to reduce symptoms. The initial treatment of choice for symptomatic PAD is supervised exercise therapy as a class I recommendation [6, 7]. Several randomized control trials have shown that supervised exercise programs improve walking distance for patients with symptomatic PAD [16]. In a recently published meta-analysis, supervised exercise therapy improved walking performance more than did lower extremity revascularization up to 18 months out, however, the combination of the two showed the greatest response [17]. The greatest barrier to supervised exercise is availability and as such, self-guided home exercise regimens can be considered.

4.2 Medical Management

The cornerstone of medical therapy involves anti-platelet and anti-thrombotic therapy. Though the effect of aspirin in all patients with PAD is not well-established, using either aspirin (75–325 mg/day) or clopidogrel (75 mg/day) is a class Ia recommendation for patients with symptomatic PAD to reduce the risk of MI, stroke, and vascular death [6, 7]. A large meta-analysis of 287 studies showed that anti-platelet agents, most commonly low dose aspirin (75–150 mg daily), in high-risk symptomatic patients reduced the risk of non-fatal myocardial infarction, non-fatal stroke, or vascular death [18]. The CLIPS (Critical Leg Ischemia Prevention Study) trial found that aspirin, when compared to placebo, reduced the rates of MACCE and critical limb ischemia (6.5% for aspirin vs. 15.5% for placebo) at 2 years in 366 symptomatic and asymptomatic PAD patients [19]. The net benefit of aspirin, however, has not been seen in asymptomatic PAD patients [20, 21]. Cilostazol is a phosphodiesterase inhibitor with anti-platelet properties that has been shown to improve symptoms in those with PAD and intermittent claudication. A Cochrane Database Systematic Review showed that the addition of cilostazol resulted in an overall improvement in claudication free walking distance, however, no significant difference in MACE was noted [22]. Cilostazol has a class I recommendation for intermittent claudication [7], though it should be avoided in those with congestive heart failure.

P2Y12 receptor inhibitors have been shown to lower the rates of MACE and MALE in symptomatic PAD patients. In the CAPRIE trial, aspirin (325 mg/day) was compared with clopidogrel in those with cardiovascular disease and demonstrated a 23.8% relative risk reduction for stroke, MI or vascular death in the clopidogrel arm compared with the aspirin arm with superior safety as well [23, 24]. Ticagrelor is another P2Y12 receptor inhibitor that was shown to reduce MACE with similar bleeding outcomes compared to clopidogrel in the EUCLID trial [25]. Combination therapy with aspirin and clopidogrel can be considered for high-risk patients, however at a cost of increased risk of bleeding as seen in the CHARISMA trial [26]. In the PLATO trial, a subgroup analysis of PAD patients showed an insignificant difference between ticagrelor and aspirin compared to clopidogrel and aspirin in the reduction of MACCE, however, patients with PAD were noted to have a 2.5-fold increased rate of events when compared to patients without PAD [24].

The factor Xa inhibitor rivaroxaban has shown benefit in secondary prevention in those with PAD. In the COMPASS trial, patients with stable atherosclerotic vascular disease were randomized to receive low dose rivaroxaban (2.5 mg twice daily) in addition to low dose aspirin (100 mg daily), low dose rivaroxaban (5 mg twice daily) plus aspirin placebo, or low dose aspirin (100 mg daily) plus rivaroxaban placebo. The low dose rivaroxaban plus aspirin arm experienced lower rates of MACE and MALE compared with the other arms, however with an increased hazard of non-fatal bleeding [27]. The VOYAGER PAD trial revealed that this benefit holds true in patients who have undergone revascularization for PAD with significant and sustained reduction in event rates at 3 years of follow up [28].

Hypertension management with ACE inhibitors or ARBs should be considered to reduce ischemic events in patients with PAD and has a class IIa recommendation [7]. In patients with either symptomatic or ABI positive PAD, the use of ramipril for hypertension management reduced the absolute risk of cardiovascular mortality, MI, and stroke by more than 5% over 4.5 years of follow-up [6].

Lipid-lowering therapy has also shown benefits in the symptomatic PAD population, reducing the risk of MACE and MALE. The HMG-CoA reductase inhibitors, or "statins", have a class I indication per the ACC/AHA guidelines [7]. The possible mechanisms of action of statins include plaque stabilization prevention of plaque rupture and decrease further plaque formation, as well as improved vasomotor effects [2]. In an analysis of the REACH registry, symptomatic PAD patients taking statins had fewer symptoms, a reduced need for revascularization and amputation, and lower rates of MACE [29]. Statin intolerance can be a barrier to attaining recommended lipid-lowering goals and in those patients, ezetimibe may be considered.

Recent studies of the proprotein convertase subtilisin/kexin type 9 (PCSK9) inhibitor evolocumab on lipid levels and cardiovascular outcomes in patients with atherosclerotic cardiovascular disease have been noteworthy [30, 31], including the FOURIER trial which showed significant reductions in MACE and MALE in the sub-group with symptomatic PAD [32].

5 Revascularization

While medical and exercise therapy are the cornerstones of PAD management and are effective in a majority of patients, revascularization may be necessary to improve quality of life and to reduce MACE and MALE in selected patients and should be considered for disabling, medically refractory intermittent claudication, critical limb ischemia, or for limb salvage. Surgical intervention has long been a mainstay of management in patients with medically refractory PAD, however endovascular therapy is being used with greater frequency as techniques and devices have improved [33]. Comparative meta-analyses of surgical and endovascular therapies for PAD show similar degrees improvement in quality of life, symptoms and walking distance in patients with intermittent claudication [34]. The decision to proceed with a surgical versus endovascular approach is typically dependent on multiple factors including surgical risk, vascular anatomy, and complexity of disease [35, 36].

5.1 Surgical Management

If a patient is deemed an appropriate surgical candidate, with a low operative risk and good anatomical targets, bypass surgery with autogenous vein grafts as compared with prosthetic grafts has been shown to have longer durability and patency at 5-year follow up [37].

5.2 Endovascular Management

Percutaneous balloon angioplasty with or without stenting can be used in symptomatic PAD in selected cases. More recently, drug-coated balloons as well as plaque and calcium modification devices such as laser, excisional or rotational atherectomy, and plaque scoring or cutting balloons have shown promise, though the long-term benefits are not well established and often dependent upon patient factors and disease anatomy or complexity [38–43]. Intravascular lithotripsy using a novel balloon that emits high-frequency ultrasonic pressure waves to modify and fracture calcium, has shown great promise in early clinical trials of calcific PAD [44, 45].

6 Conclusions

PAD is common and is vastly underdiagnosed [3] and undertreated [46] and can lead to significant disability and cardiovascular morbidity and mortality. Earlier diagnosis and the initiation of medical therapy coupled with either endovascular or surgical revascularization if indicated is essential to improve the overall cardiovascular and limb outcomes in those with PAD.

References

1. Fowkes FG, Rudan D, Rudan I, Aboyans V, Denenberg JO, McDermott MM, et al. Comparison of global estimates of prevalence and risk factors for peripheral artery disease in 2000 and 2010: a systematic review and analysis. Lancet. 2013;382(9901):1329–40. https://doi.org/10.1016/S0140-6736(13)61249-0.
2. Aburahma A, Bergan JJ. Noninvasive peripheral arterial diagnosis.
3. Ohman EM, Bhatt DL, Steg PG, Goto S, Hirsch AT, Liau CS, Mas JL, Richard AJ, Röther J, Wilson PW, REACH Registry Investigators. The REduction of Atherothrombosis for

Continued Health (REACH) Registry: an international, prospective, observational investigation in subjects at risk for atherothrombotic events-study design. Am Heart J. 2006;151(4):786. e1–10. https://doi.org/10.1016/j.ahj.2005.11.004.

4. Khan NA, Rahim SA, Anand SS, Simel DL, Panju A. Does the clinical examination predict lower extremity peripheral arterial disease? JAMA. 2006;295(5):536–46. https://doi.org/10.1001/jama.295.5.536.

5. Aboyans V, Criqui MH, Abraham P, Allison MA, Creager MA, Diehm C, et al. Measurement and interpretation of the ankle-brachial index: a scientific statement from the American Heart Association. Circulation. 2012;126(24):2890–909. https://doi.org/10.1161/CIR.0b013e318276fbcb.

6. Kithcart AP, Beckman JA. ACC/AHA versus ESC Guidelines for diagnosis and management of peripheral artery disease: JACC Guideline Comparison.

7. Gerhard-Herman MD, Gornik HL, Barrett C, Barshes NR, Corriere MA, Drachman DE, et al. 2016 AHA/ACC guideline on the management of patients with lower extremity peripheral artery disease: executive summary: a report of the American College of Cardiology/American Heart Association Task Force on Clinical Practice Guidelines. Circulation. 2017;135(12):e686–725. https://doi.org/10.1161/CIR.0000000000000470.

8. Martinelli O, Alunno A, Drudi FM, Malaj A, Irace L. Duplex ultrasound versus CT angiography for the treatment planning of lower-limb arterial disease. J Ultrasound. 2020; https://doi.org/10.1007/s40477-020-00534-y.

9. Burbelko M, Augsten M, Kalinowski MO, Heverhagen JT. Comparison of contrast-enhanced multi-station MR angiography and digital subtraction angiography of the lower extremity arterial disease. J Magn Reson Imaging. 2013;37(6):1427–35. https://doi.org/10.1002/jmri.23944.

10. Shareghi S, Gopal A, Gul K, Matchinson JC, Wong CB, Weinberg N, et al. Diagnostic accuracy of 64 multidetector computed tomographic angiography in peripheral vascular disease. Catheter Cardiovasc Interv. 2010;75(1):23–31. https://doi.org/10.1002/ccd.22228.

11. Willigendael EM, Teijink JA, Bartelink ML, Kuiken BW, Boiten J, Moll FL, et al. Influence of smoking on incidence and prevalence of peripheral arterial disease. J Vasc Surg. 2004;40(6):1158–65. https://doi.org/10.1016/j.jvs.2004.08.049.

12. Joosten MM, Pai JK, Bertoia ML, Rimm EB, Spiegelman D, Mittleman MA, et al. Associations between conventional cardiovascular risk factors and risk of peripheral artery disease in men. JAMA. 2012;308(16):1660–7. https://doi.org/10.1001/jama.2012.13415.

13. Hennrikus D, Joseph AM, Lando HA, Duval S, Ukestad L, Kodl M, et al. Effectiveness of a smoking cessation program for peripheral artery disease patients: a randomized controlled trial. J Am Coll Cardiol. 2010;56(25):2105–12. https://doi.org/10.1016/j.jacc.2010.07.031.

14. Kawachi I, Colditz GA, Stampfer MJ, Willett WC, Manson JE, Rosner B, et al. Smoking cessation and time course of decreased risks of coronary heart disease in middle-aged women. Arch Intern Med. 1994;154(2):169–75.

15. Kawachi I, Colditz GA, Stampfer MJ, Willett WC, Manson JE, Rosner B, et al. Smoking cessation and decreased risk of stroke in women. JAMA. 1993;269(2):232–6.

16. Fakhry F, van de Luijtgaarden KM, Bax L, den Hoed PT, Hunink MG, Rouwet EV, et al. Supervised walking therapy in patients with intermittent claudication. J Vasc Surg. 2012;56(4):1132–42. https://doi.org/10.1016/j.jvs.2012.04.046.

17. Biswas MP, Capell WH, McDermott MM, Jacobs DL, Beckman JA, Bonaca MP, et al. Exercise training and revascularization in the management of symptomatic peripheral artery disease. JACC Basic Transl Sci. 2021;6(2):174–88. https://doi.org/10.1016/j.jacbts.2020.08.012.

18. Antithrombotic Trialists Collaboration. Collaborative meta-analysis of randomised trials of antiplatelet therapy for prevention of death, myocardial infarction, and stroke in high risk patients. BMJ. 2002;324(7329):71–86. https://doi.org/10.1136/bmj.324.7329.71.

19. Critical Leg Ischaemia Prevention Study Group, Catalano M, Born G, Peto R. Prevention of serious vascular events by aspirin amongst patients with peripheral arterial disease: randomized, double-blind trial. J Intern Med. 2007;261(3):276–84. https://doi.org/10.1111/j.1365-2796.2006.01763.x.

20. Belch J, MacCuish A, Campbell I, Cobbe S, Taylor R, Prescott R, et al. The prevention of progression of arterial disease and diabetes (POPADAD) trial: factorial randomised placebo controlled trial of aspirin and antioxidants in patients with diabetes and asymptomatic peripheral arterial disease. BMJ. 2008;337:a1840. https://doi.org/10.1136/bmj.a1840.
21. Fowkes FG, Price JF, Stewart MC, Butcher I, Leng GC, Pell AC, et al. Aspirin for prevention of cardiovascular events in a general population screened for a low ankle brachial index: a randomized controlled trial. JAMA. 2010;303(9):841–8. https://doi.org/10.1001/jama.2010.221.
22. Bedenis R, Stewart M, Cleanthis M, Robless P, Mikhailidis DP, Stansby G. Cilostazol for intermittent claudication. Cochrane Database Syst Rev. 2014;(10):CD003748. https://doi.org/10.1002/14651858.CD003748.pub4.
23. CAPRIE Steering Committee. A randomised, blinded, trial of clopidogrel versus aspirin in patients at risk of ischaemic events (CAPRIE). CAPRIE Steering Committee. Lancet. 1996;348(9038):1329–39. https://doi.org/10.1016/s0140-6736(96)09457-3.
24. Sattur S. Chapter 5 – Peripheral arterial disease – a different kind of arterial disease? The role of antiplatelet therapy in the prevention and treatment of limb ischemia. In: Brener SJ, editor. Dual antiplatelet therapy for coronary and peripheral arterial disease. San Diego: Academic; 2021.
25. Hiatt WR, Fowkes FG, Heizer G, Berger JS, Baumgartner I, Held P, et al. Ticagrelor versus clopidogrel in symptomatic peripheral artery disease. N Engl J Med. 2017;376(1):32–40. https://doi.org/10.1056/NEJMoa1611688.
26. Bhatt DL, Flather MD, Hacke W, Berger PB, Black HR, Boden WE, et al. Patients with prior myocardial infarction, stroke, or symptomatic peripheral arterial disease in the CHARISMA trial. J Am Coll Cardiol. 2007;49(19):1982–8. https://doi.org/10.1016/j.jacc.2007.03.025.
27. Anand SS, Bosch J, Eikelboom JW, Connolly SJ, Diaz R, Widimsky P, et al. Rivaroxaban with or without aspirin in patients with stable peripheral or carotid artery disease: an international, randomised, double-blind, placebo-controlled trial. Lancet. 2018;391(10117):219–29. https://doi.org/10.1016/S0140-6736(17)32409-1.
28. Bonaca MP, Bauersachs RM, Anand SS, Debus ES, Nehler MR, Patel MR, et al. Rivaroxaban in peripheral artery disease after revascularization. N Engl J Med. 2020;382(21):1994–2004. https://doi.org/10.1056/NEJMoa2000052.
29. Kumbhani DJ, Steg PG, Cannon CP, Eagle KA, Smith SC Jr, Goto S, et al. Statin therapy and long-term adverse limb outcomes in patients with peripheral artery disease: insights from the REACH registry. Eur Heart J. 2014;35(41):2864–72. https://doi.org/10.1093/eurheartj/ehu080.
30. Sabatine MS, Giugliano RP, Keech AC, Honarpour N, Wiviott SD, Murphy SA, et al. Evolocumab and clinical outcomes in patients with cardiovascular disease. N Engl J Med. 2017;376(18):1713–22. https://doi.org/10.1056/NEJMoa1615664.
31. Schwartz GG, Steg PG, Szarek M, Bhatt DL, Bittner VA, Diaz R, et al. Alirocumab and cardiovascular outcomes after acute coronary syndrome. N Engl J Med. 2018;379(22):2097–107. https://doi.org/10.1056/NEJMoa1801174.
32. Bonaca MP, Nault P, Giugliano RP, Keech AC, Pineda AL, Kanevsky E, et al. Low-density lipoprotein cholesterol lowering with evolocumab and outcomes in patients with peripheral artery disease: insights from the FOURIER Trial (Further Cardiovascular Outcomes Research With PCSK9 Inhibition in Subjects With Elevated Risk). Circulation. 2018;137(4):338–50. https://doi.org/10.1161/CIRCULATIONAHA.117.032235.
33. Cull DL, Langan EM, Gray BH, Johnson B, Taylor SM. Open versus endovascular intervention for critical limb ischemia: a population-based study. J Am Coll Surg. 2010;210(5):555–61, 61–3. https://doi.org/10.1016/j.jamcollsurg.2009.12.019.
34. Malgor RD, Alahdab F, Elraiyah TA, Rizvi AZ, Lane MA, Prokop LJ, et al. A systematic review of treatment of intermittent claudication in the lower extremities. J Vasc Surg. 2015;61(3 Suppl):54S–73S. https://doi.org/10.1016/j.jvs.2014.12.007.
35. Society for Vascular Surgery Lower Extremity Guidelines Writing Group, Conte MS, Pomposelli FB, Clair DG, Geraghty PJ, McKinsey JF, et al. Society for Vascular Surgery practice guidelines for atherosclerotic occlusive disease of the lower extremities: management

of asymptomatic disease and claudication. J Vasc Surg. 2015;61(3 Suppl):2S–41S. https://doi.org/10.1016/j.jvs.2014.12.009.

36. Conte MS, Bradbury AW, Kolh P, White JV, Dick F, Fitridge R, et al. Global vascular guidelines on the management of chronic limb-threatening ischemia. Eur J Vasc Endovasc Surg. 2019;58(1S):S1–S109.e33. https://doi.org/10.1016/j.ejvs.2019.05.006.

37. Ambler GK, Twine CP. Graft type for femoro-popliteal bypass surgery. Cochrane Database Syst Rev. 2018;2:CD001487. https://doi.org/10.1002/14651858.CD001487.pub3.

38. Nordanstig J, Taft C, Hensater M, Perlander A, Osterberg K, Jivegard L. Improved quality of life after 1 year with an invasive versus a noninvasive treatment strategy in claudicants: one-year results of the Invasive Revascularization or Not in Intermittent Claudication (IRONIC) Trial. Circulation. 2014;130(12):939–47. https://doi.org/10.1161/CIRCULATIONAHA.114.009867.

39. Djerf H, Millinger J, Falkenberg M, Jivegard L, Svensson M, Nordanstig J. Absence of long-term benefit of revascularization in patients with intermittent claudication: five-year results from the IRONIC randomized controlled trial. Circ Cardiovasc Interv. 2020;13(1):e008450. https://doi.org/10.1161/CIRCINTERVENTIONS.119.008450.

40. Saraidaridis JT, Ergul EA, Clouse WD, Patel VI, Cambria RP, Conrad MF. The natural history and outcomes of endovascular therapy for claudication. Ann Vasc Surg. 2017;44:34–40. https://doi.org/10.1016/j.avsg.2017.04.021.

41. Greenhalgh RM, Belch JJ, Brown LC, Gaines PA, Gao L, Reise JA, et al. The adjuvant benefit of angioplasty in patients with mild to moderate intermittent claudication (MIMIC) managed by supervised exercise, smoking cessation advice and best medical therapy: results from two randomised trials for stenotic femoropopliteal and aortoiliac arterial disease. Eur J Vasc Endovasc Surg. 2008;36(6):680–8. https://doi.org/10.1016/j.ejvs.2008.10.007.

42. Sachar R, Soga Y, Ansari MM, Kozuki A, Lopez L, Brodmann M, et al. 1-Year results from the RANGER II SFA randomized trial of the Ranger drug-coated balloon. JACC Cardiovasc Interv. 2021;14(10):1123–33. https://doi.org/10.1016/j.jcin.2021.03.021.

43. Yamamoto Y, Kawarada O, Ando H, Anzai H, Zen K, Tamura K, et al. Effects of high-speed rotational atherectomy in peripheral artery disease patients with calcified lesions: a retrospective multicenter registry. Cardiovasc Interv Ther. 2020;35(4):393–7. https://doi.org/10.1007/s12928-020-00643-9.

44. Adams G, Shammas N, Mangalmurti S, Bernardo NL, Miller WE, Soukas PA, et al. Intravascular lithotripsy for treatment of calcified lower extremity arterial stenosis: initial analysis of the Disrupt PAD III study. J Endovasc Ther. 2020;27(3):473–80. https://doi.org/10.1177/1526602820914598.

45. Brodmann M, Werner M, Holden A, Tepe G, Scheinert D, Schwindt A, et al. Primary outcomes and mechanism of action of intravascular lithotripsy in calcified, femoropopliteal lesions: results of Disrupt PAD II. Catheter Cardiovasc Interv. 2019;93(2):335–42. https://doi.org/10.1002/ccd.27943.

46. Makowsky MJ, McAlister FA, Galbraith PD, Southern DA, Ghali WA, Knudtson ML, Tsuyuki RT, Alberta Provincial Program for Outcome Assessment in Coronary Heart Disease (APPROACH) Investigators. Lower extremity peripheral arterial disease in individuals with coronary artery disease: prognostic importance, care gaps, and impact of therapy. Am Heart J. 2008;155(2):348–55. https://doi.org/10.1016/j.ahj.2007.09.005.

Arrhythmia Management in the Elderly

Ryan Wallace and Hugh Calkins

1 Introduction

Arrhythmias cause significant mortality and impair the quality of life in the elderly. The prevalence of cardiac arrhythmias and disorders of impulse formation and conduction increase with age as the myocardium is progressively replaced with fibro-fatty tissue [1–3]. As the US population ages and as cardiovascular care for coronary disease and heart failure continues to improve, the prevalence and burden of electrophysiologic disorders will continue to rise. In the American Heart Association's 2021 Update on Heart Disease and Stroke statistics, the prevalence of many common arrhythmias, including atrial fibrillation, sinoatrial node dysfunction, and atrial fibrillation, continue to increase in prevalence with increasing age and are often associated with an increase in mortality. Atrial fibrillation was measured at a prevalence of 5.2 million in 2010 and is estimated to more than 12.1 million in 2030 [4]. These disorders often require the involvement of cardiovascular specialists and can present challenging management dilemmas. The purpose of this chapter is to review the current information concerning arrhythmia management in the elderly.

1.1 Aging and the Conduction System

With normal aging, the cardiac skeleton becomes fibrotic and calcified. These changes begin to appear in pathology specimens around 30–40 years of age and can lead to the disruption of the AV node and bundle branches. Despite the high

R. Wallace · H. Calkins (✉)
Division of Cardiology, Department of Medicine, Johns Hopkins University, School of Medicine, Baltimore, MD, USA
e-mail: rwalla29@jhmi.edu; hcalkins@jhmi.edu

© The Author(s), under exclusive license to Springer Nature Switzerland AG 2023
T. M. Leucker, G. Gerstenblith (eds.), *Cardiovascular Disease in the Elderly*, Contemporary Cardiology, https://doi.org/10.1007/978-3-031-16594-8_6

prevalence of ischemic disease in the Western World, age-related increases in oxidative stress and fibrosis are the most common causes of complete atrioventricular (AV) block [5–9]. Similar changes can be observed in the atria, the sinoatrial node (SAN), and the ventricular myocardium [10]. This leads to an increase in SAN recovery time and loss of atrial voltages with aging, suggesting decreased SAN function [11]. Progressive myocardial fibrosis in the ventricles creates a substrate prone to ventricular arrhythmias. Lastly, amyloid deposition may also play a role in age-related conduction disorders, as 23% of patients over 60 years of age have evidence of amyloid deposition in the atrial myocardium [9].

1.2 Electrocardiographic Changes in the Elderly

The evaluation of the conduction system in elderly patients begins with a history, physical examination, and a resting 12-lead electrocardiogram. Despite the proliferation of other diagnostic modalities, the electrocardiogram (ECG) remains an integral noninvasive diagnostic technique for the cardiovascular evaluation of elderly individuals.

Electrocardiographic abnormalities are common in the elderly. Among 5150 adults older than 65 years old enrolled in the Cardiovascular Health Study, 29% had abnormal findings on their ECG [12]. Between 0.9% and 6.8% of elderly individuals have first-degree AV block consistent with age-related atrophy and fibrosis of the AV node [13, 14]. With respect to ventricular activation, elderly individuals exhibit a leftward shift in the QRS axis, an increased prevalence of bundle branch disease, and an increase in nonspecific repolarization abnormalities such as inverted T waves. Some of these findings, specifically Q waves, ST depressions >0.5 mm, and complete bundle branch blocks, are associated with an increase in mortality in men [15].

When evaluating the elderly, special attention should be given to electrocardiographic evidence of left ventricular hypertrophy (LVH) through either the modified Cornell criteria, the Sokolow-Lyon, or the Romhilt-Estes criteria. While the ECG is not sensitive to the detection of LVH, it is highly specific. The presence of electrocardiographic evidence of LVH is an important finding in the elderly because it is a predictor of heart failure, premature cardiovascular death, and mortality [16, 17].

2 Bradyarrhythmias

2.1 Sick Sinus Syndrome

Sick sinus syndrome (SSS) is common in elderly populations, accounts for approximately one-half of pacemaker insertions in the US, and has been associated with an increased prevalence of falls and syncope in the elderly [18–20]. The term "sick sinus syndrome" was first used by Bernard Lown in 1967 to describe the slow return of sinus node activity following DC cardioversion [21]. This bradyarrhythmic syndrome is characterized by chronic inappropriate bradycardia accompanied by symptomatic sinus pauses with an inadequate junctional escape rhythm and sinoatrial block. More than half of patients with SSS have AV conduction disturbances and tachyarrhythmias. These patients are said to have a tachycardia-bradycardia syndrome. The diagnosis of tachycardia-bradycardia syndrome in a patient with SSS is concerning because tachycardia-mediated overdrive suppression can lead to long sinus pauses following the termination of an atrial arrhythmia.

The bradyarrhythmia in SSS can be due to either impaired impulse initiation or impaired impulse propagation. SSS can be caused by several pathological processes, including infiltrative processes such as sarcoidosis, amyloidosis or hemochromatosis, inflammatory pericardial processes, and metabolic disorders such as hypothyroidism. However, it is most commonly caused by the progressive and degenerative fibrous replacement of the SA node [22]. This same fibrosis underlies the atrial tachyarrhythmias that often accompany sinoatrial node dysfunction.

In patients suspected of having bradyarrhythmia and/or sinus node dysfunction, the main goal of their evaluation is to determine if the patient has symptomatic bradyarrhythmia. This is most readily accomplished with a 24 Holter monitor, an event monitor, or in-hospital telemetry monitoring. Although EP testing can also be used to evaluate sinus node function, its sensitivity is low. For this reason, EP testing is typically only used to evaluate sinus node function among patients with syncope in whom an obvious cause of syncope cannot be identified and who have significant cardiac disease. Pacemaker placement is recommended for treating most patients with symptomatic bradyarrhythmia unless the bradyarrhythmia is due to a transient and reversible cause (e.g. recent initiation of beta-blocker therapy where the indication for beta-blocker therapy is not compelling). Otherwise, patients who are asymptomatic can be followed over time and monitored for the development of symptoms attributable to bradycardia, which would prompt pacemaker placement. In those for whom pacemaker placement is pursued, the type of pacing used should be guided by a number of factors, such as the presence of AV conduction abnormalities, age, and comorbidities of heart failure with reduced ejection fraction [23]. More often than not, DDD(R) pacing should be the first choice over VVIR in patients with sinus node dysfunction, as it leads to lower rates of AF and reduces HF symptoms [24, 25]. DDD(R) also showed benefit over AAIR in terms of reduced incidence of paroxysmal AF and reduced rates of reoperation because of the development of AV block [20].

2.2 *Atrioventricular Block*

Following atrial activation, the electrical impulse must be propagated through the AV node and the bundle of His before it can activate the bundle branches. It has long been observed that AV conduction is prolonged with age. The AV node is the first part of the conduction system to be affected by age-related fibrosis, as fatty infiltrates and collagen interposition in AV nodal tissues begin to appear at 30 years of age [26]. Over time, these changes lead to delayed impulse propagation and predispose to the fractionation of AV conduction and subsequent reentry. These age-related delays in AV conduction are primarily localized to the AV node and the proximal portion of the His bundle [26].

Patients with impaired AV conduction may be asymptomatic or may present with syncope, light-headedness, and fatigue. AV conduction block can be classified as first-degree, second-degree, and third-degree atrioventricular block (also known as complete heart block). The differential diagnosis of AV block includes primary and secondary AV block. Conditions associated with secondary AV block include myocardial ischemia, enhanced vagal tone, drug effect (including digitalis intoxication, beta blockers, non-dihydropyridine calcium channel blockers, and class I antiarrhythmics), Lyme disease, syphilis, calcific aortic stenosis, aortic valve ring abscesses, and infiltrative disorders which include hemochromatosis, amyloidosis, and sarcoidosis.

First-degree AV block is defined by a PR interval longer than 200 ms. The incidence of primary first-degree heart block increases with age and is associated with a moderate increase in the PR interval (200–230 ms). First-degree AV block has been associated with increased rates of atrial fibrillation, heart failure, all-cause mortality, and pacemaker implantation [27, 28].

Second-degree AV block includes Mobitz type I and Mobitz type II block. Mobitz type I or Wenckebach block is characterized by progressive lengthening of the PR interval and intermittent block. In contrast, Mobitz type II second-degree AV block is associated with an intermittent irregular block without PR interval lengthening. The key step in evaluating a patient with second-degree heart block is determining whether or not Mobitz type II block is present, as Mobitz type II indicates distal His pathology and a high risk of progression to complete heart block. Because of these high-risk features, Mobitz type II second-degree AV block, like complete heart block, is a class I indication for permanent pacemaker insertion [23]. Similar to patients with SSS, DDD(R) pacing is preferred over VVIR given lower rates of pacemaker syndrome and to minimize unnecessary ventricular pacing, which has been associated with pacing-induced cardiomyopathy and worsened LV systolic dysfunction [29].

2.3 Bundle Branch Disease

Bundle branch block (BBB) is highly age-dependent, with a prevalence of 1.2% among those aged 50 years and a prevalence of 17% among those aged 80 years [30]. A common dilemma facing clinicians is how to manage patients with chronic bifascicular block. These patients are said to be "hanging by a fascicle." Fortunately, chronic bifascicular block rarely progresses to complete heart block. In fact, among patients with BBB, only 1% per year progress to complete heart block [31].

Given the low risk for progression to heart block, it is generally agreed that asymptomatic patients with bifascicular and trifascicular block should not undergo pacemaker implantation. Class I indications for pacemaker insertion in patients with chronic bifascicular and trifascicular block include: symptomatic bradycardia, intermittent complete heart block, and intermittent type II second-degree AV block. Patients with unexplained syncope who have evidence of underlying conduction system disease can undergo an EP study. Pacemaker placement is indicated for those patients with an H-V interval greater or equal to 70 ms, or other evidence of intranodal block during the EP study [23]. EP testing is not indicated for the asymptomatic patient with an underlying bundle branch block pattern on ECG.

The presence of bundle branch block may also accompany other indications for internal cardioverter defibrillator (ICD) placement. Patients with BBB and LVEF ≤35% should undergo ICD or cardiac resynchronization therapy defibrillator (CRT-D) placement for primary prevention of sudden cardiac death (SCD). CRT-D is recommended in these patients if they are in normal sinus rhythm with a LBBB QRS morphology measuring ≥150 ms. CRT-D can be considered in those with narrower QRS of 130–149 if symptomatic, those with QRS ≥150 ms with a non-LBBB morphology [32].

3   Tachyarrhythmias

3.1   *Supraventricular Arrhythmias*

3.1.1   Paroxysmal Supraventricular Tachycardia

The term paroxysmal supraventricular tachycardia (PSVT) generally refers to a clinical syndrome characterized by a sustained regular supraventricular arrhythmia of abrupt onset and termination. Two-thirds of all cases of PSVT result from atrioventricular nodal reentrant tachycardia. The remaining one-third of patients with PSVT have an accessory pathway that provides a substrate for atrioventricular reciprocating tachycardia. In very unusual cases, PSVT may result from a reentrant atrial tachycardia, such as sinus node reentrant tachycardia, or from an ectopic atrial focus. While the incidence of PSVT peaks in the fifth decade, patients 65 years and older have five times the risk of developing PSVT compared to their younger counterparts [23, 31].

The presentation of PSVT can vary dramatically. Some patients complain of palpitations, light-headedness, neck-pounding, and fatigue, others remain asymptomatic, while a few present with syncope. If an episode of PSVT is prolonged, patients may report polyuria because of atrial stretch-mediated release of atrial natriuretic peptide. Generally, the physical examination has limited diagnostic value in the diagnosis of PSVT. This reflects the fact that most episodes of PSVT terminate spontaneously. Furthermore, the physical examination is rarely informative in the rare situation when tachycardia is ongoing.

Evaluation of a patient with PSVT should include a search for possible precipitants, including infection, hypoxemia, anemia, and metabolic disturbances. The first step in management includes an assessment of the patient's vital signs. Hemodynamically unstable PSVT, like any unstable tachyarrhythmia, should be treated with immediate DC cardioversion; otherwise, attempts should be made to obtain an ECG and abort the arrhythmia with vagal maneuvers.

If PSVT does not terminate with vagal maneuvers, therapeutic and diagnostic administration of adenosine is recommended. Adenosine should be administered in a rapid bolus with an initial dose of 6 mg (3 mg if given through central venous access). If the tachycardia persists, 12 mg of adenosine should be administered (6 mg if given through central venous access). The only contraindications to adenosine are a history of severe bronchospastic pulmonary disease or second or third AV block. Adenosine should never be administered unless the patient is being monitored and a defibrillator is present. Rarely, on termination of PSVT, atrial fibrillation appears. If a patient has a rapidly conducting accessory pathway, this may lead to ventricular fibrillation. Rarely, adenosine administration will result in the persistence of tachycardia with AV block. This finding excludes an arrhythmia involving the AV node and strongly suggests that the underlying arrhythmia is either atrial tachycardia or atrial flutter. If the arrhythmia does not terminate with adenosine, a calcium channel blocker or beta blocker can be considered.

Once PSVT has been terminated, either spontaneously or following adenosine, a long-term treatment strategy can be developed. In general, the approach to treatment depends on the severity and frequency of symptoms and patient preference. Catheter ablation is considered appropriate first-line therapy for PSVT, particularly among patients with frequent tachycardic episodes, hemodynamic intolerance, or who have failed an attempt at empiric therapy with a beta blocker or calcium channel blocker. As discussed below, catheter ablation is also recommended for all patients with PSVT that occurs in the setting of the Wolff-Parkinson-White Syndrome. For patients who are not interested in catheter ablation, alternate treatment strategies include clinical follow-up without specific therapy, empiric treatment with a calcium channel blocker or beta blocker, or rarely a class 1c anti-arrhythmic agent such as flecainide or propafenone [33] (Fig. 1).

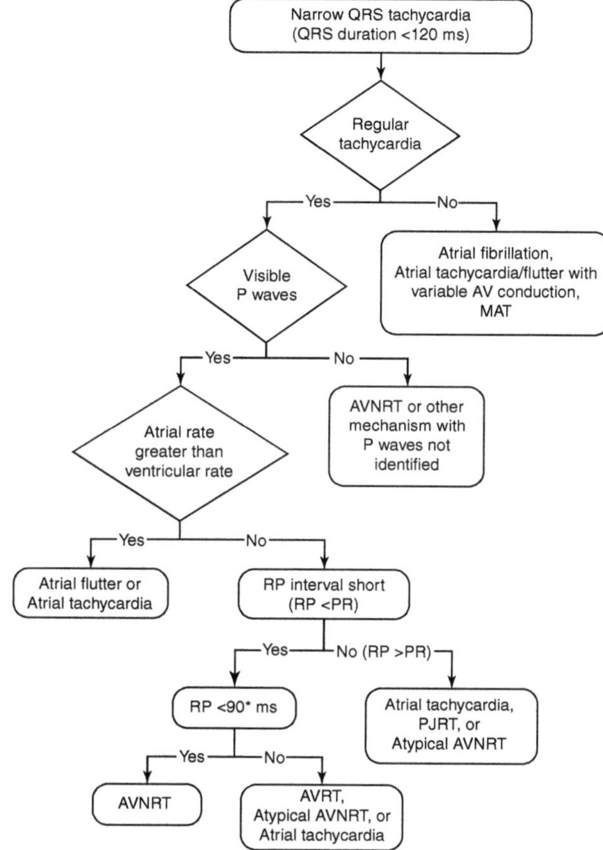

Fig. 1 Diagnostic algorithm for narrow QRS tachycardias. (Adapted from [33])

3.2 AV Nodal Reentrant Tachycardia

AV nodal reentrant tachycardia (AVNRT) is the most common cause of PSVT in the elderly, accounting for approximately two-thirds of all cases [34, 35]. The presence of a narrow complex tachycardia with a regular RR interval at a rate of 140–250 beats per minute without P waves or with retrograde P waves in the ST segment suggests the presence of AVNRT.

The AV node is a compact bundle of atrial tissue located at the apex of the triangle of Koch. In AVNRT, the presence of a second conducting pathway (with a different refractory period) adjacent to the AV node enables a unidirectional block and formation of a reentrant circuit involving both the fast and slow pathways. This unique anatomic relationship enables the adjacent slow pathway to be safely ablated with a success rate in excess of 95% [36]. Since the elderly are at the greatest risk for adverse events related to long-term oral anti-arrhythmic therapy, radio frequency ablation should be considered first-line therapy in all active elderly individuals who

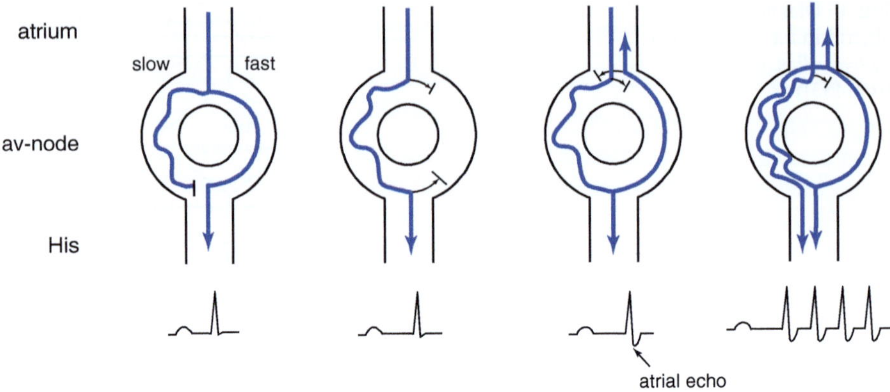

Fig. 2 Cartoon of dual pathway physiology in AVNRT with accompanying ECG

are willing to accept the less than 1% risk of AV block associated with catheter ablation of AVNRT [36, 37].

Often, ECG changes are observed during an episode of AVNRT or shortly thereafter. Significant ST-segment depressions can be seen during tachycardia in 25–50% of patients with AVNRT; however, these changes are not predictive of ischemia [38]. Additionally, there is no correlation between the rate of tachycardia and the presence or extent of ST segment changes. Other ECG changes may be seen during or after the termination of AVNRT. Newly acquired T wave inversion after the termination of AVNRT, commonly in anterior or inferior leads, can be present in nearly 40% of patients [39]. Despite the concern that is often raised with these ECG changes, there is no significant association between AVNRT and underlying structural heart disease (Fig. 2). Furthermore, ST depressions and elevated troponin I were not associated with either coronary artery disease or acute coronary syndrome [40, 41].

3.3   *Accessory Pathway Tachycardias*

Accessory pathways are anatomically distinct atrioventricular connections that form due to incomplete separation of the myocardium during development. These connections bypass the AV node and can lead to premature excitation of the ventricle. Accessory pathways can conduct from the atrium to the ventricle, from the ventricle to the atrium, or both. Accessory pathways that only conduct from the ventricle to the atrium are not apparent on a 12-lead ECG and are referred to as "concealed" pathways. In contrast, anterograde conducting accessory pathways result in premature activation of the ventricle and give the typical pattern of preexcitation on the ECG. Features of preexcitation include a short PR interval, a slurred QRS upstroke (delta wave), and a widened QRS complex. The

Wolff-Parkinson-White syndrome is an accessory pathway syndrome characterized by the presence of delta-waves on the 12 lead ECG in conjunction with supraventricular arrhythmias. Because patients with Wolff-Parkinson-White syndrome have an increased risk of sudden death, catheter ablation is considered the standard of care for these patients.

Among patients with an accessory pathway, the most common arrhythmia is orthodromic atrioventricular reciprocating tachycardia (AVRT). This tachycardia involves anterograde conduction through the AV node to the ventricles and retrograde conduction from the ventricles to the atrium via the accessory pathway. Orthodromic AV reciprocating tachycardia typically presents as a narrow complex tachycardia. Antidromic AVRT, a less common arrhythmia, involves the same reentrant circuit, but the wavefront travels anterogradely from the atrium to the ventricle via the accessory pathway and results in a wide complex tachycardia.

3.4 Sinus Tachycardia

Elderly individuals frequently present with sinus tachycardia. Sinus tachycardia is marked by a gradual onset and termination and its diagnosis requires electrocardiographic evidence of sinus rhythm. Sinus activation results in a P wave vector between $0°$ and $90°$ with positive deflections in leads I, II, and aVF and a negative deflection in lead aVR. The presence of sinus tachycardia almost always represents an appropriate physiologic response to a demand stressor. In the elderly, the differential diagnosis is broad, but consideration should be given to hyperthyroidism, occult gastro intestinal bleeding, pulmonary embolism, and infection. Since this rhythm represents an appropriate physiologic response, treatment should be directed at the underlying etiology. Inappropriate sinus tachycardia is defined as sinus tachycardia in the absence of a physiologic stimulus. This condition is rare and virtually never occurs in the elderly.

3.5 Multifocal Atrial Tachycardia

Multifocal atrial tachycardia (MAT) is an uncommon arrhythmia seen in critically ill elderly inpatients, with a mean age at diagnosis of about 70 years [42]. MAT is rare, but when it does occur, it is usually in the setting of an intensive care unit admission due to an exacerbation of underlying pulmonary disease (especially chronic obstructive pulmonary disease). MAT portends an ominous prognosis with an in-hospital mortality rate of 45% [43]. This high mortality rate likely reflects the severity of the underlying disease, not the presence of MAT itself [44]. Clinically, MAT is often mistaken for atrial fibrillation because it is an irregular narrow complex rhythm. The diagnosis of MAT rests on an atrial rate greater than 100 beats per minute, the presence of three unique P wave morphologies, and irregular R-R intervals. Like sinus tachycardia, the treatment is directed at reversing the underlying cause; however, previous studies have shown that metoprolol and verapamil can be useful for rate-control [42].

3.6 Atrial Flutter

Atrial flutter occurs 100 times more often in those aged 80 years and older as compared to younger persons [45]. Risk factors for atrial flutter include advancing age, heart failure, and chronic obstructive pulmonary disease. Among patients who present with supraventricular tachycardia, approximately 10% will have an atrial flutter [46]. Atrial flutter is a macroreentrant atrial tachycardia distinguished by its atrial rate—which typically ranges from 250 to 350 bpm. The reentrant circuit in atrial flutter is almost always located in the right atrium, commonly involving the cavotricuspid isthmus, an isolated area of slowed conduction anatomically bound by the coronary sinus, the inferior vena cava, the tricuspid annulus, and the eustachian ridge. Also known as typical flutter or type 1 flutter, this common type of atrial flutter is characterized by a counterclockwise wavefront in the right atrium that gives rise to negative flutter waves in leads II, III, and aVF, with positive atrial deflections in lead V1. Reverse atrial flutter involves the same reentrant circuit, but the wavefront travels in a clockwise direction leading to the opposite orientation of the flutter waves. In contrast to type 1 atrial flutter, atypical or type 2 atrial flutter is a more rapid arrhythmia that results from functional reentry. Atrial flutter is commonly associated with the presence of structural heart disease; thus, patients with no known structural heart disease should undergo an investigative echocardiogram to evaluate cardiac function and left atrial size [47].

The management of atrial flutter consists of two main strategies. Because atrial flutter is associated with an increased risk of stroke, systemic anticoagulation is recommended for all patients with atrial flutter who have other risk factors for stroke (including age >75 years). The 2019 Focused Update from American Heart Association (AHA)/American College of Cardiology (ACC)/Heart Rhythm Society (HRS) Guidelines recommended a preference for direct oral anticoagulants (DOACs) over warfarin in patients eligible for DOACs [48]. If a patient has symptomatic atrial flutter, treatment to restore sinus rhythm is indicated. This can involve a cardioversion procedure in the short term. However, a previous randomized clinical trial demonstrated that catheter ablation is superior to pharmacologic therapy in the maintenance of sinus rhythm in patients with atrial flutter [49]. For this reason, catheter ablation is considered first-line therapy if in line with patient preference. Catheter ablation can be performed on an outpatient basis and is associated with a greater than 90% efficacy and a <1% risk of major complications [50, 51]. If a patient prefers pharmacologic therapy, a rate control strategy can be pursued with beta blockers or calcium channel blockers. Additionally, class 1c (in the absence of structural heart disease) or class 3 anti-arrhythmics can be considered if pursuing a rhythm control strategy. The selection of an anti-arrhythmic agent is generally based on the drug's side effect profile. Pharmacologic therapy is successful in the long-term suppression of atrial flutter in approximately 50% of patients.

3.7 *Atrial Fibrillation*

Atrial fibrillation (AF) is a reentrant supraventricular tachycardia that is confined to the atrium. This tachyarrhythmia is characterized by (1) the absence of organized atrial activity, (2) the presence of irregular oscillations or fibrillatory waves, and (3) an irregularly irregular ventricular rate. AF is by far the most common and clinically important supraventricular tachycardia. AF prevalence was estimated at 5.2 million Americans in 2010, a figure that is expected to increase to 12.1 million in 2030 in the next 50 years [52]. Not surprisingly, the prevalence of AF increases with age. Starting at age 65 years, the prevalence of AF increases by 5% per year [53]. Patients who were without AF at age 55 years were followed and found to have a cumulative incidence of AF by age 90 years ranging from one in five to as high as one in three depending on risk profile [54]. Among patients undergoing cardiac surgery, older age was a predictor of postoperative AF (POAF), and this was associated with an increased risk for stroke [55, 56]. Patients who already have a history of AF and are undergoing cardiac surgery may be considered for left atrial appendage occlusion to reduce ischemic stroke risk [57].

Although AF is common, it is not a benign rhythm and is associated with considerable morbidity and mortality. Most importantly, AF increases the risk of stroke, accounts for approximately one-sixth of all strokes in the United States, and particularly increases stroke risk in elderly patients [58, 59]. In the Framingham Heart Study, patients with AF had a two- to threefold increase in cardiovascular mortality (Fig. 3) [60]. Patients with lone AF over the age of 60 years have been found to have a marked increase in cardiovascular events [61].

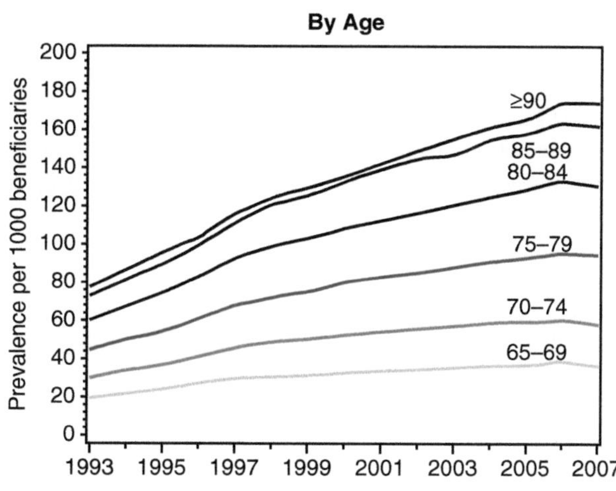

Fig. 3 Bar graph—Prevalence of atrial fibrillation by age [53, 60]

Once initiated, AF is composed of multiple reentrant circuits with a cycle length between 150 and 300 ms. The decremental conduction properties of the AV node prevent most of these atrial impulses from reaching the ventricle. AF facilitates its own propagation by shortening the atrial refractory period, mostly through reductions in L-type calcium channel current. Previously, it has been taught that the initiation of AF, much like sustained AF, was not a focal process. Associations with hyperthyroidism and ethanol consumption appeared to support this hypothesis. However, it has become clear that the spontaneous initiation of AF is often due to isolated rapidly firing foci that are found in the right atrium, left atrium, superior vena cava, the coronary sinus, and most commonly, the pulmonary vein ostia [62]. Over the past decades, it has been demonstrated that ectopic foci in the pulmonary vein ostia are amenable to ablation techniques and that pulmonary vein ablation can be a very effective treatment for AF.

The management of AF includes: (1) an evaluation of underlying etiology and risk stratification, (2) selecting a rhythm versus rate-control strategy, and (3) stroke prophylaxis [47, 48]. Patients suspected of having AF should undergo 24-hour Holter monitoring. All patients with a new diagnosis of atrial fibrillation should undergo echocardiography to evaluate the presence of any structural heart disease and to identify high-risk features for stroke. The size of the left atrium provides a general assessment of how long a patient has been in atrial fibrillation and the probability that sinus rhythm can be restored and maintained. The chance of successful conversion in a patient with a left atrial size greater than six cm is extremely small. Chest radiography should be obtained if there is suspicion of pulmonary disease as a contributing factor in the development of AF. Thyroid function should also be assessed, as AF may be the only presenting symptom of thyroid disease. Other blood work, including blood counts, renal and hepatic function, as well as electrolytes, should be obtained to evaluate for other possible inciting factors.

When a patient presents with AF, the onset and duration of the arrhythmia must be determined. Patients who present within 48 hours of onset are candidates for immediate pharmacologic or electrical conversion. However, more recent data suggest an increased risk for stroke in those greater than 75 years old, as well as in those where cardioversion was delayed >12 hours [63, 64]. Patients who otherwise present with AF longer than 48 hours must be anticoagulated for three weeks prior to cardioversion. The clinician can also pursue trans-esophageal echocardiography (TEE) guided cardioversion. If a patient has no evidence of LAA thrombi or spontaneous echo contrast on TEE examination, they can safely undergo cardioversion without increased risk of cardioembolic stroke. Conversely, all patients with AF for longer than 48 hours duration, regardless of their pre-cardioversion care, must be anticoagulated for four weeks following resumption of sinus rhythm. This strategy is necessary because there is a paradoxical increase in the rate of stroke in the first 48 hours following cardioversion due to LA stunning (localized tachycardia-mediated atrial cardiomyopathy) following the termination of AF.

While many debate the relative merits of rate-control and rhythm control, it is reasonable to give every patient at least one chance at cardioversion, regardless of their risk for recurrence. Cardioversion has an 86% success rate at 72 hours [65].

However, it is important to note that 68% of patients who present with AF of less than 72 hours duration will spontaneously convert to normal sinus rhythm [66]. Risk factors for arrhythmia recurrence include age greater than 75 years, LA diameter greater than 45 mm, AF >four weeks, presence of heart failure, LV systolic dysfunction, a history of prior cardioversion, greater $CHA_2DS_2S\text{-}VAS_c$, metabolic syndrome, and sleep apnea [67–70]. Utilization of a biphasic waveform achieves cardioversion at lower energy levels when compared with monophasic waveform defibrillation [71]. Anterior–posterior application of defibrillator leads are associated with increased cardioversion efficacy [72]. Lastly, maximum-fixed energy shocks may be more effective than starting with low energy shocks and escalating energy levels when cardioverting atrial fibrillation [73].

A central debate in clinical cardiology is whether patients with AF should be managed with rate-control or rhythm-based strategies. As mentioned previously, AF is not a benign rhythm. The presence of AF impairs cardiovascular hemodynamics through several mechanisms. Loss of synchronous atrial contraction results in impaired ventricular filling and elevation of left atrial end-diastolic pressures. Inappropriate tachycardia in AF decreases the diastolic filling interval, while irregular RR intervals are associated with decreased cardiac output, elevated pulmonary capillary wedge pressures, and elevated right atrial pressures. These alterations can lead to adverse cardiac remodeling and impaired LV function. Older patients with poor vascular compliance and diastolic dysfunction may not tolerate these changes as well as younger individuals, thus leading to impaired ventricular function and heart failure. Maintenance of sinus rhythm has several advantages, including relief of symptoms and improved hemodynamics. The considerations that should be given to each approach are discussed below [74–78].

Despite the common perception that rate control represents a "simpler" strategy, rate control can often be difficult to achieve, especially in patients with LV dysfunction. The target heart rate in a rate control strategy has been previously debated, but the RACE trial found that a lenient resting heart rate target of less than 110 versus less than 80 had similar rates of cardiovascular events [79]. This target HR should be adjusted based on the patient's symptoms and if there are signs of worsening LV function at more lenient heart rates. First-line rate control agents include beta-blockers and non-dihydropyridine calcium channel blockers. Digitalis preparations are rarely as adequate as monotherapy, especially in active individuals or those with high sympathetic drive, because digitalis lowers heart rate through a vagotonic mechanism. Digoxin has also been associated with higher rates of mortality in patients with AF, regardless of heart failure status [80]. The DIGIT-HF randomized control trial is currently underway to further investigate these findings, specifically in patients with heart failure [81].

When considering a rhythm control strategy, it is important to note that pharmacologic cardioversion is most successful when attempted within seven days of AF onset [82]. Although several drugs have been shown to limit the recurrence of AF, amiodarone appears to be more effective than sotalol and class I agents at maintaining sinus rhythm [83–85]. Selection of an initial anti-arrhythmic agent in AF should focus on the patient's underlying pathophysiology and comorbidities. For those patients without structural heart disease, flecainide, propafenone, and sotalol are all reasonable choices, given their tolerability and lower incidence of complications. The presence of ischemic heart disease is a relative contraindication for class 1c anti-arrhythmic drugs like flecainide or propafenone. A "pill in the pocket" approach can be considered with a self-administered dose of oral flecainide or propafenone in patients with infrequent paroxysmal AF episodes [86]. In young patients, disopyramide is often recommended for the treatment of vagally mediated atrial fibrillation, as well as for those with hypertrophic cardiomyopathy (HCM). However, it is important to note that disopyramide may exacerbate bladder outlet obstruction in elderly men and, therefore, should be avoided in this clinical situation. Similarly, beta-blockers should be considered in those patients with adrenergically mediated AF. Amiodarone is generally reserved for patients who have failed other anti-arrhythmic drugs and/or those with severe underlying cardiomyopathy. Although amiodarone has been shown to have the greatest efficacy for the treatment of atrial fibrillation, it is associated with important side effects, including thyroid disease, pulmonary disease, and peripheral neuropathy. Amiodarone may also result in impairment of vision. For these reasons, screening is required to allow for early detection of amiodarone-induced side effects.

Several randomized controlled trials have compared a primary strategy of rate control versus rhythm control [87–90]. These studies have been limited by selection bias, exclusion criteria, limited follow-up duration, and varying efficacy in the rhythm control arm. The data from these studies suggested that in the short term (i.e. one–three years of follow-up), rate-control is not inferior to a rhythm control strategy. However, the recent EAST-AF trial showed not only a reduction in stroke but also cardiovascular mortality and heart failure hospitalization in those with early AF and in whom an early rhythm control strategy was pursued. Early AF was defined as new onset AF within 12 months of diagnosis [78]. Otherwise, it has been observed that the maintenance of sinus rhythm may be difficult to achieve, as only 40–60% of the patients in the rhythm control arms actually were in sinus rhythm at the conclusion of these older trials. Also, in several of the trials, most of the cardioembolic events occurred in the rhythm control groups. Patients with risk factors for stroke should continue to receive anticoagulation even after sinus rhythm is maintained. Lastly and not unexpectedly, exercise tolerance was better in patients managed with rhythm control.

In addition to the findings of the EAST-AF trial, there is growing evidence of potential situations when rhythm control strategy may be beneficial. The recent CASTLE-AF trial found that in patients with heart failure with reduced ejection fraction (HFrEF), a rhythm control strategy through catheter ablation was superior to medical management (either rate or rhythm control) in reducing mortality, hospitalizations for heart failure while showing a greater improvement in LVEF and greater maintenance of sinus rhythm [91]. Catheter ablation was also superior to amiodarone in maintaining sinus rhythm in patients with a history of HFrEF and persistent AF [92]. On the other hand, the results of the CABANA trial found there were no reductions in cardiovascular outcomes with catheter ablation in a more generalizable patient population [76]. Taken together, and given the progressive nature of atrial fibrillation ("atrial fibrillation begets atrial fibrillation"), the evidence showing benefit in early rhythm control, and the effectiveness of catheter ablation to achieve and maintain rhythm control, it may be reasonable to pursue an initial trial of rhythm control through an ablation [93, 94].

If a patient has asymptomatic atrial fibrillation, rate control and systemic anticoagulation are considered the standard of care. However, attempts at cardioversion could be considered if this is the patient's first episode of atrial fibrillation. In contrast, rhythm control with catheter-based therapy should be considered for patients with symptomatic atrial fibrillation. Anti-arrhythmic therapy is generally the first step. As discussed earlier, the selection of anti-arrhythmic agents is based largely on the drug's side effect profile and potential for proarrhythmia. Amiodarone is an effective pharmacologic agent but is associated with many potential side effects. For this reason, it is rarely considered first-line therapy. Catheter ablation of atrial fibrillation has made tremendous strides over the past several years. Catheter ablation is indicated for patients with highly symptomatic atrial fibrillation, which has been refractory to attempts at pharmacologic therapy. The one-year efficacy of this procedure for patients with paroxysmal atrial fibrillation is approximately 75%.

4 Ventricular Arrhythmias

4.1 Monomorphic Ventricular Tachycardia

There are two important types of reentrant ventricular arrhythmias, ventricular tachycardia (VT) and ventricular fibrillation (VF). VT can be further subdivided based on its morphology into monomorphic VT and polymorphic VT. These descriptive labels are very helpful from a diagnostic standpoint because they shed light on the etiology behind each dysrhythmia. To be more specific, monomorphic VT is caused by fixed reentry, and polymorphic VT is caused by dynamic reentry. Therefore, after examining the patient's rhythm strip, the clinician is immediately clued into the possible etiologies of the ventricular arrhythmia.

Sustained monomorphic ventricular tachycardia (SMVT) is usually due to the presence of a fixed reentrant circuit in the ventricle. Almost all patients with this type of VT have some form of structural heart disease which accounts for the presence of this abnormal reentrant circuit, most commonly prior to myocardial infarction (MI). The border zone of an MI is often characterized by an island of fibrosis surrounded by living tissue. Myocardial scar enables unidirectional block and establishes the milieu necessary for reentry. Sustained VT in the setting of structural heart disease (and, therefore, not idiopathic) is associated with an increased risk of SCD. VT requires aggressive evaluation and treatment, often with ICD implantation for secondary prevention.

VT must be differentiated from aberrantly conducted supraventricular arrhythmias. ECG features that suggest ventricular origin include A/V dissociation (apparent in 30%), QRS complex duration longer than 160 ms, a shift in the QRS axis, and the presence of fusion beats. While these features are helpful, the patient's history may be more informative. In patients with a history of coronary artery disease (CAD), greater than 95% of wide complex tachycardia represents VT.

4.2 Polymorphic Ventricular Tachycardia

Polymorphic ventricular tachycardia is a form of VT in which there is variation in the axis and morphology of the QRS complex. Unlike monomorphic VT, which is usually caused by a fixed reentrant circuit, polymorphic VT is due to heterogeneity in ventricular repolarization. Polymorphic VT is most commonly seen under the following situations; (1) long QT syndrome resulting in torsade de pointes, (2) pro-arrhythmia resulting from a drug-induced prolongation of the QT interval and torsade, (3) severe dilated cardiomyopathy, and (4) severe ischemic disease with ongoing ischemia (e.g., left main CAD).

4.3 Ventricular Fibrillation

VF is a rapid, irregular tachycardia arising in the ventricles that results from multiple reentrant circuits. The ECG features of VF include a rapid (>250 bpm) and very irregular wide complex tachycardia.

Ventricular fibrillation may occur as a primary arrhythmia or may result from degeneration of VT to VF. As VF continues, global myocardial ischemia ensues, and post-repolarization refractoriness and conduction delay increase [78, 95]. Unless terminated, VF results rapidly in SCD. Most patients who experience VF have cardiac disease, especially CAD. Although VF can occur within 24 hours of acute myocardial infarction, the vast majority of VF does not.

4.4 Evaluation of Ventricular Arrhythmias in the Elderly

The evaluation of a patient who has experienced a sustained or nonsustained ventricular arrhythmia involves several steps. In the case of VT, the first step is to determine if the event was sustained or not. Sustained VT is defined as VT lasting longer than 30 s, hemodynamic instability, or severely symptomatic (chest pain, shortness of breath, dizziness). On the other hand, asymptomatic nonsustained VT lasts less than 30 s and rarely requires further treatment unless otherwise indicated. There are exceptions to this rule. Patients with cardiomyopathy may benefit from ICD placement for primary prevention of SCD, which is discussed later in this chapter. The second step in the evaluation of a patient with ventricular arrhythmia involves an ischemic evaluation. Elderly patients without structural heart disease or exercise-induced NSVT do not appear to have an increased risk of sudden death [96].

4.5 Management of Ventricular Arrhythmias

Management of patients with ventricular arrhythmias is focused on assessing the severity of symptoms and risk for sudden death. The role of defibrillator therapy in the primary and secondary prevention of sudden death is discussed later. For patients who are not at high risk of sudden death, the treatment of ventricular arrhythmias is directed at reducing symptoms and episodes. Treatment options include pharmacologic agents such as beta blockers and anti-arrhythmic agents, as well as catheter ablation. The success of catheter ablation is highly dependent on the arrhythmia being ablated. Among patients with idiopathic VT arising from the right ventricular outflow tract, catheter ablation is associated with efficacy greater than 90%. In contrast, the success of catheter ablation in cases of scar-related VT is much more dependent on the ability to obtain accurate electroanatomical or substrate mapping to guide ablation.

4.6 Secondary Prevention of Sudden Cardiac Death

In the late 1970s, Michel Mirokski pioneered the development of the ICD at Sinai Hospital in Baltimore. His work led to the first implantation of an ICD at the Johns Hopkins Hospital in 1980 [97]. Since that time, the number of ICDs implanted per annum has increased significantly.

Patients with a history of sustained VT and prior myocardial infarction are at high risk for future SCD. The survival rate to discharge for out-of-hospital cardiac arrest is low; however, this has improved from 5.7% in 2005 to 20.8% in 2012 and has been largely attributed to a focus in early CPR [98, 99]. As a result, the ICD became the focus of several clinical trials aimed at secondary prevention of sudden cardiac death due to the risk of proarrhythmia with drug treatment and the association between time-to-defibrillation and survival. The Anti-arrhythmics Versus Implantable Defibrillators (AVID) trial randomized 1016 survivors of cardiac arrest (455 patients had VT, 561 patients had VF) to conventional anti-arrhythmic treatment versus ICD implantation. When the investigators found a significant reduction in mortality in the ICD group (15.8% versus 24.0%) after 18.2 months of follow-up, the trial was terminated prematurely [100]. The mortality benefit in AVID seemed to be restricted to those patients with an LVEF <35%, confirming the predictive power of LV dysfunction for SCD. The results of this trial were soon confirmed by two other secondary prevention trials: the Canadian Implantable Defibrillator Study (CIDS) and the Cardiac Arrest Study Hamburg (CASH). A meta-analysis of approximately 900 patients enrolled in randomized controlled trials (RCTs) of secondary prevention found a 27% risk reduction for SCD after ICD implantation [101]. Consistent with the results of these studies, ICDs are indicated as secondary prevention for the treatment of almost all survivors of sudden cardiac death due to VT/VF. ICDs are also recommended for the treatment of sustained ventricular arrhythmias that occur in the setting of structural heart disease, in those with ischemic heart disease who present with cardiac syncope and an LVEF <35% or with inducible VA on EP study [102]. Patients whose physicians recommend foregoing ICD placement include those with identified reversible causes (e.g. drug-related ischemia).

4.7 *Primary Prevention of Sudden Cardiac Death*

While our attempts at secondary prevention have been successful, patients with a history of lethal ventricular arrhythmia only account for only 5–10% of sudden cardiac death victims in the US [103]. Primary prevention varies based on the underlying disease that places the patient at risk for SCD and VT/VF. In ischemic heart disease, the amount of MI plays a pivotal role in determining whether a patient would benefit from ICD placement. Based on the results of the MADIT-II and SCD-HeFT trial, patients who are greater than 40 days from MI and greater than 90 days from revascularization and have either an LVEF of <30% with NYHA class I symptoms or LVEF <35% with NYHA II or III symptoms reduces all-cause mortality [104, 105]. If it has been less than 40 days since MI, an ICD should not be implanted as it has not been shown to reduce all-cause mortality [106]. Instead, goal directed medical therapy (GDMT) should be pursued, and LVEF should be reevaluated past 40 days since the MI and 90 days post revascularization. Wearable cardioverter defibrillators can be considered in the immediate post-MI period (up to 40 days), but they have not been shown to reduce arrhythmic death [107].

ICDs also have a role to play in the primary prevention of nonischemic dilated cardiomyopathy. Current guidelines recommend ICD placement in patients with non-ischemic cardiomyopathy (NICM) who have LVEF <35% and NYHA class II or III symptoms despite GDMT. Multiple RCTs have contributed to the formation of these guidelines. The DANISH and DEFINITE trials did not find any difference in all-cause mortality but did find a reduction in SCD in those with ICDs. However, a meta-analysis including these trials and multiple other RCTs investigating ICD use in NICM showed reductions in all-cause mortality with ICD use [108].

EP testing has a limited role in both ischemic cardiomyopathy (ICM) and NICM. For ICM, the presence of sustained inducible VT would prompt ICD placement. For NICM, syncope has been associated with higher mortality. Given syncopal episodes may be possibly cardiac in origin, an EP study can be used to further investigate if syncope is due to a VA. If EP study shows inducible VA, ICD should be considered (Figs. 4 and 5) [102].

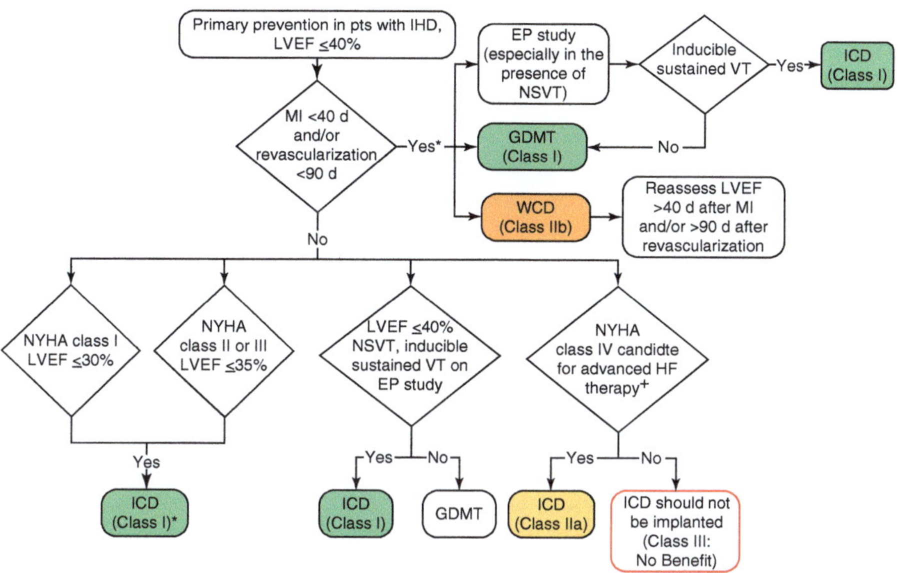

Fig. 4 AHA/ACC/HRS Primary Prevention in Ischemic Heart Disease ICD implantation guidelines [102]

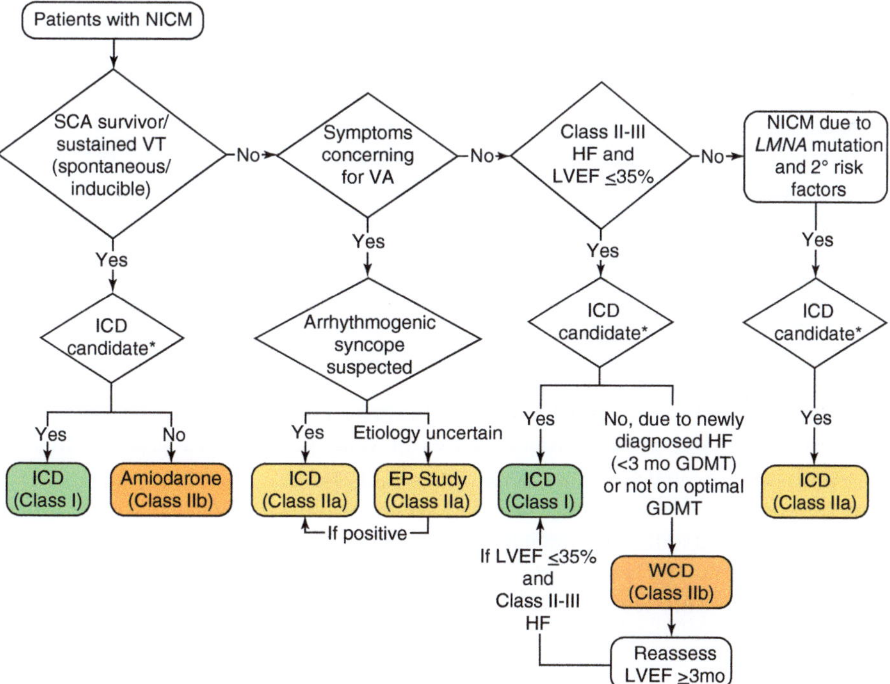

Fig. 5 AHA/ACC/HRS Primary and Secondary Prevention in NICM ICD implantation guidelines [102]

Lastly, it is important to note that ICD placement is an invasive procedure that comes with risks and benefits. These must be considered and discussed with patients. In all cases of ICD placement, life expectancy with a reasonable quality of life should be greater than one year.

5 Syncope

Syncope is a sudden transient loss of consciousness and postural tone with complete spontaneous recovery. Loss of consciousness results from a reduction of blood flow to the reticular activating system located in the brain stem and does not require electrical or chemical therapy for reversal. Cessation of cerebral blood flow leads to loss of consciousness within approximately 10 seconds. Syncope is an important clinical problem because it is a common, costly, and often disabling problem. Syncope may be the only warning sign before SCD [109]. First incidence of syncope has a trimodal distribution, with one of the peaks occurring in the elderly [110]. Elderly persons have anywhere from a 2–6% annual incidence of syncope and a 20–30% recurrence rate [111, 112]. The annual cost of evaluating and treating patients with syncope has been estimated to be about $5.4 billion dollars [113].

The causes of syncope can be classified into three primary groups: reflex, orthostatic, and cardiac. Reflex syncope, previously also known as neutrally-mediated or neuroreflex syncope, is further subdivided into vasovagal (long periods of standing, emotional triggers), situational (micturition), or carotid sinus syndrome (due to carotid sinus hypersensitivity). Orthostatic hypotension can be due to multiple etiologies, such as drug side effects, hypovolemia, or autonomic dysfunction. Lastly, cardiac syncope can be due to an arrhythmia, structural disorders (valve disease), or vascular causes (pulmonary embolism). Despite this framework, up to a third of patients admitted for syncope never have a cause identified [115].

5.1 Orthostatic Syncope

Syncope in elderly individuals is often multifactorial in origin. Reflex and orthostatic are by far the most common causes of syncope, accounting for as high as two-thirds of syncopal episodes in one study in the elderly but about one-third in the general population (Table 1) [111, 114]. When a person stands, 500–800 mL of blood is displaced to the abdomen and lower extremities, resulting in an abrupt drop in venous return to the heart. This leads to a decrease in cardiac output and therefore blood pressure. This leads to stimulation of aortic, carotid, and cardiopulmonary baroreceptors that trigger a reflex increase in sympathetic outflow and a decrease in parasympathetic activity. As a result, heart rate, cardiac contractility, and vascular resistance increase to maintain stable systemic blood pressure on standing [111, 116]. Orthostatic hypotension is defined as a 20-mmHg drop in systolic blood

Table 1 Etiology and prevalence of syncope in different elderly populations [114]

Etiology of syncope	All (*n* = 231)	65–74 (*n* = 71)	≥75 (*n* = 160)	*P*-value[a]
	n(%)			
Cardiac	34 (14.7)	8 (11.3)	26 (16.3)	0.06
Neuroreflex	102 (44.1)	44 (62)	58 (36.3)	<0.001
Orthostatic	52 (22.5)	3 (4.2)	49 (30.5)	<0.001
Drug-induced	11 (4.8)	3 (4.2)	8 (5)	0.33
Multifactorial	8 (3.5)	3 (4.2)	5 (3.1)	0.21
Unexplained	24 (10.4)	10 (14.1)	14 (8.8)	0.10

[a] *P*-value for difference between age groups, chi square

pressure or a 10-mmHg drop in diastolic blood pressure within three minutes of standing, resulting from a defect in any portion of this blood pressure control system [114]. Orthostatic hypotension may be asymptomatic or may be associated with symptoms such as light-headedness, dizziness, blurred vision, weakness, palpitations, tremulousness, and syncope. These symptoms are often worse immediately arising in the morning and/or after meals or exercise. Syncope that occurs after meals, particularly in the elderly, may result from a redistribution of blood to the gut. A decline in systolic blood pressure of about 20 mmHg approximately one hour after eating has been reported in up to one in four elderly patients [114, 117]. Although usually asymptomatic, it may result in light-headedness or syncope.

Drugs that either cause volume depletion or result in vasodilation are common causes of orthostatic hypotension. Elderly patients are particularly susceptible to the hypotensive effects of drugs because of reduced baroreceptor sensitivity, decreased cerebral blood flow, and age-related renal sodium wasting [118]. Orthostatic hypotension may also result from neurogenic causes, including primary and secondary autonomic failure.

Postural orthostatic tachycardia syndrome (POTS) is a milder form of chronic autonomic failure and orthostatic intolerance characterized by the presence of symptoms of orthostatic intolerance for at least six months, a 30-beats/minute or greater increase in heart rate within 5–10 minutes of assuming an upright position without a significant change in blood pressure, and no identified etiology [119]. POTS appears to result from a failure of the peripheral vasculature to appropriately vasoconstriction under orthostatic stress.

5.2 Reflex-Mediated Syncope

Reflex-mediated syncopal syndromes are characterized by an increased vagal tone and the withdrawal of peripheral sympathetic tone, leading to bradycardia, vasodilation, and, ultimately, hypotension, presyncope, or syncope. What distinguishes these causes of syncope are the specific triggers. For example, micturition syncope results from activation of mechanoreceptors in the bladder; defecation syncope results from neural inputs from gut wall tension receptors; and swallowing syncope results from afferent neural impulses arising from the upper gastrointestinal tract. The two most common types of reflex-mediated syncope are vasovagal syncope and carotid sinus hypersensitivity.

Vasovagal syncope, also known as neurocardiogenic, vasodepressor, and as "fainting," has been used to describe a common abnormality of blood pressure regulation characterized by the abrupt onset of hypotension with or without bradycardia. Triggers associated with the development of vasovagal syncope are those that either reduce ventricular filling (prolonged standing, a warm environment, or hot shower) or increase catecholamine secretion (sight of blood, pain, and stressful situations). Under these types of situations, patients with this condition develop severe light-headedness and/or syncope. It has been proposed that these clinical phenomena result from a paradoxical reflex that is initiated when ventricular preload is reduced by venous pooling. This leads to a reduction in cardiac output and blood pressure, which is sensed by arterial baroreceptors. The resultant increased catecholamine levels, combined with reduced venous filling, lead to a vigorously contracting volume-depleted ventricle. This hypercontractile state leads a paradoxical bradycardia and a decrease in peripheral vascular resistance, resulting in hypotension and syncope [120]. Neurally-mediated syncope is far more common among young individuals than among the elderly.

Syncope due to carotid sinus hypersensitivity results from stimulation of carotid sinus baroreceptors. Carotid sinus hypersensitivity is diagnosed by applying gentle pressure over the carotid pulsation just below the angle of the jaw, where the carotid bifurcation is located. After listening for a carotid bruit, pressure should be applied unilaterally for approximately five seconds. The sensitivity of diagnosing carotid sinus hypersensitivity can be increased, with no change in specificity, by performing carotid sinus massage during upright position in addition to supine position [121]. The normal response to carotid sinus massage is a transient decrease in the sinus rate and/or slowing of atrioventricular (AV) conduction. Three types of abnormal responses have been described: (1) the cardioinhibitory response, characterized by marked bradycardia (>three-second pause) or AV block; (2) the vasodepressor type, characterized by a 50-mmHg fall in the systolic blood pressure in the absence of bradycardia; and (3) the mixed response. It is important to recognize that carotid sinus hypersensitivity is also commonly observed in asymptomatic elderly patients. One study found that about 39% of participants had carotid sinus hypersensitivity, but only about half of these were symptomatic cases of carotid sinus hypersensitivity [122]. Because of this, the diagnosis of carotid sinus hypersensitivity should be approached cautiously after excluding alternative causes of syncope.

5.3 Cardiac Syncope

Cardiac causes of syncope, particularly tachyarrhythmias and bradyarrhythmias, are the second most common causes, accounting for about 10% of syncopal episodes [111]. Ventricular tachycardia is the most common tachyarrhythmia that causes syncope. Supraventricular arrhythmias can also cause syncope, although the great majority of patients with supraventricular arrhythmias present with less severe symptoms such as palpitations, dyspnea, and light-headedness. Bradyarrhythmias that can result in syncope include sick sinus syndrome as well as AV block. Anatomical causes of syncope result from obstruction to blood flow, such as a massive pulmonary embolus, an atrial myxoma, and aortic stenosis.

5.4 Neurologic Causes of Syncope

Neurological causes of syncope are surprisingly uncommon, accounting for less than 10% of all cases of syncope [111]. The majority of patients in whom a "neurological" cause of syncope is established are found, in fact, to have had a seizure rather than true syncope [111, 123]. Syncope, as an isolated symptom, is rarely due to a neurological cause. As a result, widespread use of tests to screen for neurologic conditions rarely are diagnostic. In many institutions, computed tomography, electroencephalography, and carotid duplex scans are overused, being obtained in more than 50% of patients with syncope. A diagnosis is almost never uncovered that was not first suspected based on a careful history and neurologic examination [124]. One study indicated that 29% of patients with treatment-resistant epilepsy or suspected nonepileptic seizures have an underlying cardiovascular cause of syncope such as neutrally-mediated hypotension, carotid sinus hypersensitivity, or transient AV block [125].

5.4.1 Metabolic/Miscellaneous Causes of Nonsyncope

Metabolic causes of syncope are rare, and their presentations are usually considered nonsyncopal in nature. Their mechanism differs from that of hypoperfusion in typical syncope and typically presents with altered consciousness instead of transient loss of consciousness in typical syncope. The most common metabolic causes of nonsyncope include hypoglycemia, hypoxia, and hyperventilation. The establishment of hypoglycemia as the cause of nonsyncope requires demonstration of hypoglycemia during the episode. Psychiatric disorders may also cause nonsyncope. About one percent of patients who initially had a diagnosis of syncope were found to have psychogenic syncope [126]. However, appropriate evaluation should be undertaken prior to determining nonsyncopal etiology, given the not uncommon side effect of orthostasis seen with many psychiatric drugs.

5.4.2 Prognosis in Syncope

The prognosis of patients with syncope varies greatly with diagnosis. Vasovagal syncope is generally associated with a benign prognosis, with life expectancy similar to those without a history of syncope. Orthostatic syncope may be associated with greater mortality, likely reflecting the comorbidities that usually accompany orthostasis in the elderly [127]. In contrast, syncope due to a cardiac cause is associated with a 50% mortality at five years [111].

5.5 Diagnostic Testing

Identification of the precise cause of syncope is often challenging [128]. The history and physical examination are the most important components of the evaluation of a patient with syncope. When taking a clinical history, particular attention should then be focused on (1) determining if the patient experienced true syncope as compared with a transient alteration in consciousness without loss of postural tone; (2) determining if the patient has a history of cardiac disease and if a family history of cardiac disease, syncope, or sudden death exists; (3) identifying medications that may have played a role in syncope; (4) quantifying the number and chronicity of prior episodes; (5) identifying precipitating factors including body position; and (6) quantifying the type and duration of prodromal and recovery symptoms. Much of this information may be obtained by interviewing witnesses of the event and is important in elucidating possible etiologies. After obtaining a careful history, evaluation should continue with a physical examination, including determining vital orthostatic signs, defining the patient's level of hydration, ECG, and a thorough examination [129].

Tilt-table testing (TTT) is a standard diagnostic test for evaluating patients with syncope. Despite its limitations, tilt-table testing is generally considered the "gold standard" for establishing a diagnosis of reflex-mediated or orthostatic syncope. Upright TTT is performed for 30–45 minutes at an angle of approximately 70°. In general, a positive response to TTT is defined as the development of syncope or presyncope in association with hypotension and/or bradycardia. The sensitivity of the test can be increased, with an associated fall in specificity, by the use of longer tilt durations, steeper tilt angles, and provocative agents such as isoproterenol, nitroglycerin, or edrophonium. The specificity of TTT is highly dependent on the ability to correlate a positive test to the patients' clinical presentation. There is general agreement that upright tilt-table testing is indicated in patients with (1) recurrent syncope or a single syncopal episode in a high-risk patient who either has no evidence of structural heart disease or in whom other causes of syncope have been excluded, (2) evaluation of patients in whom the causes of syncope have been determined (e.g., asystole) but in whom the presence of vasovagal or orthostatic mediated syncope on upright tilt would influence treatment, and (3) as part of the evaluation of patients with exercise-related syncope. There is also general agreement that upright TTT is not necessary for patients who have experienced only a single syncopal episode that was highly typical for vasovagal syncope and during which no injury occurred. Tilt-table testing is not useful in establishing a diagnosis of situation syncope (i.e., postmicturition syncope) [130].

Although echocardiograms are commonly used in the evaluation of patients with syncope, little objective evidence exists to support their use in patients without a history of heart disease, and with a normal physical examination and normal ECG [131]. The rationale for obtaining an echocardiogram in patients with syncope is to risk the patient by excluding the possibility of occult cardiac disease not apparent after the history, physical examination, and electrocardiography. If detected, the presence of impaired ventricular function or significant valvular dysfunction would suggest a cardiac cause of syncope and, therefore, a worse long-term prognosis.

Myocardial ischemia is an unlikely cause of syncope and, when present, is usually accompanied by angina. The use of stress tests in the evaluation of a patient with syncope is best reserved for patients in whom the clinical suspicion of ischemia is high, i.e. syncope or presyncope that occurred during or immediately after exertion or in association with chest pain. Even among patients with syncope during exertion, it is highly unlikely that exercise stress testing will trigger another event. Patients suspected of having severe aortic stenosis or obstructive hypertrophic cardiomyopathy should not undergo exercise stress testing because it may precipitate a cardiac arrest.

The 12-lead ECG is a standard component in the workup of a patient with syncope. With history and physical examination, this combination can lead to a diagnosis in 24–40% of patients [132]. Specific findings that may identify the probable cause of syncope include QT prolongation (long QT syndrome), the presence of a short PR interval, and a delta wave (Wolff-Parkinson-White syndrome), evidence of acute myocardial infarction, and high-grade AV block. Less specific findings that may suggest potential causes of syncope include evidence of prior myocardial infarction, bundle branch block, ventricular hypertrophy, and ventricular premature beats. These findings can be confirmed later with direct testing. T wave inversion in the right precordial leads to an incomplete right bundle branch block pattern, suggesting a diagnosis of right ventricular dysplasia. Persistent ST-segment elevation in leads V_1 to V_3 with an incomplete RBBB pattern suggests a Brugada syndrome diagnosis. These hereditary disorders are associated with a high incidence of SCD. Although more common in younger patients, they can present in the elderly [133]. The finding of a normal ECG suggests that a cardiac cause of syncope is unlikely.

Continuous ECG monitoring using telemetry, Holter monitor, loop, or patch recorders is commonly performed in patients with syncope. The information provided by ECG recording at the time of syncope is extremely valuable because it allows an arrhythmic cause of syncope to be established or excluded. The type of monitoring device should be selected based on the frequency of syncopal episodes. Because of the infrequent and sporadic nature of syncope, the diagnostic yield of Holter recording may be low and may not be cost-effective. The likelihood of experiencing an episode of syncope while wearing a Holter recorder in an unselected population of patients with syncope is generally low. Detection of asymptomatic sinus bradycardia, AV block, or nonsustained supraventricular or ventricular arrhythmias on Holter monitoring can suggest an arrhythmic cause of syncope, but it is important to recognize that unless syncope or presyncope accompanies these arrhythmias, they are likely to be incidental findings and should not be assumed to be the cause of syncope. For these reasons, the clinical situation in which Holter recording is most likely to be diagnostic is when used in the occasional patient with very frequent (i.e., daily) episodes of syncope or presyncope. Alternatively, external loop or patch recorders are especially useful for patients with infrequent episodes of presyncope or syncope, particularly once potentially malignant causes of syncope have been excluded. These have been shown to have increased diagnostic yield compared to Holter monitors, likely given the longer time of monitoring with loop recorders [134].

5.5.1 Electrophysiology Testing

The results of an EP study (EPS) can be useful in establishing a diagnosis of sick sinus syndrome, heart block, supraventricular tachycardia, or ventricular tachycardia in patients with syncope. The indications for EPS in the evaluation of patients with syncope have been established based on AHA/ACC/HRS guidelines [135]. There is general agreement that EPS can be useful in patients in whom syncope is suspected to be due to an arrhythmia. The diagnostic yield of EPS is highest in those suspected or known structural heart disease and unexplained syncope (COR IIa). If an arrhythmia is not suspected in patients with normal ECG and no history of cardiac disease, EPS is not recommended as the diagnostic yield is low [136].

5.6 Management of the Syncope Patient

The approach to the treatment of a patient with syncope depends largely on the diagnosis that is established. For example, the appropriate treatment of a patient with syncope due to AV block or sick sinus syndrome would likely involve placement of a permanent pacemaker; treatment of a patient with syncope due to the Wolff-Parkinson White syndrome would likely involve catheter ablation; and treatment of a patient with syncope due to VT would likely involve placement of an ICD. For other types of syncope, optimal patient management may involve discontinuation of an offending pharmacological agent, increased salt intake, or patient education.

6 Special Issues in Management

6.1 AF Screening in the Elderly

AF screening remains a controversial topic. Mass screening in an elderly population showed an increase in detection by about 33%, which highlights the large amounts of asymptomatic AF in the elderly [137]. Furthermore, multiple devices now exist that can detect silent AF. These range from patient-purchased smartwatches to physician-implanted cardiac monitors. Certain smartwatches can detect possible AF with relatively decent accuracy and can lead to the diagnosis of AF when conventional cardiac monitoring with physician review confirms the diagnosis [138, 139]. The detection of AF was superior to conventional monitoring in the case of implanted cardiac monitors [140]. The large amount of data provided from these screenings has created a new area for the investigation that identifies patients who would benefit most from AF screening. The higher prevalence of AF in the elderly and the associated higher risk for stroke may identify this group as one that would benefit greater from AF screening. However, more investigation is needed regarding the pros and cons of AF screening in the elderly. Greater screening may lead to more misdiagnosis cases, as well as unnecessary and possibly harmful and therapeutic interventions.

6.2 Anticoagulation in the Elderly

Anticoagulation for stroke prophylaxis represents a special challenge in the elderly. While the aged benefit the most from anticoagulation, they also are at the highest risk for iatrogenic bleeding events, including intracranial bleeding.

AF is an independent risk factor for stroke and is associated with a fivefold increased risk of stroke [141]. AF leads to atrial stasis and the formation of LA thrombi, which may embolize the cerebral vasculature. Among patients with atrial fibrillation, the risk of stroke is approximately five percent per year. Non-paroxysmal AF has a higher stroke risk than paroxysmal AF [142].

Risk stratification and cardioembolic stroke prophylaxis represent a cornerstone in managing AF patients. Patients at a high risk of stroke benefit the most from systemic anticoagulation. The $CHA_2 DS_2$-VASc is a well-known stroke risk calculator used to aid in decision-making regarding anticoagulation [143]. This risk calculator uses age, specifically age from 65 to 74 years and greater than 75 years as markers of increased risk. The other risk factors included in this calculator that increase risk for stroke are sex, congestive heart failure, hypertension, stroke/transient ischemic attack (TIA)/thromboembolism, vascular disease (such as MI or peripheral artery disease), and diabetes. Many of these risks are more common as we age, reflecting the increased risk of stroke the elderly have.

Anticoagulation in AF is based on their individual CHA_2 DS_2-VASc score. For men, a score of two or greater, and for women, a score of three or greater indicate that anticoagulation should be recommended for stroke prevention. The current options for anticoagulation include coumadin and the more recent class of DOACs. Coumadin was the first anticoagulant used to prevent stroke in AF [144, 145]. As expected, the trade-off of stroke prevention with anticoagulation is an increased risk of bleeding events. In the last decade, DOACs have risen in favor mainly due to noninferiority and sometimes superiority over coumadin in stroke prevention, as well as similar or decreased risk for bleeding [146–149]. The most recent AHA/ACC/HRS guidelines reflect the favorability of DOACs over coumadin in patients with AF, with the exception of patients with valvular AF (defined as AF in the setting of mechanical valves or moderate to severe mitral stenosis) [48, 150].

Multiple authorities have questioned the role of anticoagulation in the oldest old (those 85 years and older). RCTs studying coumadin in octogenarians have suggested benefits from coumadin use in this patient population [151, 152]. Current observational studies and post-hoc analysis of DOAC RCTs suggest that anticoagulation prevents stroke risk with an expected increase in bleeding events but that there was a net positive benefit from anticoagulation. Furthermore, these studies seem to suggest that the benefit was increased in elderly patients taking DOACs as compared to coumadin [48, 153–155]. Stroke prophylaxis should still be tailored to the individual patient and guided by the patient's risk profile and functional status. If the patient has both high risk and good functional status (i.e. their quality of life would be impaired by a disabling stroke), then they should be anticoagulated, regardless of their age. Despite these data suggesting the benefit of DOACs, they are less often prescribed for AF stroke prevention in the elderly. Instead, antiplatelets are more often prescribed for AF-related stroke prevention in the elderly, despite data suggesting no benefit, and possibly even harm, in those on aspirin monotherapy [156, 157].

6.3 Left Atrial Appendage Occlusion Devices

Given that the vast majority of AF-related stroke is related to the formation of LAA thrombus, occlusion of the appendage can reduce stroke risk. The most common implanted device, the WATCHMAN is placed transeptally into the LAA, occluding it and preventing thrombus from embolizing from the LAA. In the PROTECT-AF trial, the WATCHMAN device was shown to have noninferiority to coumadin in ischemic stroke prevention [158]. A follow-up trial, PREVAIL-AF, also showed noninferiority to coumadin in ischemic stroke prevention [159]. Metanalysis from the PROTECT-AF trial and PREVAIL-AF trial demonstrated lower rates of hemorrhagic stroke when compared to coumadin, as well as lower rates of ischemic stroke when periprocedural strokes were excluded [160]. Other risks besides periprocedural stroke include procedure-related pericardial effusions and device-related thrombus, which are associated with increased risk for stroke [161]. WATCHMAN implantation still requires at least 45 days of anticoagulation to allow time for device endothelialization. Whether or not patients may benefit from antiplatelet therapy instead of anticoagulation after WATCHMAN implantation is currently being investigated. Oral anticoagulation is still the preferred treatment for AF, but LAA occlusion may be a reasonable alternative in those with nonvalvular AF and a contraindication to anticoagulation.

6.4   Anti-arrhythmics in the Elderly

Elderly patients are more likely to suffer complications and side effects from anti-arrhythmic medications. For example, in the Cardiac Arrhythmia Suppression Trial (CAST), older age was an independent predictor of adverse events in patients taking flecainide [162]. Additionally, left atrial size increases with age, and LAE has been associated with the recurrence of AF after rhythm control strategies [163]. Given these concerns, the current practice seems to favor rate control over rhythm control strategy [157]. However, data regarding outcomes between rate versus rhythm control in the elderly remains controversial, with some suggesting no difference and others the suggesting superiority of either approach [164–166].

There are several age-associated changes that make pharmacotherapy in the elderly more challenging. Glomerular filtration rate declines with age, limiting therapeutic options like sotalol and dofetilide, which are renally cleared. Decreased drug clearance and decreases in lean body mass lead to an increased half-life and volume of distribution of amiodarone in elderly patients and have been associated with increased rates of pacemaker insertion due to bradyarrhythmias [167]. With regard to amiodarone, it is important to remember that its side effects include corneal deposits and photosensitivity, in addition to the better-known thyroid, hepatic, and pulmonary complications. Routine monitoring for patients on amiodarone should include thyroid function testing, serum transaminase determination, and a chest X-ray at baseline and every 6–12 months when stable. Pulmonary function testing is the most sensitive test for amiodarone-associated pulmonary fibrosis and should be done annually or whenever patients complain of dyspnea on exertion [167].

6.5   Radiofrequency and Cryoablation

Radiofrequency and cryoablation destroy arrhythmogenic tissue through the thermal disruption of cardiac membranes. While catheter ablation is an invasive procedure and is associated with procedural risk, ablative termination often liberates patients from anti-arrhythmic medications which carry significant side effects, especially in the elderly population. Both RFA and cryoablation have similar safety profiles and similar outcomes compared to younger populations and should not be avoided in elderly patients who would benefit from ablation [168–171].

According to the 2017 HRS AF ablation guidelines, AF ablation is recommended for symptomatic paroxysmal AF refractory or intolerant to at least one class I or III anti-arrhythmic, and reasonable for symptomatic paroxysmal AF prior to trial of pharmacotherapy or for persistent AF. Ablation can still be considered in those with long-standing AF [172]. These guidelines also note that these recommendations can be reasonably applied to patients greater than 75 years old. Other forms of SVT, including AVNRT, AV junction, isthmus-dependent atrial flutter, and accessory pathways, have success rates in excess of 85% [50, 173]. The overall risk of thromboembolic complications after catheter ablation is less than one percent [174–176]. This risk increases with left heart involvement and the ablation of ventricular tachycardias [177].

6.6   Device Therapy in the Elderly

The incidence of sinus node dysfunction, atrioventricular block, heart failure, and sudden cardiac death all increase with age. Among octagenarians and nonagenarians, atrioventricular block, SSS, and chronic AF complicated by bradycardia are the most common indications for a pacemaker placement. Accordingly, most patients who require pacemaker or ICD implantation are older. Given the finite resources of our health care system and the disproportionate expenditure of health care dollars in the later years of life, many have examined the efficacy of device therapy in the elderly. Several studies have shown that although device therapy in the elderly may have higher rates of perioperative complications, in general, age is not associated with exceedingly high complication rates [178–182]. Age alone should not be a contraindication to devise therapy, but strong consideration should be given to life expectancy and comorbidities, as elderly patients over 75 years old may not as much benefit from secondary prevention ICD compared to younger cohorts, and the degree of benefit remains controversial for primary prevention ICDs [183–185]. Pacemaker implantation does relieve symptoms in about three-fourths of elderly patients, and elderly patients receiving ICD have similar quality of live (QOL) to patients with major cardiac disease [186]. Much like any therapeutic intervention, treatment should be tailored to the individual patient after consideration of the potential risks and benefits. While device therapy is a safe and effective intervention in the functional elderly patient, more research is needed regarding patient selection among the oldest-old. Further investigations regarding newer pacing approaches, such as leadless pacemakers and His bundle pacing, are also needed in elderly populations.

Lastly, ICD management at the end of life is particularly important in elderly patients. About 20% of patients receive ICD shocks in the last week of their lives. This can significantly affect the QOL of both patients and their families. The majority of patients with ICDs express a desire for ICD deactivation during the end of life care. Despite this, ICD management at end of life is infrequently discussed between patients and families [186]. Additionally, ICD management during the end of life requires integration of multiple ethical principles, including patients' right to refuse care and surrogate decision-making in cases of incapacitated patients [187]. Focus should be made on improving communication between physicians and patients regarding end-of-life ICD decision-making and highlights a significant area for improvement.

7 Conclusion

The prevalence of cardiac arrhythmias and conduction disorders increases with age and impart significant morbidity and mortality in the elderly population, especially among those with compromised left ventricular function and heart failure. Fortunately, over the past decade, numerous safe and effective therapies have been developed to treat dysrhythmia and prevent sudden cardiac death. As with any condition, treatment should be tailored to the individual patient. However, age should not preclude functional elderly patients from anticoagulation, catheter ablation, device therapy, or other interventional strategies. These patients have much to gain from symptomatic relief and stand to benefit the most from avoiding the side effects of anti-arrhythmic medications.

References

1. Chow GV, Marine JE, Fleg JL. Epidemiology of arrhythmias and conduction disorders in older adults. Clin Geriatr Med. 2012;28(4):539–53. https://www.clinicalkey.es/playcontent/1-s2.0-S0749069012000717. https://doi.org/10.1016/j.cger.2012.07.003.
2. Feinberg WM, Blackshear JL, Laupacis A, Kronmal R, Hart RG. Prevalence, age distribution, and gender of patients with atrial fibrillation: analysis and implications. Arch Intern Med (1960). 1995;155(5):469–73. https://doi.org/10.1001/archinte.1995.00430050045005.
3. Go AS, Hylek EM, Phillips KA, et al. Prevalence of diagnosed atrial fibrillation in adults: national implications for rhythm management and stroke prevention: The AnTicoagulation and risk factors in atrial fibrillation (ATRIA) study. JAMA. 2001;285(18):2370–5. https://doi.org/10.1001/jama.285.18.2370.
4. Benjamin E, Muntner P, Alonso A, et al. Heart disease and stroke Statistics—2019 update: a report from the American Heart Association. Circulation (New York, NY). 2019;139(10):e56–66. https://www.ncbi.nlm.nih.gov/pubmed/30700139. https://doi.org/10.1161/CIR.0000000000000659.
5. Lev M. Anatomic basis for atrioventricular block. Am J Med. 1964;37(5):742–8. https://doi.org/10.1016/0002-9343(64)90022-1.
6. Davies MJ. Pathology of chronic A-V block. Acta Cardiol. 1976;Suppl 21:19–30. https://www.ncbi.nlm.nih.gov/pubmed/1087803
7. Zoob M, Smith KS. Aetiology of complete heart-block. Br Med J. 1963;2(5366):1149–53. https://doi.org/10.1136/bmj.2.5366.1149.
8. North B, Sinclair D. The intersection between aging and cardiovascular disease. Circ Res. 2012;110(8):1097–108. http://ovidsp.ovid.com/ovidweb.cgi?T=JS&NEWS=n&CSC=Y

&PAGE=fulltext&D=ovft&AN=00003012-201204130-00013.   https://doi.org/10.1161/CIRCRESAHA.111.246876.

9. Hodkinson HM, Pomerance A. The clinical significance of senile cardiac amyloidosis: a prospective clinico-pathological study. QJM. 1977;46(3):381–7. https://api.istex.fr/ark:/67375/HXZ-MQ895V3B-P/fulltext.pdf. https://doi.org/10.1093/oxfordjournals.qjmed.a067513.

10. Lev M. Aging changes in the human sinoatrial node. J Gerontol. 1954;9:1–8.

11. Kistler PM, Sanders P, Fynn SP, et al. Electrophysiologic and electroanatomic changes in the human atrium associated with age. J Am Coll Cardiol. 2004;44(1):109–16. https://doi.org/10.1016/j.jacc.2004.03.044.

12. Furberg CD, Manolio TA, Psaty BM, et al. Major electrocardiographic abnormalities in persons aged 65 years and older (the cardiovascular health study). Cardiovascular Health Study Collaborative Research Group. Am J Cardiol. 1992;69(16):1329–35. https://www.ncbi.nlm.nih.gov/pubmed/1585868

13. Östör E, Jensen G, Nyboe J, Hansen AT. Electrocardiographic findings and their association with mortality in the Copenhagen City Heart Study. Eur Heart J. 1981;2(4):317–28. https://api.istex.fr/ark:/67375/HXZ-MD03WLW2-K/fulltext.pdf. https://doi.org/10.1093/oxfordjournals.eurheartj.a061212.

14. Caird FI, Campbell A, Jackson TF. Significance of abnormalities of electrocardiogram in old people. Br Heart J. 1974;36(10):1012–8. https://doi.org/10.1136/hrt.36.10.1012.

15. Molander U, Kumar Dey D, Sundh V, Steen B. ECG abnormalities in the elderly: prevalence, time and generation trends and association with mortality. Aging Clin Exp Res. 2003;15(6):488–93.   https://www.ncbi.nlm.nih.gov/pubmed/14959952.   https://doi.org/10.1007/BF03327371.

16. Sundstrom J, Lind L, Arnlov J, Zethelius B, Andren B, Lithell HO. Echocardiographic and electrocardiographic diagnoses of left ventricular hypertrophy predict mortality independently of each other in a population of elderly men. Circulation. 2001;103(19):2346–51. http://circ.ahajournals.org/cgi/content/abstract/103/19/2346.   https://doi.org/10.1161/01.CIR.103.19.2346.

17. Kannel WB, Dannenberg AL, Levy D. Population implications of electrocardiographic left ventricular hypertrophy. Am J Cardiol. 1987;60(17):85–93. https://doi.org/10.1016/0002-9149(87)90466-8.

18. Seifer C, Kenny RA. The prevalence of falls in older persons paced for atrioventricular block and sick sinus syndrome. Am J Geriatr Cardiol. 2003;12(5):298–305. https://onlinelibrary.wiley.com/doi/abs/10.1111/j.1076-7460.2003.01854.x. https://doi.org/10.1111/j.1076-7460.2003.01854.x.

19. Lamas GA, Pashos CL, Normand ST, McNeil B. Permanent pacemaker selection and subsequent survival in elderly Medicare pacemaker recipients. Circulation. 1995;91(4):1063–9. http://circ.ahajournals.org/cgi/content/abstract/91/4/1063.   https://doi.org/10.1161/01.CIR.91.4.1063.

20. Cosedis Nielsen J, Thomsen PEB, Christensen PD, et al. A comparison of single-lead atrial pacing with dual-chamber pacing in sick sinus syndrome. Eur Heart J. 2011;32(6):686–96. https://www.ncbi.nlm.nih.gov/pubmed/21300730. https://doi.org/10.1093/eurheartj/ehr022.

21. Lown B. Electrical reversion of cardiac arrhythmias. Br Heart J. 1967;29(4):469–89. https://doi.org/10.1136/hrt.29.4.469.

22. Csepe TA, Kalyanasundaram A, Hansen BJ, Zhao J, Fedorov VV. Fibrosis: a structural modulator of sinoatrial node physiology and dysfunction. Front Physiol. 2015;6:37. https://www.ncbi.nlm.nih.gov/pubmed/25729366. https://doi.org/10.3389/fphys.2015.00037.

23. Kusumoto FM, Schoenfeld MH, Barrett C, et al. 2018 ACC/AHA/HRS guideline on the evaluation and management of patients with bradycardia and cardiac conduction delay: a report of the American College of Cardiology/American Heart Association task force on clinical practice guidelines and the Heart Rhythm Society. Heart Rhythm. 2019;16(9):e128–226. https://www.ncbi.nlm.nih.gov/pubmed/30412778. https://doi.org/10.1016/j.hrthm.2018.10.037.

24. Lamas GA, Lee KL, Sweeney MO, et al. Ventricular pacing or dual-chamber pacing for sinus-node dysfunction. N Engl J Med. 2002;346(24):1854–62. http://content.nejm.org/cgi/content/abstract/346/24/1854. https://doi.org/10.1056/NEJMoa013040.
25. Sweeney MO, Bank AJ, Nsah E, et al. Minimizing ventricular pacing to reduce atrial fibrillation in sinus-node disease. N Engl J Med. 2007;357(10):1000–8. http://content.nejm.org/cgi/content/abstract/357/10/1000. https://doi.org/10.1056/NEJMoa071880.
26. Song Y, Yao Q, Zhu J, Luo B, Liang S. Age-related variation in the interstitial tissues of the cardiac conduction system; and autopsy study of 230 Han Chinese. Forensic Sci Int. 1999;104(2):133–42. https://doi.org/10.1016/S0379-0738(99)00103-6.
27. Cheng S, Keyes MJ, Larson MG, et al. Long-term outcomes in individuals with prolonged PR interval or first-degree atrioventricular block. JAMA. 2009;301(24):2571–7. https://doi.org/10.1001/jama.2009.888.
28. Kwok CS, Rashid M, Beynon R, et al. Prolonged PR interval, first-degree heart block and adverse cardiovascular outcomes: a systematic review and meta-analysis. Heart. 2016;102(9):672–80. https://doi.org/10.1136/heartjnl-2015-308956.
29. Tayal B, Fruelund P, Sogaard P, et al. Incidence of heart failure after pacemaker implantation: a nationwide Danish Registry-based follow-up study. Eur Heart J. 2019;40(44):3641–8. https://www.ncbi.nlm.nih.gov/pubmed/31504437. https://doi.org/10.1093/eurheartj/ehz584.
30. Eriksson P, Hansson P, Eriksson H, Dellborg M. Bundle-branch block in a general male population: the study of men born 1913. Circulation. 1998;98(22):2494–500. http://circ.ahajournals.org/cgi/content/abstract/98/22/2494. https://doi.org/10.1161/01.CIR.98.22.2494.
31. McAnulty JH, Rahimtoola SH, Murphy E, et al. Natural history of "high-risk" bundle-branch block: final report of a prospective study. N Engl J Med. 1982;307(3):137–43. http://content.nejm.org/cgi/content/abstract/307/3/137. https://doi.org/10.1056/NEJM198207153070301.
32. 2021 ESC guidelines on cardiac pacing and cardiac resynchronization therapy. Eur Heart J. 2021;42(35):3427–520. https://search.proquest.com/docview/2566265368. https://doi.org/10.1093/eurheartj/ehab364.
33. Page RL, Joglar JA, Caldwell MA, et al. 2015 ACC/AHA/HRS guideline for the management of adult patients with supraventricular tachycardia: a report of the American College of Cardiology/American Heart Association task force on clinical practice guidelines and the Heart Rhythm Society. J Am Coll Cardiol. 2016;67(13):e27–e115. https://www.ncbi.nlm.nih.gov/pubmed/26409259. https://doi.org/10.1016/j.jacc.2015.08.856.
34. Wu D, Denes P, Amat-Y-Leon F, et al. Clinical, electrocardiographic and electrophysiologic observations in patients with paroxysmal supraventricular tachycardia. Am J Cardiol. 1978;41(6):1045–51. https://doi.org/10.1016/0002-9149(78)90856-1.
35. Brembilla-Perrot B, Houriez P, Beurrier D, et al. Influence of age on the electrophysiological mechanism of paroxysmal supraventricular tachycardias. Int J Cardiol. 2001;78(3):293–8. https://doi.org/10.1016/S0167-5273(01)00392-8.
36. Chrispin J, Misra S, Marine JE, et al. Current management and clinical outcomes for catheter ablation of atrioventricular nodal re-entrant tachycardia. Europace (London, England). 2018;20(4):e51–9. https://www.ncbi.nlm.nih.gov/pubmed/28541507. https://doi.org/10.1093/europace/eux110.
37. Katritsis DG, Zografos T, Siontis KC, et al. Endpoints for successful slow pathway catheter ablation in typical and Atypical Atrioventricular nodal re-entrant tachycardia: a contemporary, multicenter study. JACC Clin Electrophysiol. 2019;5(1):113–9. https://www.ncbi.nlm.nih.gov/pubmed/30678775. https://doi.org/10.1016/j.jacep.2018.09.012.
38. Nelson SD, Kou WH, Annesley T, de Buitleir M, Morady F. Significance of ST segment depression during paroxysmal supraventricular tachycardia. J Am Coll Cardiol. 1988;12(2):383. http://content.onlinejacc.org/cgi/content/abstract/12/2/383
39. Paparella N, Ouyang F, Fucă G, Kuck K, Cappato R, Alboni P. Significance of newly acquired negative T waves after interruption of paroxysmal reentrant supraventricular tachycardia with narrow QRS complex. Am J Cardiol. 2000;85(2):261–3. https://doi.org/10.1016/S0002-9149(99)00633-5.

40. Zaman S, Sayami LA, Rahim MA, et al. Significance of ST-segment depression during paroxysmal supraventricular tachycardia. Cardiovasc J. 2015;7(2):93–7. https://doi.org/10.3329/cardio.v7i2.22249.

41. Bukkapatnam RN, Robinson M, Turnipseed S, Tancredi D, Amsterdam E, Srivatsa UN. Relationship of myocardial ischemia and injury to coronary artery disease in patients with supraventricular tachycardia. Am J Cardiol. 2010;106(3):374–7. https://www.clinicalkey.es/playcontent/1-s2.0-S0002914910007848. https://doi.org/10.1016/j.amjcard.2010.03.035.

42. Kastor JA. Multifocal atrial tachycardia. Card Electrophysiol Rev. 2001;5(2):294. https://search.proquest.com/docview/213614786. https://doi.org/10.1023/A:1011430227366.

43. McCord J, Borzak S. Multifocal atrial tachycardia. Chest. 1998;113(1):203–9. https://doi.org/10.1378/chest.113.1.203.

44. Lazaros G, Chrysohoou C, Oikonomou E, et al. The natural history of multifocal atrial rhythms in elderly outpatients: insights from the "Ikaria Study". Ann Noninvasive Electrocardiol. 2014;19(5):483–9. https://api.istex.fr/ark:/67375/WNG-H0S6WCB6-8/fulltext.pdf. https://doi.org/10.1111/anec.12165.

45. Granada J, Uribe W, Chyou P, et al. Incidence and predictors of atrial flutter in the general population. J Am Coll Cardiol. 2000;36(7):2242–6. https://doi.org/10.1016/S0735-1097(00)00982-7.

46. Hall BW, Bialy DJ, Lehmann MH. Hospitalizations for arrhythmias in the United States, 1985 through 1999: importance of atrial fibrillation. J Am Coll Cardiol. 2002;39:89. https://doi.org/10.1016/S0735-1097(02)80382-5.

47. January C, Wann L, Alpert J, et al. 2014 AHA/ACC/HRS guideline for the management of patients with atrial fibrillation: executive summary: a report of the American College of Cardiology/American Heart Association task force on practice guidelines and the Heart Rhythm Society. Circulation (New York, NY). 2014;130(23):2071–104. https://www.ncbi.nlm.nih.gov/pubmed/24682348. https://doi.org/10.1161/CIR.0000000000000040.

48. January CT, Wann LS, Calkins H, et al. 2019 AHA/ACC/HRS focused update of the 2014 AHA/ACC/HRS guideline for the management of patients with atrial fibrillation: a report of the American College of Cardiology/American Heart Association task force on clinical practice guidelines and the Heart Rhythm Society. J Am Coll Cardiol. 2019;74(1):104–32. https://www.ncbi.nlm.nih.gov/pubmed/30703431. https://doi.org/10.1016/j.jacc.2019.01.011.

49. Natale A, Newby KH, Pisanó E, et al. Prospective randomized comparison of antiarrhythmic therapy versus first-line radiofrequency ablation in patients with atrial flutter. J Am Coll Cardiol. 2000;35(7):1898–904. https://doi.org/10.1016/S0735-1097(00)00635-5.

50. Spector P, Reynolds MR, Calkins H, et al. Meta-analysis of ablation of atrial flutter and supraventricular tachycardia. Am J Cardiol. 2009;104(5):671–7. https://www.clinicalkey.es/playcontent/1-s2.0-S000291490901008X. https://doi.org/10.1016/j.amjcard.2009.04.040.

51. Perez FJ, Schubert CM, Parvez B, Pathak V, Ellenbogen KA, Wood MA. Long-term outcomes after catheter ablation of cavo-tricuspid isthmus dependent atrial flutter: a meta-analysis. Circ Arrhythm Electrophysiol. 2009;2(4):393–401. http://circep.ahajournals.org/cgi/content/abstract/2/4/393. https://doi.org/10.1161/CIRCEP.109.871665.

52. Virani SS, Alonso A, Aparicio HJ, et al. Heart disease and stroke statistics-2021 update: a report from the American Heart Association. Circulation (New York, NY). 2021;143(8):e254–743. https://www.ncbi.nlm.nih.gov/pubmed/33501848. https://doi.org/10.1161/CIR.0000000000000950.

53. Piccini JP, Hammill BG, Sinner MF, et al. Incidence and prevalence of atrial fibrillation and associated mortality among Medicare beneficiaries, 1993–2007. Circ Cardiovasc Qual Outcomes. 2012;5(1):85–93. https://www.ncbi.nlm.nih.gov/pubmed/22235070. https://doi.org/10.1161/CIRCOUTCOMES.111.962688.

54. Staerk L, Wang B, Preis SR, et al. Lifetime risk of atrial fibrillation according to optimal, borderline, or elevated levels of risk factors: cohort study based on longitudinal data from the Framingham Heart Study. BMJ. 2018;361:k1453. https://doi.org/10.1136/bmj.k1453.

55. Helgadottir S, Sigurdsson MI, Ingvarsdottir IL, Arnar DO, Gudbjartsson T. Atrial fibrillation following cardiac surgery: risk analysis and long-term survival. J Cardiothorac Surg. 2012;7(1):87. https://www.ncbi.nlm.nih.gov/pubmed/22992266. https://doi.org/10.1186/1749-8090-7-87.

56. Lin M, Kamel H, Singer D, Wu Y, Lee M, Ovbiagele B. Perioperative/postoperative atrial fibrillation and risk of subsequent stroke and/or mortality: a meta-analysis. Stroke (1970). 2019;50(6):1364–71. https://doi.org/10.1161/STROKEAHA.118.023921.

57. Whitlock RP, Belley-Cote EP, Paparella D, et al. Left atrial appendage occlusion during cardiac surgery to prevent stroke. N Engl J Med. 2021;384(22):2081–91. https://doi.org/10.1056/NEJMoa2101897.

58. Wolf PA, Abbott RD, Kannel WB. Atrial fibrillation as an independent risk factor for stroke: the Framingham Study. Stroke. 1991;22(8):983–8. http://stroke.ahajournals.org/cgi/content/abstract/22/8/983. https://doi.org/10.1161/01.STR.22.8.983.

59. Risk factors for stroke and efficacy of antithrombotic therapy in atrial fibrillation: analysis of pooled data from five randomized controlled trials. Arch Intern Med (1960). 1994;154(13):1449–57. https://doi.org/10.1001/archinte.1994.00420130036007.

60. Kannel WB, Abbott RD, Savage DD, McNamara PM. Epidemiologic features of chronic atrial fibrillation: the Framingham Study. N Engl J Med. 1982;306(17):1018–22. http://content.nejm.org/cgi/content/abstract/306/17/1018. https://doi.org/10.1056/NEJM198204293061703.

61. Kopecky SL, Gersh BJ, McGoon MD, et al. Lone atrial fibrillation in elderly persons: a marker for cardiovascular risk. Arch Intern Med (1960). 1999;159(10):1118–22. https://doi.org/10.1001/archinte.159.10.1118.

62. Haissaguerre M, Jais P, Shah DC, et al. Spontaneous initiation of atrial fibrillation by ectopic beats originating in the pulmonary veins. N Engl J Med. 1998;339(10):659–66. http://content.nejm.org/cgi/content/abstract/339/10/659. https://doi.org/10.1056/NEJM199809033391003.

63. Bah A, Nuotio I, Grönberg T, Ylitalo A, Airaksinen KEJ, Hartikainen JEK. Sex, age, and time to cardioversion. Risk factors for cardioversion of acute atrial fibrillation from the FinCV study. Ann Med (Helsinki). 2017;49(3):254–9. https://doi.org/10.1080/07853890.2016.1267869.

64. Nuotio I, Hartikainen JEK, Grönberg T, Biancari F, Airaksinen KEJ. Time to cardioversion for acute atrial fibrillation and thromboembolic complications. JAMA. 2014;312(6):647–9. https://doi.org/10.1001/jama.2014.3824.

65. Lundstrom T, Ryden L. Chronic atrial fibrillation: long term results of direct current conversion. Acta Med Scand. 1988;223(1):53–9. https://www.ncbi.nlm.nih.gov/pubmed/3348103. https://doi.org/10.1111/j.0954-6820.1988.tb15764.x.

66. Danias PG, Caulfield TA, Weigner MJ, Silverman DI, Manning WJ. Likelihood of spontaneous conversion of atrial fibrillation to sinus rhythm. J Am Coll Cardiol. 1998;31(3):588–92. https://doi.org/10.1016/S0735-1097(97)00534-2.

67. Flaker GC, Fletcher KA, Rothbart RM, Halperin JL, Hart RG. Clinical and echocardiographic features of intermittent atrial fibrillation that predict recurrent atrial fibrillation. Stroke Prevention in Atrial Fibrillation (SPAF) Investigators. Am J Cardiol. 1995;76(5):355–8. https://www.ncbi.nlm.nih.gov/pubmed/7639159

68. Dittrich HC, Pearce LA, Asinger RW, et al. Left atrial diameter in nonvalvular atrial fibrillation: an echocardiographic study. Stroke Prevention in Atrial Fibrillation Investigators. Am Heart J. 1999;137(3):494–9. https://www.ncbi.nlm.nih.gov/pubmed/10047632

69. Duytschaever M, Haerynck F, Tavernier R, Jordaens L. Factors influencing long term persistence of sinus rhythm after a first electrical cardioversion for atrial fibrillation. Pacing Clin Electrophysiol. 1998;21(1):284–7. https://api.istex.fr/ark:/67375/WNG-BV7TG2Z0-8/fulltext.pdf. https://doi.org/10.1111/j.1540-8159.1998.tb01105.x.

70. Lau DH, Nattel S, Kalman JM, Sanders P. Modifiable risk factors and atrial fibrillation. Circulation (New York, NY). 2017;136(6):583–96. https://www.ncbi.nlm.nih.gov/pubmed/28784826. https://doi.org/10.1161/CIRCULATIONAHA.116.023163.

71. Mittal S, Ayati S, Stein KM, et al. Transthoracic cardioversion of atrial fibrillation: comparison of rectilinear biphasic versus damped sine wave monophasic shocks. Circulation. 2000;101(11):1282–7. http://circ.ahajournals.org/cgi/content/abstract/101/11/1282. https://doi.org/10.1161/01.CIR.101.11.1282.

72. Kirchhof P, Eckardt L, Loh P, et al. Anterior-posterior versus anterior-lateral electrode positions for external cardioversion of atrial fibrillation: a randomised trial. The Lancet (British edition). 2002;360(9342):1275–9. https://doi.org/10.1016/S0140-6736(02)11315-8.

73. Schmidt AS, Lauridsen KG, Torp P, Bach LF, Rickers H, Løfgren B. Maximum-fixed energy shocks for cardioverting atrial fibrillation. Eur Heart J. 2020;41(5):626–31. https://www.ncbi.nlm.nih.gov/pubmed/31504412. https://doi.org/10.1093/eurheartj/ehz585.

74. Bunch TJ, Crandall BG, Weiss JP, et al. Patients treated with catheter ablation for atrial fibrillation have long-term rates of death, stroke, and dementia similar to patients without atrial fibrillation. J Cardiovasc Electrophysiol. 2011;22(8):839–45. https://api.istex.fr/ark:/67375/WNG-DDNS3844-7/fulltext.pdf. https://doi.org/10.1111/j.1540-8167.2011.02035.x.

75. Reynolds MR, Gunnarsson CL, Hunter TD, et al. Health outcomes with catheter ablation or antiarrhythmic drug therapy in atrial fibrillation: results of a propensity-matched analysis. Circ Cardiovasc Qual Outcomes. 2012;5(2):171–81. https://www.ncbi.nlm.nih.gov/pubmed/22373904. https://doi.org/10.1161/CIRCOUTCOMES.111.963108.

76. Packer DL, Mark DB, Robb RA, et al. Effect of catheter ablation vs antiarrhythmic drug therapy on mortality, stroke, bleeding, and cardiac arrest among patients with atrial fibrillation: the CABANA randomized clinical trial. JAMA. 2019;321(13):1261–74. https://doi.org/10.1001/jama.2019.0693.

77. Hunter RJ, McCready J, Diab I, et al. Maintenance of sinus rhythm with an ablation strategy in patients with atrial fibrillation is associated with a lower risk of stroke and death. Heart. 2012;98(1):48–53. https://doi.org/10.1136/heartjnl-2011-300720.

78. Kirchhof P, Camm AJ, Goette A, et al. Early rhythm-control therapy in patients with atrial fibrillation. N Engl J Med. 2020;383(14):1305–16. https://doi.org/10.1056/NEJMoa2019422.

79. Van Gelder IC, Groenveld HF, Crijns HJGM, et al. Lenient versus strict rate control in patients with atrial fibrillation. N Engl J Med. 2010;362(15):1363–73. https://doi.org/10.1056/NEJMoa1001337.

80. Lopes RD, Rordorf R, De Ferrari GM, et al. Digoxin and mortality in patients with atrial fibrillation. J Am Coll Cardiol. 2018;71(10):1063–74. https://doi.org/10.1016/j.jacc.2017.12.060.

81. Bavendiek U, Berliner D, Dávila LA, et al. Rationale and design of the DIGIT-HF trial (DIGitoxin to improve ouTcomes in patients with advanced chronic heart failure): a randomized, double-blind, placebo-controlled study. Eur J Heart Fail. 2019;21(5):676–84. https://onlinelibrary.wiley.com/doi/abs/10.1002/ejhf.1452. https://doi.org/10.1002/ejhf.1452.

82. Kochiadakis GE, Igoumenidis NE, Solomou MC, Kaleboubas MD, Chlouverakis GI, Vardas PE. Efficacy of amiodarone for the termination of persistent atrial fibrillation. Am J Cardiol. 1999;83(1):58–61. https://doi.org/10.1016/S0002-9149(98)00783-8.

83. Roy D, Talajic M, Dorian P, et al. Amiodarone to prevent recurrence of atrial fibrillation. N Engl J Med. 2000;342(13):913–20. http://content.nejm.org/cgi/content/abstract/342/13/913. https://doi.org/10.1056/NEJM200003303421302.

84. Singh BN, Singh SN, Reda DJ, et al. Amiodarone versus sotalol for atrial fibrillation. N Engl J Med. 2005;352(18):1861–72. http://content.nejm.org/cgi/content/abstract/352/18/1861. https://doi.org/10.1056/NEJMoa041705.

85. Dorian P, Mangat I. Maintenance of sinus rhythm in patients with atrial fibrillation: an AFFIRM substudy of the first antiarrhythmic drug. J Am Coll Cardiol. 2003;42(1):20–32. http://content.onlinejacc.org/cgi/content/abstract/42/1/20. https://doi.org/10.1016/S0735-1097(03)00559-X.

86. Alboni P, Botto GL, Baldi N, et al. Outpatient treatment of recent-onset atrial fibrillation with the "pill-in-the-pocket" approach. N Engl J Med. 2004;351(23):2384–91. http://content.nejm.org/cgi/content/abstract/351/23/2384. https://doi.org/10.1056/NEJMoa041233.

87. Hohnloser SH, Kuck K, Lilienthal J. Rhythm or rate control in atrial fibrillation—pharmacological intervention in atrial fibrillation (PIAF): a randomised trial. Lancet. 2000;356(9244):1789–94. https://doi.org/10.1016/S0140-6736(00)03230-X.

88. Jo C, Miketic S, Windeler J, et al. Randomized trial of rate-control versus rhythm-control in persistent atrial fibrillation: the strategies of treatment of Atrial Fibrillation (STAF) Study. J Am Coll Cardiol. 2003;41(10):1690–6. http://content.onlinejacc.org/cgi/content/abstract/41/10/1690. https://doi.org/10.1016/S0735-1097(03)00332-2.

89. Wyse DG, Waldo AL, DiMarco JP, et al. A comparison of rate control and rhythm control in patients with atrial fibrillation. N Engl J Med. 2002;347(23):1825–33. http://content.nejm.org/cgi/content/abstract/347/23/1825. https://doi.org/10.1056/NEJMoa021328.

90. Van Gelder IC, Hagens VE, Bosker HA, et al. A comparison of rate control and rhythm control in patients with recurrent persistent atrial fibrillation. N Engl J Med. 2002;347(23):1834–40. http://content.nejm.org/cgi/content/abstract/347/23/1834.   https://doi.org/10.1056/NEJMoa021375.

91. Marrouche NF, Brachmann J, Andresen D, et al. Catheter ablation for atrial fibrillation with heart failure. N Engl J Med. 2018;378(5):417–27. https://doi.org/10.1056/NEJMoa1707855.

92. Di Biase L, Mohanty P, Mohanty S, et al. Ablation versus amiodarone for treatment of persistent atrial fibrillation in patients with congestive heart failure and an implanted device: results from the AATAC multicenter randomized trial. Circulation (New York, NY). 2016;133(17):1637–44.   https://www.ncbi.nlm.nih.gov/pubmed/27029350.   https://doi.org/10.1161/CIRCULATIONAHA.115.019406.

93. Wazni OM, Dandamudi G, Sood N, et al. Cryoballoon ablation as initial therapy for atrial fibrillation. N Engl J Med. 2021;384(4):316–24. https://doi.org/10.1056/NEJMoa2029554.

94. Andrade JG, Wells GA, Deyell MW, et al. Cryoablation or drug therapy for initial treatment of atrial fibrillation. N Engl J Med. 2021;384(4):305–15. https://doi.org/10.1056/NEJMoa2029980.

95. Kimura S, Bassett AL, Kohya T, Kozlovskis PL, Myerburg RJ. Simultaneous recording of action potentials from endocardium and epicardium during ischemia in the isolated cat ventricle: relation of temporal electrophysiologic heterogeneities to arrhythmias. Circulation. 1986;74(2):401–9.   http://circ.ahajournals.org/cgi/content/abstract/74/2/401.   https://doi.org/10.1161/01.CIR.74.2.401.

96. Fleg JL, Lakatta EG. Prevalence and prognosis of exercise-induced nonsustained ventricular tachycardia in apparently healthy volunteers. Am J Cardiol. 1984;54(7):762–4. https://doi.org/10.1016/S0002-9149(84)80204-0.

97. Mirowski M, Reid PR, Mower MM, et al. Termination of malignant ventricular arrhythmias with an implanted automatic defibrillator in human beings. N Engl J Med. 1980;303(6):322–4. https://doi.org/10.1056/NEJM198008073030607.

98. Hasselqvist-Ax I, Riva G, Herlitz J, et al. Early cardiopulmonary resuscitation in out-of-hospital cardiac arrest. N Engl J Med. 2015;372(24):2307–15. https://doi.org/10.1056/NEJMoa1405796.

99. Chan P, McNally B, Tang F, Kellermann A. Recent trends in survival from out-of-hospital cardiac arrest in the United States. Circulation (New York, NY). 2014;130(21):1876–82. http://ovidsp.ovid.com/ovidweb.cgi?T=JS&NEWS=n&CSC=Y&PAGE=fulltext&D=ovft&AN=00003017-201411180-00008. https://doi.org/10.1161/CIRCULATIONAHA.114.009711.

100. The Antiarrhythmics versus Implantable Defibrillators (AVID) Investigators. A comparison of antiarrhythmic-drug therapy with implantable defibrillators in patients resuscitated from near-fatal ventricular arrhythmias. N Engl J Med. 1997;337(22):1576–84. http://content.nejm.org/cgi/content/abstract/337/22/1576. https://doi.org/10.1056/NEJM199711273372202.

101. Connolly SJ, Hallstrom AP, Cappato R, et al. Meta-analysis of the implantable cardioverter defibrillator secondary prevention trials. AVID, CASH and CIDS studies. Antiarrhythmics vs Implantable Defibrillator Study. Cardiac Arrest Study Hamburg. Canadian Implantable Defibrillator Study. Eur Heart J. 2000;21(24):2071–8. https://www.ncbi.nlm.nih.gov/pubmed/11102258

102. Al-Khatib SM, Stevenson WG, Ackerman MJ, et al. 2017 AHA/ACC/HRS guideline for management of patients with ventricular arrhythmias and the prevention of sudden cardiac death: a report of the American College of Cardiology/American Heart Association task force on clinical practice guidelines and the Heart Rhythm Society. J Am Coll Cardiol. 2018;72(14):e91–e220. https://www.ncbi.nlm.nih.gov/pubmed/29097296. https://doi.org/10.1016/j.jacc.2017.10.054.

103. Myerburg RJ, Interian A, Mitrani RM, Kessler KM, Castellanos A. Frequency of sudden cardiac death and profiles of risk. Am J Cardiol. 1997;80(5):10F–9F. https://doi.org/10.1016/S0002-9149(97)00477-3.

104. Moss AJ, Zareba W, Hall WJ, et al. Prophylactic implantation of a defibrillator in patients with myocardial infarction and reduced ejection fraction. N Engl J Med. 2002;346(12):877–83. http://content.nejm.org/cgi/content/abstract/346/12/877. https://doi.org/10.1056/NEJMoa013474.

105. Bardy GH, Lee KL, Mark DB, et al. Amiodarone or an implantable cardioverter-defibrillator for congestive heart failure. N Engl J Med. 2005;352(3):225–37. http://content.nejm.org/cgi/content/abstract/352/3/225. https://doi.org/10.1056/NEJMoa043399.

106. Hohnloser SH, Kuck KH, Dorian P, et al. Prophylactic use of an implantable cardioverter-defibrillator after acute myocardial infarction. N Engl J Med. 2004;351(24):2481–8. http://content.nejm.org/cgi/content/abstract/351/24/2481. https://doi.org/10.1056/NEJMoa041489.

107. Olgin JE, Pletcher MJ, Vittinghoff E, et al. Wearable Cardioverter–Defibrillator after myocardial infarction. N Engl J Med. 2018;379(13):1205–15. https://doi.org/10.1056/NEJMoa1800781.

108. Golwala H, Bajaj N, Arora G, Arora P. Implantable cardioverter-defibrillator for non-ischemic cardiomyopathy: an updated meta-analysis. Circulation (New York, NY). 2017;135(2):201–3. https://www.ncbi.nlm.nih.gov/pubmed/27993908. https://doi.org/10.1161/CIRCULATIONAHA.116.026056.

109. Koene RJ, Adkisson WO, Benditt DG. Syncope and the risk of sudden cardiac death: evaluation, management, and prevention. J Arrhythmia. 2017;33(6):533–44. https://onlinelibrary.wiley.com/doi/abs/10.1016/j.joa.2017.07.005. https://doi.org/10.1016/j.joa.2017.07.005.

110. Ruwald MH, Hansen ML, Lamberts M, et al. The relation between age, sex, comorbidity, and pharmacotherapy and the risk of syncope: a Danish Nationwide Study. Europace (London, England). 2012;14(10):1506–14. https://www.ncbi.nlm.nih.gov/pubmed/22588456. https://doi.org/10.1093/europace/eus154.

111. Soteriades ES, Evans JC, Larson MG, et al. Incidence and prognosis of syncope. N Engl J Med. 2002;347(12):878–85. http://content.nejm.org/cgi/content/abstract/347/12/878. https://doi.org/10.1056/NEJMoa012407.

112. Nyman JA, Krahn AD, Bland PC, Griffiths S, Manda V. The costs of recurrent syncope of unknown origin in elderly patients. Pacing Clin Electrophysiol. 1999;22(9):1386–94. https://api.istex.fr/ark:/67375/WNG-T03F67DT-J/fulltext.pdf. https://doi.org/10.1111/j.1540-8159.1999.tb00633.x.

113. Sun BC, Emond JA, Camargo CA. Direct medical costs of syncope-related hospitalizations in the United States. Am J Cardiol. 2005;95(5):668–71. https://doi.org/10.1016/j.amjcard.2004.11.013.

114. Ungar A, Mussi C, Del Rosso A, et al. Diagnosis and characteristics of syncope in older patients referred to geriatric departments. J Am Geriatr Soc. 2006;54(10):1531–6. https://api.istex.fr/ark:/67375/WNG-FSMZQ4HN-K/fulltext.pdf. https://doi.org/10.1111/j.1532-5415.2006.00891.x.

115. D'Ascenzo F, Biondi-Zoccai G, Reed MJ, et al. Incidence, etiology and predictors of adverse outcomes in 43,315 patients presenting to the emergency department with syncope: an international meta-analysis. Int J Cardiol. 2011;167(1):57–62. https://www.clinicalkey.es/playcontent/1-s2.0-S0167527311021401. https://doi.org/10.1016/j.ijcard.2011.11.083.

116. Kaufmann H, Norcliffe-Kaufmann L, Palma J. Baroreflex dysfunction. N Engl J Med. 2020;382(2):163–78. https://doi.org/10.1056/NEJMra1509723.

117. Barochiner J, Alfie J, Aparicio LS, et al. Postprandial hypotension detected through home blood pressure monitoring: a frequent phenomenon in elderly hypertensive patients. Hypertens Res. 2014;37(5):438–43. https://www.ncbi.nlm.nih.gov/pubmed/24108236. https://doi.org/10.1038/hr.2013.144.

118. Kenny RA. Syncope in the elderly: diagnosis, evaluation, and treatment. J Cardiovasc Electrophysiol. 2003;14(9 Suppl):S74–7. https://www.ncbi.nlm.nih.gov/pubmed/12950524. https://doi.org/10.1046/j.1540-8167.14.s9.8.x.

119. Bryarly M, Phillips LT, Fu Q, Vernino S, Levine BD. Postural orthostatic Tachycardia Syndrome: JACC focus seminar. J Am Coll Cardiol. 2019;73(10):1207–28. https://www.ncbi.nlm.nih.gov/pubmed/30871704. https://doi.org/10.1016/j.jacc.2018.11.059.

120. Grubb BP. Neurocardiogenic syncope. N Engl J Med. 2005;352(10):1004–10. http://content.nejm.org/cgi/content/extract/352/10/1004. https://doi.org/10.1056/NEJMcp042601.

121. Puggioni E, Guiducci V, Brignole M, et al. Results and complications of the carotid sinus massage performed according to the "method of symptoms". Am J Cardiol. 2002;89(5):599–601. https://doi.org/10.1016/S0002-9149(01)02303-7.

122. Kerr SRJ, Pearce MS, Brayne C, Davis RJ, Kenny RA. Carotid sinus hypersensitivity in asymptomatic older persons: implications for diagnosis of syncope and falls. Arch Intern Med (1960). 2006;166(5):515–20. https://doi.org/10.1001/archinte.166.5.515.

123. Kapoor WN. Evaluation and outcome of patients with syncope. Medicine (Baltimore). 1990;69(3):160–75. https://www.ncbi.nlm.nih.gov/pubmed/2189056. https://doi.org/10.1097/00005792-199005000-00004.

124. Quinn JV. Yield of diagnostic tests in evaluating syncopal episodes in older patients—Invited commentary. Arch Intern Med (1960). 2009;169(14):1305–6. https://doi.org/10.1001/archinternmed.2009.203.

125. Zaidi A, Clough P, Cooper P, Scheepers B, Fitzpatrick AP. Misdiagnosis of epilepsy: many seizure-like attacks have a cardiovascular cause. J Am Coll Cardiol. 2000;36(1):181–4. https://doi.org/10.1016/S0735-1097(00)00700-2.

126. Brignole M, Ungar A, Casagranda I, et al. Prospective multicentre systematic guideline-based management of patients referred to the syncope units of general hospitals. Europace (London, England). 2010;12(1):109–18. https://www.ncbi.nlm.nih.gov/pubmed/19948566. https://doi.org/10.1093/europace/eup370.

127. Ricci F, Fedorowski A, Radico F, et al. Cardiovascular morbidity and mortality related to orthostatic hypotension: a meta-analysis of prospective observational studies. Eur Heart J. 2015;36(25):1609–17. https://www.ncbi.nlm.nih.gov/pubmed/25852216. https://doi.org/10.1093/eurheartj/ehv093.

128. Calkins H, Shyr Y, Frumin H, Schork A, Morady F. The value of the clinical history in the differentiation of syncope due to ventricular tachycardia, atrioventricular block, and neurocardiogenic syncope. Am J Med. 1995;98(4):365–73. https://doi.org/10.1016/S0002-9343(99)80315-5.

129. Brignole M, Moya A, de Lange FJ, et al. 2018 ESC guidelines for the diagnosis and management of syncope. Eur Heart J. 2018;39(21):1883–948. https://www.narcis.nl/publication/RecordID/oai:pure.amc.nl:publications%2F5c0f3843-e414-4a01-8ce6-7b56a0f15f17. https://doi.org/10.1093/eurheartj/ehy037.

130. Sumiyoshi M, Nakata Y, Mineda Y, et al. Response to head-up tilt testing in patients with situational syncope. Am J Cardiol. 1998;82(9):1117–8. https://doi.org/10.1016/S0002-9149(98)00561-X.

131. Sarasin FP, Junod A, Carballo D, Slama S, Unger P, Louis-Simonet M. Role of echocardiography in the evaluation of syncope: a prospective study. Heart. 2002;88(4):363–7. https://doi.org/10.1136/heart.88.4.363.

132. Van Dijk N, Boer KR, Colman N, et al. High diagnostic yield and accuracy of history, physical examination, and ECG in patients with transient loss of consciousness in FAST: the fainting assessment study. J Cardiovasc Electrophysiol. 2008;19(1):48–55. https://api.istex.

fr/ark:/67375/WNG-XJ7GFVVL-S/fulltext.pdf. https://doi.org/10.1111/j.1540-8167.2007. 00984.x.

133. More D, O'Brien K, Shaw J. Arrhythmogenic right ventricular dysplasia in the elderly. Pacing Clin Electrophysiol. 2002;25(8):1266–9. https://onlinelibrary.wiley.com/doi/abs/10.1046/ j.1460-9592.2002.01266.x. https://doi.org/10.1046/j.1460-9592.2002.01266.x.

134. Sivakumaran S, Krahn AD, Klein GJ, et al. A prospective randomized comparison of loop recorders versus Holter monitors in patients with syncope or presyncope. Am J Med. 2003;115(1):1–5. https://doi.org/10.1016/S0002-9343(03)00233-X.

135. Shen W, Sheldon RS, Benditt DG, et al. 2017 ACC/AHA/HRS guideline for the evaluation and management of patients with syncope: a report of the American College of Cardiology/American Heart Association task force on clinical practice guidelines, and the Heart Rhythm Society. Heart Rhythm. 2017;14(8):e155–217. https://www.ncbi.nlm.nih.gov/ pubmed/28286247. https://doi.org/10.1016/j.hrthm.2017.03.004.

136. Gatzoulis KA, Karystinos G, Gialernios T, et al. Correlation of noninvasive electrocardiography with invasive electrophysiology in syncope of unknown origin: implications from a large syncope database. Ann Noninvasive Electrocardiol. 2009;14(2):119–27. http://www. ingentaconnect.com/content/bsc/anec/2009/00000014/00000002/art00003. https://doi. org/10.1111/j.1542-474X.2009.00286.x.

137. Svennberg E, Engdahl J, Al-Khalili F, Friberg L, Frykman V, Rosenqvist M. Mass screening for untreated atrial fibrillation: the STROKESTOP Study. Circulation (New York, NY). 2015;131(25):2176–84. https://www.ncbi.nlm.nih.gov/pubmed/25910800. https://doi. org/10.1161/CIRCULATIONAHA.114.014343.

138. Perez MV, Mahaffey KW, Hedlin H, et al. Large-scale assessment of a smartwatch to identify atrial fibrillation. N Engl J Med. 2019;381(20):1909–17. https://doi.org/10.1056/ NEJMoa1901183.

139. Bumgarner JM, Lambert CT, Hussein AA, et al. Smartwatch algorithm for Automated Detection of atrial fibrillation. J Am Coll Cardiol. 2018;71(21):2381–8. https://doi. org/10.1016/j.jacc.2018.03.003.

140. Sanna T, Diener H, Passman RS, et al. Cryptogenic stroke and underlying atrial fibrillation. N Engl J Med. 2014;370(26):2478–86. https://doi.org/10.1056/NEJMoa1313600.

141. Hinicks G, Potpara T, Dagres N, et al. 2020 ESC guidelines for the diagnosis and management of atrial fibrillation developed in collaboration with the European Association for Cardio-Thoracic Surgery (EACTS). Eur Heart J. 2021;42(5):373–498. https://www.narcis.nl/publication/RecordID/oai:pure.rug.nl:publications%2F3317b4ce-3ccc-4eb2-afb1-abd471c1daca. https://doi.org/10.1093/eurheartj/ehaa612.

142. Ganesan AN, Chew DP, Hartshorne T, et al. The impact of atrial fibrillation type on the risk of thromboembolism, mortality, and bleeding: a systematic review and meta-analysis. Eur Heart J. 2016;37(20):1591–602. https://www.ncbi.nlm.nih.gov/pubmed/26888184. https:// doi.org/10.1093/eurheartj/ehw007.

143. Lip GYH, Nieuwlaat R, Pisters R, Lane DA, Crijns HJGM. Refining clinical risk stratification for predicting stroke and thromboembolism in atrial fibrillation using a novel risk factor-based approach the Euro Heart Survey on atrial fibrillation. Chest. 2010;137(2):263–72. https://www. narcis.nl/publication/RecordID/oai:cris.maastrichtuniversity.nl:publications%2F23809ce3-ed44-4fdb-88be-b83946b1f602. https://doi.org/10.1378/chest.09-1584.

144. Blackshear JL, Halperin JL, Hart RG, Laupacis A. Adjusted-dose warfarin versus low-intensity, fixed-dose warfarin plus aspirin for high-risk patients with atrial fibrillation. The Lancet (British edition). 1996;348(9028):633. https://search.proquest.com/docview/198969540

145. EAFT (European Atrial Fibrillation Trial) Study Group. Secondary prevention in non-rheumatic atrial fibrillation after transient ischaemic attack or minor stroke. The Lancet (British edition). 1993;342(8882):1255–62. https://doi.org/10.1016/0140-6736(93)92358-Z.

146. Granger CB, Alexander JH, McMurray JJV, et al. Apixaban versus warfarin in patients with atrial fibrillation. N Engl J Med. 2011;365(11):981–92. https://doi.org/10.1056/ NEJMoa1107039.

147. Niessner A, Rose A, Rosenstein R, et al. Rivaroxaban versus warfarin in nonvalvular atrial fibrillation. N Engl J Med. 2011;365(24):2333–5. https://doi.org/10.1056/NEJMc1112233.
148. Houston DS, Zarychanski R, Tomoda H, et al. Dabigatran versus warfarin in patients with atrial fibrillation. N Engl J Med. 2009;361(27):2671–5. http://content.nejm.org/cgi/content/extract/361/27/2671. https://doi.org/10.1056/NEJMc0909962.
149. Giugliano RP, Ruff CT, Braunwald E, et al. Edoxaban versus warfarin in patients with atrial fibrillation. N Engl J Med. 2013;369(22):2093–104. https://doi.org/10.1056/NEJMoa1310907.
150. Eikelboom JW, Connolly SJ, Brueckmann M, et al. Dabigatran versus warfarin in patients with mechanical heart valves. N Engl J Med. 2013;369(13):1206–14. https://doi.org/10.1056/NEJMoa1300615.
151. Rash A, Downes T, Portner R, Yeo WW, Morgan N, Channer KS. A randomised controlled trial of warfarin versus aspirin for stroke prevention in octogenarians with atrial fibrillation (WASPO). Age Ageing. 2007;36(2):151–6. https://api.istex.fr/ark:/67375/HXZ-GQMDGZ50-D/fulltext.pdf. https://doi.org/10.1093/ageing/afl129.
152. Mant J, Hobbs FR, Fletcher K, et al. Warfarin versus aspirin for stroke prevention in an elderly community population with atrial fibrillation (the Birmingham Atrial Fibrillation Treatment of the Aged Study, BAFTA): a randomised controlled trial. The Lancet (British edition). 2007;370(9586):493–503. https://www.clinicalkey.es/playcontent/1-s2.0-S0140673607612331. https://doi.org/10.1016/S0140-6736(07)61233-1.
153. Chao T, Liu C, Lin Y, et al. Oral anticoagulation in very elderly patients with atrial fibrillation: a nationwide cohort study. Circulation (New York, NY). 2018;138(1):37–47. https://www.ncbi.nlm.nih.gov/pubmed/29490992. https://doi.org/10.1161/CIRCULATIONAHA.117.031658.
154. Halvorsen S, Atar D, Yang H, et al. Efficacy and safety of apixaban compared with warfarin according to age for stroke prevention in atrial fibrillation: observations from the ARISTOTLE trial. Eur Heart J. 2014;35(28):1864–72. https://www.ncbi.nlm.nih.gov/pubmed/24561548. https://doi.org/10.1093/eurheartj/ehu046.
155. Halperin JL, Hankey GJ, Paolini JF, et al. Efficacy and safety of rivaroxaban compared with warfarin among elderly patients with nonvalvular atrial fibrillation in the rivaroxaban once daily, oral, direct factor Xa inhibition compared with vitamin K antagonism for prevention of stroke and embolism trial in atrial fibrillation (ROCKET AF). Circulation (New York, NY). 2014;130(2):138–46. https://www.ncbi.nlm.nih.gov/pubmed/24895454. https://doi.org/10.1161/CIRCULATIONAHA.113.005008.
156. Själander S, Själander A, Svensson PJ, Friberg L. Atrial fibrillation patients do not benefit from acetylsalicylic acid. Europace (London, England). 2014;16(5):631–8. https://www.ncbi.nlm.nih.gov/pubmed/24158253. https://doi.org/10.1093/europace/eut333.
157. Fumagalli S, Said SAM, Laroche C, et al. Age-related differences in presentation, treatment, and outcome of patients with Atrial fibrillation in Europe: The EORP-AF general pilot registry (EURObservational Research programme-atrial fibrillation). JACC Clin Electrophysiol. 2015;1(4):326–34. https://www.ncbi.nlm.nih.gov/pubmed/29759321. https://doi.org/10.1016/j.jacep.2015.02.019.
158. Reddy VY, Doshi SK, Sievert H, et al. Percutaneous left atrial appendage closure for stroke prophylaxis in patients with atrial fibrillation: 2.3-year follow-up of the PROTECT AF (watchman left atrial appendage system for embolic protection in patients with atrial fibrillation) trial. Circulation (New York, NY). 2013;127(6):720–9. https://www.ncbi.nlm.nih.gov/pubmed/23325525. https://doi.org/10.1161/CIRCULATIONAHA.112.114389.
159. Belgaid DR, Khan Z, Zaidi M, Hobbs A. Prospective randomized evaluation of the watchman left atrial appendage closure device in patients with atrial fibrillation versus long-term warfarin therapy: the PREVAIL trial. Int J Cardiol. 2016;219:177–9. https://www.ncbi.nlm.nih.gov/pubmed/27343417. https://doi.org/10.1016/j.ijcard.2016.06.041.
160. Holmes J, David R, Doshi SK, Kar S, et al. Left atrial appendage closure as an alternative to warfarin for stroke prevention in atrial fibrillation: a patient-level meta-analysis. J Am Coll

Cardiol. 2015;65(24):2614–23. https://www.ncbi.nlm.nih.gov/pubmed/26088300. https://doi.org/10.1016/j.jacc.2015.04.025.

161. Dukkipati S, Kar S, Holmes D, et al. Device-related thrombus after left atrial appendage closure: incidence, predictors, and outcomes. Circulation (New York, NY). 2018;138(9):874–85. https://www.ncbi.nlm.nih.gov/pubmed/29752398. https://doi.org/10.1161/CIRCULATIONAHA.118.035090.

162. Echt DS, Liebson PR, Mitchell LB, et al. Mortality and morbidity in patients receiving encainide, flecainide, or placebo. The Cardiac Arrhythmia Suppression Trial. N Engl J Med. 1991;324(12):781–8. http://content.nejm.org/cgi/content/abstract/324/12/781. https://doi.org/10.1056/NEJM199103213241201.

163. Zemrak F, Ambale-Venkatesh B, Captur G, et al. Left atrial structure in relationship to age, sex, ethnicity, and cardiovascular risk factors: MESA (multi-ethnic study of atherosclerosis). Circ Cardiovasc Imaging. 2017;10(2) https://www.ncbi.nlm.nih.gov/pubmed/28196797 https://doi.org/10.1161/CIRCIMAGING.116.005379.

164. Paciullo F, Proietti M, Bianconi V, et al. Choice and outcomes of rate control versus rhythm control in elderly patients with atrial fibrillation: a report from the REPOSI study. Drugs Aging. 2018;35(4):365–73. https://www.ncbi.nlm.nih.gov/pubmed/29564755. https://doi.org/10.1007/s40266-018-0532-8.

165. Shariff N, Desai RV, Patel K, et al. Rate-control versus rhythm-control strategies and outcomes in septuagenarians with atrial fibrillation. Am J Med. 2013;126(10):887–93. https://www.clinicalkey.es/playcontent/1-s2.0-S0002934313004993. https://doi.org/10.1016/j.amjmed.2013.04.021.

166. Purmah Y, Proietti M, Laroche C, et al. Rate vs. rhythm control and adverse outcomes among European patients with atrial fibrillation. Europace (London, England). 2018;20(2):243–52. https://www.ncbi.nlm.nih.gov/pubmed/28160483. https://doi.org/10.1093/europace/euw421.

167. Essebag V, Hadjis T, Platt RW, Pilote L. Amiodarone and the risk of bradyarrhythmia requiring permanent pacemaker in elderly patients with atrial fibrillation and prior myocardial infarction. J Am Coll Cardiol. 2003;41(2):249–54. https://doi.org/10.1016/S0735-1097(02)02709-2.

168. Abdin A, Yalin K, Lyan E, et al. Safety and efficacy of cryoballoon ablation for the treatment of atrial fibrillation in elderly patients. Clin Res Cardiol. 2019;108(2):167–74. https://www.ncbi.nlm.nih.gov/pubmed/30187178. https://doi.org/10.1007/s00392-018-1336-x.

169. Heeger C, Bellmann B, Fink T, et al. Efficacy and safety of cryoballoon ablation in the elderly: a multicenter study. Int J Cardiol. 2019;278:108–13. https://doi.org/10.1016/j.ijcard.2018.09.090.

170. Metzner I, Wissner E, Tilz RR, et al. Ablation of atrial fibrillation in patients >/=75 years: long-term clinical outcome and safety. Europace (London, England). 2016;18(4):543–9. https://www.ncbi.nlm.nih.gov/pubmed/26826139. https://doi.org/10.1093/europace/euv229.

171. Bulava A, Hanis J, Dusek L. Clinical outcomes of radiofrequency catheter ablation of atrial fibrillation in octogenarians-10-year experience of a one high-volume center. J Geriatr Cardiol. 2017;14(9):575–81. https://www.ncbi.nlm.nih.gov/pubmed/29056956. https://doi.org/10.11909/j.issn.1671-5411.2017.09.007.

172. Calkins H, Hinicks G, Cappato R, et al. 2017 HRS/EHRA/ECAS/APHRS/SOLAECE expert consensus statement on catheter and surgical ablation of atrial fibrillation: Executive summary. Europace (London, England). 2018;20(1):157–208. https://www.narcis.nl/publication/RecordID/oai:repub.eur.nl:104197. https://doi.org/10.1093/europace/eux275.

173. Langberg JJ, Calkins H, Kim Y, et al. Recurrence of conduction in accessory atrioventricular connections after initially successful radiofrequency catheter ablation. J Am Coll Cardiol. 1992;19(7):1588–92. https://doi.org/10.1016/0735-1097(92)90622-T.

174. Kornej J, Hindricks G, Kosiuk J, et al. Renal dysfunction, stroke risk scores (CHADS2, CHA2DS2-VASc, and R2CHADS2), and the risk of thromboembolic events after catheter ablation of atrial fibrillation: The Leipzig Heart Center AF Ablation Registry. Circ Arrhythm Electrophysiol. 2013;6(5):868–74. http://ovidsp.ovid.com/ovidweb.cgi?T=JS&N

EWS=n&CSC=Y&PAGE=fulltext&D=ovft&AN=01337493-201310000-00008. https://doi. org/10.1161/CIRCEP.113.000869.

175. Saad E, d'Avila A, Costa I, et al. Very low risk of thromboembolic events in patients undergoing successful catheter ablation of atrial fibrillation with a CHADS2 score ≤3: a long-term outcome study. Circ Arrhythm Electrophysiol. 2011;4(5):615–21. http://ovidsp.ovid.com/ ovidweb.cgi?T=JS&NEWS=n&CSC=Y&PAGE=fulltext&D=ovft&AN=01337493-201110 000-00005. https://doi.org/10.1161/CIRCEP.111.963231.

176. Kosiuk J, Kornej J, Bollmann A, et al. Early cerebral thromboembolic complications after radiofrequency catheter ablation of atrial fibrillation: incidence, characteristics, and risk factors. Heart Rhythm. 2014;11(11):1934–40. https://www.clinicalkey.es/playcontent/1-s2.0-S1547527114008121. https://doi.org/10.1016/j.hrthm.2014.07.039.

177. Calkins H, Epstein A, Packer D, et al. Catheter ablation of ventricular tachycardia in patients with structural heart disease using cooled radiofrequency energy: results of a prospective multicenter study. J Am Coll Cardiol. 2000;35(7):1905–14. http://content.onlinejacc.org/cgi/ content/abstract/35/7/1905

178. Mandawat A, Curtis JP, Mandawat A, Njike VY, Lampert R. Safety of pacemaker implantation in nonagenarians an analysis of the healthcare cost and utilization Project—Nationwide inpatient sample. Circulation (New York, NY). 2013;127(14):1453–65. https://www.ncbi. nlm.nih.gov/pubmed/23513066. https://doi.org/10.1161/CIRCULATIONAHA.113.001434.

179. Geelen P, Lorga Filho A, Primo J, Wellens F, Brugada P. Experience with implantable cardioverter defibrillator therapy in elderly patients. Eur Heart J. 1997;18(8):1339–42. https://api. istex.fr/ark:/67375/HXZ-VRMC5JPL-K/fulltext.pdf. https://doi.org/10.1093/oxfordjournals. eurheartj.a015447.

180. Armaganijan LV, Toff WD, Nielsen JC, et al. Are elderly patients at increased risk of complications following pacemaker implantation? A meta-analysis of randomized trials. Pacing Clin Electrophysiol. 2012;35(2):131–4. https://api.istex.fr/ark:/67375/WNG-QWZ3B0MM-X/ fulltext.pdf. https://doi.org/10.1111/j.1540-8159.2011.03240.x.

181. Tsai V, Goldstein MK, Hsia HH, Wang Y, Curtis J, Heidenreich PA. Influence of age on perioperative complications among patients undergoing implantable cardioverter-defibrillators for primary prevention in the United States. Circ Cardiovasc Qual Outcomes. 2011;4(5):549–56. https://www.ncbi.nlm.nih.gov/pubmed/21878667. https://doi. org/10.1161/CIRCOUTCOMES.110.959205.

182. Kirkfeldt RE, Johansen JB, Nohr EA, Jørgensen OD, Nielsen JC. Complications after cardiac implantable electronic device implantations: an analysis of a complete, nationwide cohort in Denmark. Eur Heart J. 2014;35(18):1186–94. https://www.ncbi.nlm.nih.gov/ pubmed/24347317. https://doi.org/10.1093/eurheartj/eht511.

183. Healey JS, Hallstrom AP, Kuck K, et al. Role of the implantable defibrillator among elderly patients with a history of life-threatening ventricular arrhythmias. Eur Heart J. 2007;28(14):1746–9. https://www.ncbi.nlm.nih.gov/pubmed/17283003. https://doi. org/10.1093/eurheartj/ehl438.

184. Yung D, Birnie D, Dorian P, et al. Survival after implantable cardioverter-defibrillator implantation in the elderly. Circulation (New York, NY). 2013;127(24):2383–92. http://ovidsp.ovid. com/ovidweb.cgi?T=JS&NEWS=n&CSC=Y&PAGE=fulltext&D=ovft&AN=00003017-20 1306180-00008. https://doi.org/10.1161/CIRCULATIONAHA.113.001442.

185. Køber L, Thune JJ, Nielsen JC, et al. Defibrillator implantation in patients with nonischemic systolic heart failure. N Engl J Med. 2016;375(13):1221–30. https://doi.org/10.1056/ NEJMoa1608029.

186. Lampert R. Quality of life and end-of-life issues for older patients with implanted cardiac rhythm devices. Clin Geriatr Med. 2012;28(4):693–702. https://www.clinicalkey.es/ playcontent/1-s2.0-S0749069012000730. https://doi.org/10.1016/j.cger.2012.07.005.

187. Lampert R, Hayes DL, Annas GJ, et al. HRS expert consensus statement on the management of cardiovascular implantable electronic devices (CIEDs) in patients nearing end of life or requesting withdrawal of therapy. Heart Rhythm. 2010;7(7):1008–26. https:// www.clinicalkey.es/playcontent/1-s2.0-S154752711000408X. https://doi.org/10.1016/j. hrthm.2010.04.033.

Percutaneous Interventions for Structural Heart Disease in the Elderly

Faisal Rahman, Jon R. Resar, and Matthew J. Czarny

1 Introduction

The life expectancy in the United States continues to rise, and as a result, the incidence of cardiovascular disease will also increase. Advancing age is also associated with a higher risk of cardiovascular morbidity, a higher risk of complications of cardiovascular procedures, and a higher likelihood of comorbidities that reduce treatment options for cardiovascular disease [1]. Because of the lower invasiveness and resultant lower procedural hemodynamic stresses, the rapidly growing field of Structural Interventional Cardiology has expanded elderly patients' access to treatment that reduces both the morbidity and mortality of cardiovascular disease as well as minimizes the periprocedural risks. This chapter will provide an overview of the transcatheter treatment of structural heart disease in the elderly.

2 Aortic Stenosis

Calcific degenerative aortic valve stenosis (AS) is the most common form of acquired valvular heart disease in the elderly, and with the aging population, the number of patients with severe AS will only increase [2]. Low-grade chronic inflammation potentially related to or exacerbated by mechanical stress results in aortic valvular fibrosis, calcification, and subsequent progressive restriction of leaflet motion [2, 3]. Mild or moderate AS does not usually cause symptoms, and it is not uncommon that even patients with severe AS are asymptomatic. However, the progressive and relentless pressure overload conferred upon the left ventricle

F. Rahman · J. R. Resar · M. J. Czarny (✉)
Division of Cardiology, Johns Hopkins University School of Medicine, Baltimore, MD, USA
e-mail: jresar@jhmi.edu; mczarny@jhmi.edu

T. M. Leucker, G. Gerstenblith (eds.), *Cardiovascular Disease in the Elderly*, Contemporary Cardiology, https://doi.org/10.1007/978-3-031-16594-8_7

by the severely stenotic aortic valve eventually results in an inability to sufficiently augment cardiac output to exertional demands, which produces the typical symptoms of fatigue, exertional dyspnea, exertional angina, syncope, and eventually, heart failure. In their seminal paper in *Circulation* in the 1960s, Drs. Ross and Braunwald demonstrated that survival of patients with severe AS was excellent until angina, syncope, or heart failure developed, with an average survival of five, three, or two years, respectively [4]. This study also suggested that medical management does not modify disease trajectory, which remains true to this day. The role of medical therapy in the management of severe symptomatic AS is limited to temporary symptomatic relief in those awaiting definitive aortic valve replacement (AVR) and palliation in patients who are not suitable for more definitive treatments.

2.1 Balloon Aortic Valvuloplasty

Balloon aortic valvuloplasty (BAV) is a procedure during which a balloon catheter is percutaneously inserted into the aortic valve and inflated, increasing the aortic valve area by a modest amount, with retrospective studies reporting an increase from $0.5 \, cm^2$ to $0.7 \, cm^2$ in the mean or median aortic valve area [5–7]. BAV was first reported in a case series in 1986 by Cribier et al. as an alternative to surgical aortic valve replacements (SAVR) in patients who were elderly and, therefore, at high risk for surgery [8]. Initial data demonstrated early symptomatic relief with the hope of improved survival, but on long-term follow-up, early restenosis was evident, and there did not seem to be an improvement in hospitalizations or mortality compared to medical management [6, 7]. As a result of this and subsequent confirmatory studies, utilization subsequently decreased considerably, and BAV was thereby relegated to a primarily palliative role.

In recent decades, however, BAV use has increased as the advent of transcatheter aortic valve replacement (TAVR) has expanded the potential patients eligible for definitive AS therapy. In current practice, BAV is most frequently used to bridge patients who are not presently candidates for AVR to AVR candidacy. Examples include patients in cardiogenic shock because of critical AS for whom BAV may enable recovery to a point where AVR can be considered, as well as for patients with cancer and an unknown survival who require aortic valve intervention to tolerate cancer therapies and enable subsequent estimation of cancer-related survival and therefore AVR candidacy. Less frequently, BAV may be used to assess the possibility of symptom improvement with aortic valve intervention in patients with severe comorbidities and symptoms to which the contribution of AS is unclear (e.g., patients with severe oxygen-dependent chronic obstructive pulmonary disease (COPD) and low-flow low-gradient severe AS). However, it is important to consider the risks of BAV alone and the safety of simply waiting to perform AVR without any intervention. Data from the National Inpatient Sample showed that BAV has a procedural mortality of 1.4%, in-hospital mortality of 8.5%, stroke rate of 1.8%, and a vascular complication rate of 7.6% [9]. As a result, BAV is rarely used for palliation. Current American College of Cardiology (ACC)/American Heart Association (AHA) guidelines give BAV a Class IIb recommendation as a bridge to SAVR or TAVR [10].

2.2 Transcatheter Aortic Valve Replacement

TAVR is the implantation within the existing aortic valve (native or prior bioprosthesis) of a bioprosthetic aortic valve typically made of bovine or porcine pericardium, mounted on a collapsible metal frame, and delivered via a catheter-based system. This is most commonly performed through percutaneous iliofemoral access but can also be done through percutaneous axillary access or surgical femoral, apical, carotid, subclavian, or direct aortic access. Although several valves are in use or under study, the two most commonly used and only FDA-approved systems in the United States are the balloon-expandable SAPIEN™ (Edwards LifeSciences LLC, Irvine, CA; Fig. 1) and the self-expanding CoreValve™/Evolut™ valves (Medtronic, Inc., Minneapolis, MN; Fig. 2). While TAVR was initially developed as an alternative to SAVR in patients who were not surgical candidates, use has rapidly expanded to patients across the surgical risk spectrum. Importantly, the growth of TAVR has increased so much in the last decade that TAVR volume currently eclipses that of SAVR in the United States [11].

The first randomized controlled data of TAVR in the United States came from the pivotal PARTNER (Placement of AoRTic TraNscathetER) trial of the Edwards SAPIEN™ valve in patients with severe symptomatic AS. In PARTNER 1B, 358 inoperable patients were randomized to conservative therapy including BAV or TAVR (mean age 83.1 years). Patients who received TAVR had a 20% absolute risk reduction in mortality (30.7% vs. 50.7%, $p < 0.001$, number needed to treat = 5) as well as a reduction in repeat hospitalization (22.3% vs. 44.1%, $p < 0.001$) [12] with results sustained to two-year follow-up [13]. Similar results were shown with the

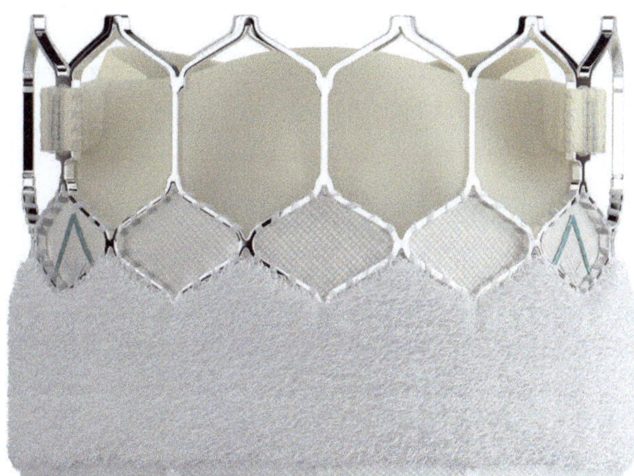

Fig. 1 The SAPIEN 3 Ultra™ transcatheter aortic valve. Image courtesy Edwards Lifesciences LLC, Irvine, CA. Edwards, the stylized E logo, Edwards SAPIEN 3, and SAPIEN 3 Ultra are trademarks of Edwards Lifesciences Corporation

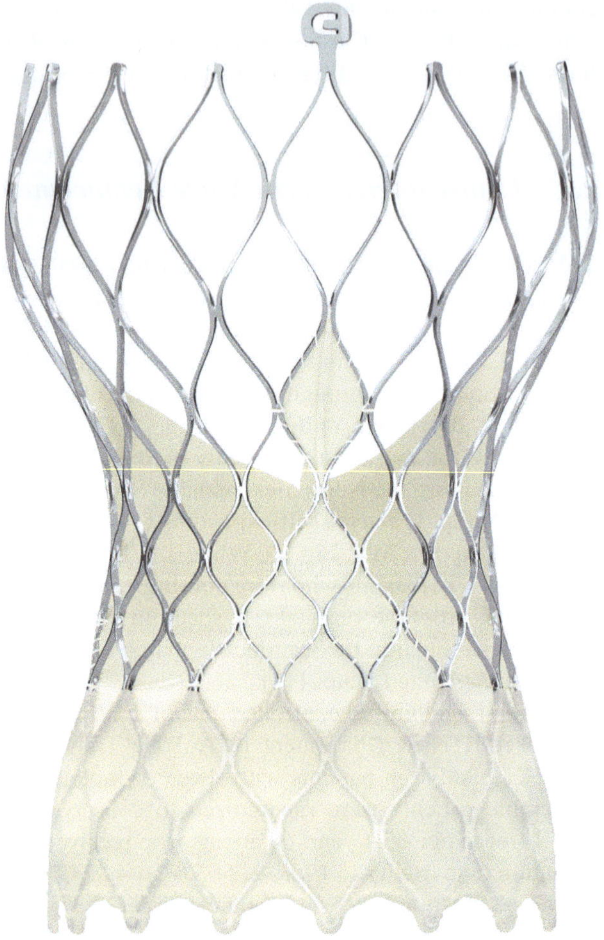

Fig. 2 The Evolut Pro™ transcatheter aortic valve. Image provided courtesy of Medtronic, Minneapolis, MN. Evolut Pro is a trademark of Medtronic

self-expanding CoreValve compared to an objective performance goal [14]. In PARTNER 1A, 699 patients at high surgical risk (STS risk score ≥ 10% or higher predicted risk of mortality ≥15%) were randomized to SAVR or transfemoral/transapical TAVR (mean age of 83.6 years). SAVR and TAVR demonstrated similar one-year mortality (24.2% vs. 26.8%), while patients in the TAVR arm had a higher rate of all vascular complications (17.0% vs. 3.8%) at 30 days and numerically higher major stroke at one year (5.1% vs. 2.4%, $p = 0.07$). Conversely, patients in the SAVR arm had higher rates of 30-day major bleeding (19.5% vs. 9.3%) and new-onset atrial fibrillation (16% vs. 8.6%) [15]. The self-expanding valve was evaluated in similar high surgical risk patients in the randomized US CoreValve High-Risk Study, where one-year mortality was significantly lower with TAVR (14.2% vs. 19.1%) [16]. Although the trials in prohibitive surgical risk patients showed that TAVR was far superior to medical management (with or without BAV) and therefore the new standard, the studies in high surgical risk patients demonstrated that

TAVR could achieve similar outcomes to SAVR with far less invasiveness. Additionally, these studies established the need for a Heart Team approach to carefully assess the surgical risk in real-world settings that included but was not limited to the Society for Thoracic Surgery (STS) predicted risk of mortality alone.

Subsequently, TAVR was shown to be safe and effective in patients at intermediate surgical risk (STS predicted risk of mortality of 4–8% or otherwise deemed at intermediate risk by a cardiac surgeon because of comorbidities). In the PARTNER 2A trial, 2000 intermediate-risk patients were randomized to TAVR with the Edwards SAPIEN XT™ or SAVR; TAVR was noninferior to SAVR for the primary endpoint of stroke or death at two years (19.3% in TAVR vs. 21% in SAVR; $p = 0.001$ for noninferiority). Importantly, patients randomized to TAVR who had transfemoral access (as opposed to transapical) had a lower rate of all-cause death or stroke than patients undergoing SAVR (HR 0.79, $p = 0.05$) [17]. Similarly, The SURTAVI study evaluated the CoreValve™ or Evolut R™ valve in intermediate-risk patients (30-day surgical risk of death estimated at 3–15%), and at 24 months, the primary endpoint of all-cause death or disabling stroke was not significantly different (12.6% for TAVR and 14% in SAVR) [18].

As data accumulated for the safety of TAVR in intermediate- and high-risk patients, the question shifted to performing TAVRs in low-risk patients, which are typically defined as patients with an STS predicted risk of mortality <4% and Heart Team consensus that the patient is at low risk of operative mortality. However, TAVR was initially studied in patients with limited life expectancy, and because enrollment in the US pivotal trials only began in 2007, limited data existed regarding transcatheter valve durability and the management of degenerated transcatheter valves. In addition, the long-term effects of paravalvular leak and TAVR-related new conduction abnormalities were unknown. These were important issues for low-risk patients who are likely to live longer. Hence, the Nordic Aortic Valve Intervention (NOTION) was an initial small, randomized control trial in a low surgical risk cohort that provided preliminary evidence of the safety and efficacy of TAVR [19] and thereby supported subsequent larger studies. In the Evolut Low-Risk Trial, non-inferiority for the primary endpoint of death or disabling stroke at 24 months was demonstrated (5.3% vs. 6.7%) [20]. In the PARTNER 3 trial with the SAPIEN 3™ valve, the primary endpoint of one-year death, stroke, or rehospitalization was significantly lower with TAVR (8.5% vs. 15.1% $p = 0.001$ for superiority) [21]. These results opened the door for TAVR in low-risk patients.

These studies of TAVR and SAVR in low-surgical risk patients highlight consistent differences between the two therapies. TAVR is associated with a lower risk of new-onset atrial fibrillation, bleeding, acute renal injury, and shorter hospital stays than SAVR [22]. Conversely, TAVR is associated with a higher rate of conduction abnormality; the new permanent pacemaker rate was 17.4% for TAVR and 6.1% for SAVR in the Evolut Low-Risk trial. Although there was no difference in one-year pacemaker rates (7.5% vs. 5.5% for TAVR and SAVR, respectively) in PARTNER 3, new left bundle branch block was more common at one year in patients undergoing TAVR (23.7% vs. 8% in SAVR). However, the long-term consequences of these findings are unknown.

As described earlier, we have a five-year follow-up of the intermediate-risk population but only up to two-year follow-up in low-risk patients to assess the durability of TAVR. Although the studies on high to inoperable risk patients are older and thus have the potential for long-term follow-up, patients in these studies have such high annual mortality that follow-up data remains sparse. The follow-up issue is also limited in low- and intermediate-risk patients where the average age was >73 years, and with US life expectancy at 79.8 years, there is still significant loss to follow-up. However, in the PARTNER 1 trials, at five years, neither TAVR nor SAVR experienced any evidence of structural valve deterioration that required repeat AVR. The long-term performance of the balloon-expandable system used was good, with a mean transvalvular gradient of 10.7 mm Hg and the estimated aortic valve area of 1.6 cm^2 at five years. However, moderate or severe aortic regurgitation was higher with TAVR (14% vs. 1%) [23]. In contrast, the five-year follow-up data from the PARTNER 2 trial showed a higher rate of valve reoperation with TAVR compared to SAVR because of progressive valve stenosis or residual aortic regurgitation (3.2% vs. 0.8%), suggesting a need for closer evaluation of durability [24]. Five-year follow-up in the PARTNER 2 trial showed some significant differences between TAVR and SAVR, including a higher rate of re-hospitalization (33.3% vs. 25.2%) with TAVR. The PARTNER 2 trial also demonstrated no difference in all-cause mortality or disabling stroke between TAVR and SAVR, although a trend towards higher death and stroke was seen between two and five years [24]. In comparison, the rate of moderate to severe structural valve deterioration was lower (4.8% vs. 24%) with TAVR with the self-expanding system compared to SAVR in the NOTION trial. Importantly, the effective orifice area was higher for TAVR than SAVR (at six years it was 1.53 cm^2 vs. 1.16 cm^2 for SAVR), consistent with greater patient-prosthesis mismatch with SAVR (28.1% vs. 12.2%; $p = 0.001$) [25]. Both the PARTNER 1 and 2 trials did not demonstrate any significant difference in all-cause mortality at five-year follow-up. Notably, the devices used in these studies have largely been replaced by later-generation devices with features aimed at decreasing paravalvular leaks. Accordingly, the applicability of these prior studies to current devices is unclear. Overall, there is no clear signal of long-term superiority of either TAVR or SAVR with regard to valve durability or survival in patients who are candidates for both.

Therefore, the decision to undertake TAVR or SAVR is a nuanced one that requires careful evaluation of each patient by the Heart Team, including both an interventional cardiologist and a cardiac surgeon, as well as a physician–patient discussion of individual preferences. Importantly, several types of patients were commonly excluded in the different randomized trials, such as those with bicuspid aortic valves, complex coronary artery disease or prohibitive risk for coronary artery occlusion, significant mitral or tricuspid valvular disease, and previous valvular surgery. In the Evolut Low Risk and PARTNER 3 trials, 14.8% and 34%, respectively, of patients evaluated were ineligible for enrollment in the studies. Observational registry data may help bridge the gap to evaluate the outcomes of TAVR in these excluded groups. However, observational studies have their own weaknesses, including selection bias as a result of unmeasured or difficult-to-measure factors by which higher-risk patients, despite low STS risk scores, receive TAVR instead of

SAVR (e.g. patients with heavy aortic calcification or marked frailty). Therefore, patient selection is a critical role of the Heart Team and is more than just the STS risk score. The 2020 ACC/AHA guidelines take a combination of surgical risk and an age/life-expectancy-based approach (Table 1). In patients who are less than 65 years old without any high-risk features, the preference should be SAVR, whereas patients between 65 and 80 years of age should be considered for SAVR or TAVR based on other comorbidities and risk, and patients who are over 80 years of age should preferably have a TAVR [10]. However, these are not hard cutoffs, and several important factors must be considered, such as the risk of coronary artery occlusion with TAVR, the need for other surgical treatment, for example, a complex

Table 1 ACC/AHA Guidelines for structural heart disease

Recommendation class	Recommendation	Guideline year
Transcatheter aortic valve implantation		
Class I	65–80 years: asymptomatic severe AS and LVEF <50%, or symptomatic severe AS with no anatomic contraindication to transfemoral AVR either SAVR or transfemoral TAVR is recommended after shared decision making	2020
Class I	Symptomatic patients with severe AS who are >80 years of age or with younger patients with a life expectancy <10 years and no CI to transfemoral access—TAVR is recommended over SAVR	2020
Class I	<65 years old or life expectancy >20 years: asymptomatic severe AS and LVEF <50%, or symptomatic severe AS–SAVR is recommended	2020
Class I	Asymptomatic severe AS and an abnormal exercise test, very severe AS, rapid progression or an elevated BNP, SAVR is recommended in preference to TAVR	2020
Class I	For patients with an indication for AVR for whom a bioprosthetic valve is preferred but valve or vascular anatomy or other factors are not suitable for transfemoral TAVR, SAVR is recommended	2020
Class I	For symptomatic patients with severe AS for whom predicted post-TAVR or post-SAVR survival is <12 months or for whom minimal improvement in quality of life is expected, palliative care is recommended after shared decision-making, including discussion of patient preferences and values	2020
Class I	For symptomatic patients of any age with severe AS and a high or prohibitive surgical risk, TAVR is recommended if the predicted post-TAVR survival is >12 months with an acceptable quality of life	2020
Class IIb	In critically ill patients with severe AS, percutaneous aortic balloon dilation may be considered as a bridge to SAVR or TAVR	2020
Class III	In patients with isolated severe AR who have indications for SAVR and are candidates for surgery, TAVR should not be performed	2020

(continued)

Table 1 (continued)

Recommendation class	Recommendation	Guideline year
Mitral stenosis		
Class I	In symptomatic patients (NYHA Class II, III, or IV) with severe rheumatic MS (mitral valve area $\leq$ 1.5 cm^2, stage D), and favorable valve morphology with less than moderate (2+) MR in the absence of LA thrombus, percutaneous mitral balloon valvotomy is recommended if it can be performed at a comprehensive valve center	2020
Class IIa	In asymptomatic patients with severe rheumatic MS (mitral valve area 1.5 cm^2, stage C) and favorable valve morphology with less than 2+ MR in the absence of LA thrombus who have elevated pulmonary pressures (pulmonary artery systolic pressure > 50 mm Hg), percutaneous mitral balloon valvotomy is reasonable if it can be performed at a comprehensive valve center	2020
Class IIb	In asymptomatic patients with severe rheumatic MS (mitral valve area 1.5 cm^2, stage C) and favorable valve morphology with less than 2+ MR in the absence of LA thrombus who have new onset of atrial fibrillation, percutaneous mitral balloon valvotomy may be considered if it can be performed at a comprehensive valve center	2020
Class IIb	In symptomatic patients (NYHA class II, III, or IV) with rheumatic MS and a mitral valve area > 1.5 cm^2, if there is evidence of hemodynamically significant rheumatic MS on the basis of a pulmonary artery wedge pressure > 25 mmHg or a mean mitral valve gradient >15 mmHg during exercise, percutaneous mitral balloon valvotomy may be considered if it can be performed at a comprehensive valve center	2020
Class IIb	In severely symptomatic patients (NYHA class III or IV) with severe rheumatic MS (mitral valve area 1.5 cm^2, stage D) who have a suboptimal valve anatomy and who are not candidates for surgery or are at high risk for surgery, primary mitral balloon valvotomy may be considered if it can be performed at a comprehensive valve center	2020
Transcatheter mitral edge-to-edge repair		
Class IIa	In severely symptomatic patients (NYHA III or IV) with primary severe MR and high or prohibitive surgical risk, transcatheter edge-to-edge repair (TEER) is reasonable if mitral valve anatomy is favorable for the repair procedure and patient life expectancy is at least 1 year	2020
Class IIa	In patients with chronic severe secondary MR related to LV systolic dysfunction (LVEF <50%) who have persistent symptoms (NYHA class II, III, or IV) while on optimal goal directed medical therapy for heart failure (stage D), TEER is reasonable in patients with appropriate anatomy as defined on transesophageal echocardiogram and with LVEF between 20% and 50%, LVESD $\leq$70 mm, and pulmonary artery systolic pressure $\leq$ 70 mm Hg	2020
Left atrial appendage occlusion		
Class IIb	Percutaneous LAA occlusion may be considered in patients with AF at increased risk of stroke who have contraindications to long-term anticoagulation	2019

coronary disease requiring bypass, other significant valvular diseases, aortic aneurysm, anatomical features that may increase risk for significant paravalvular leak, vascular access, and patient preference. Furthermore, although TAV-in-TAV has been shown to be feasible, experience with this is very limited, and concerns include increasing difficulty of future coronary access and higher rates of patient-prosthesis mismatch [26].

3 Mitral Valve Regurgitation

Similar to aortic valve disease, mitral valve disease is also increasing in prevalence, especially in the elderly [27]. Mitral valve regurgitation can be either primary (degeneration of the mitral valve apparatus) or secondary because of structural abnormalities of the left atrium or ventricle. The mitral valve is complex with an asymmetrical and saddle-shaped annulus, a complex subvalvular apparatus, and a bileaflet valvular system with three scallops in the posterior leaflet. In addition, the valve can be affected by a wide variety of pathologies that can result in mitral regurgitation or mixed disease; it lies in close proximity to the aortic valve and left ventricular outflow tract (LVOT); and can have a varying degree of calcification of the leaflets, annulus and subvalvular apparatus. Finally, the room for manipulation of devices is affected by left atrial and ventricular chamber size. These features add to the complexity of any percutaneous intervention.

3.1 Transcatheter Mitral Valve Repair

Historically mitral valve regurgitation (MR) was treated surgically with either repair or replacement. One of the surgical repair techniques is the Alfieri repair, in which the surgeon sutures the anterior and posterior leaflets together at the site of the MR jet, creating a "double-orifice" valve. Typically, this repair is combined with mitral annuloplasty to reduce the size of the mitral orifice, further reducing MR. One FDA-approved device for transcatheter mitral valve repair, the MitraClip™ system (Abbott, Abbott Park, IL, USA; Fig. 3), was developed to mimic the Alfieri repair using a clip that attaches to the anterior and posterior leaflets (Fig. 4). More broadly, this technique is known as transcatheter edge-to-edge repair (TEER).

The safety and efficacy of the MitraClip™ system have been studied in both primary and secondary MR. The Endovascular Valve Edge-to-Edge Repair Study (EVEREST I & II) trials compared MitraClip™ to surgical repair; EVEREST II enrolled predominantly primary MR patients (only 25% of patients had secondary MR) and found no difference in one-year mortality but significantly higher recurrence of MR requiring intervention in the MitraClip™ arm (20%) versus the surgical arm (2%). However, 30-day major adverse events were significantly higher in the surgery group and were associated with a decrease in 30-day quality of life

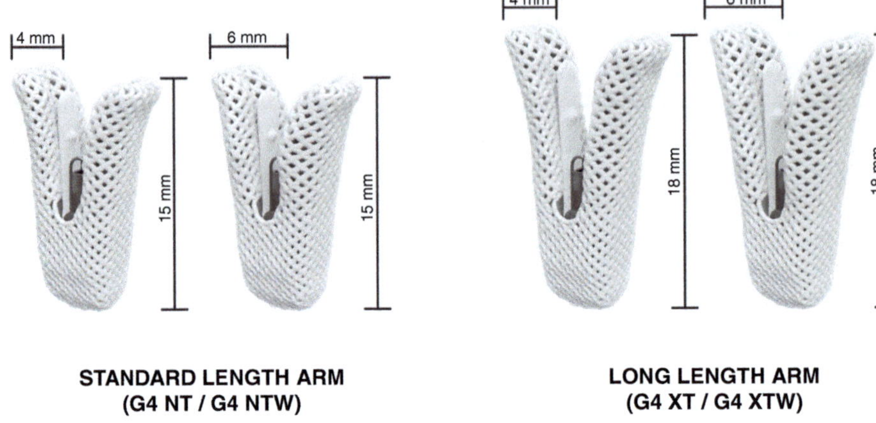

Fig. 3 The MitraClip ™ G4 family of devices. Image provided courtesy of Abbott, Abbott Park, IL. MitraClip is a trademark of Abbott

Fig. 4 Illustration of MitraClip™ implantation. The Clip Delivery System traverses the inferior vena cava, enters the right atrium, and crosses the interatrial septum into the left atrium. The MitraClip™ is illustrated in a closed, pre-deployment position after grasping both anterior and posterior mitral valve leaflets. Image provided courtesy of Abbott, Abbot Park, IL. MitraClip is a trademark of Abbott

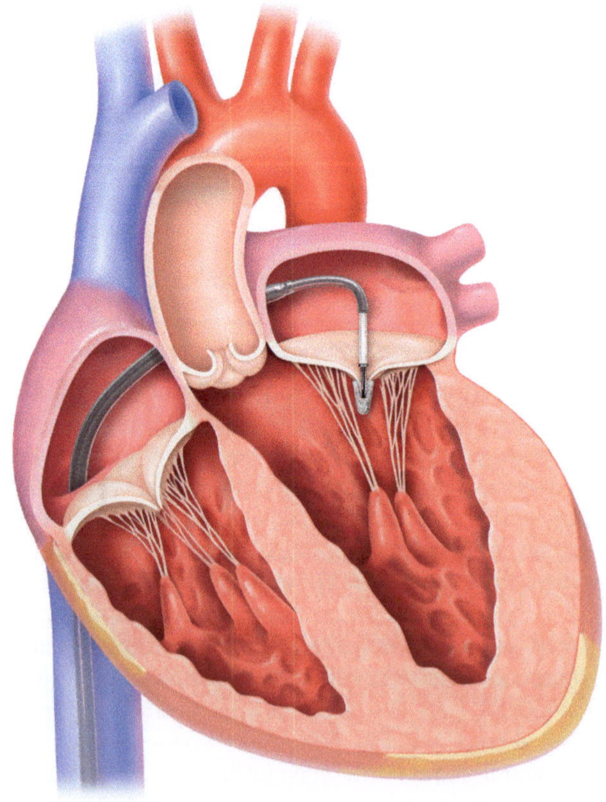

measures. At one-year, both groups showed a similar significant improvement in quality of life [28]. In retrospect, it is not surprising that MitraClip™ had a higher rate of subsequent intervention compared to surgery; MitraClip™ does not address the annulus (as most surgical repairs do), and mitral valve surgery is a well-established and very effective treatment for primary MR. Overall, the study demonstrated the effectiveness of the MitraClip™ for MR reduction and feasibility for patients who are at high surgical risk but supported surgical repair as first-line therapy in appropriate candidates. These findings were confirmed by the EVEREST High-risk Registry, where patients at high STS surgical risk (mortality risk $\geq 12\%$) demonstrated a significant reduction in heart failure hospitalization and improvement in symptoms with MitraClip™ [29].

However, the strongest data for the effectiveness of the MitraClip™ system is from more recent studies in patients with secondary MR. In the randomized controlled MITRA-FR trial, the primary composite endpoint of all-cause death and unplanned hospitalization for heart failure at 12 months did not differ between the medical therapy and MitraClip groups (51.3% vs. 54.6%, $p = 0.53$) [30]. Conversely, the COAPT study demonstrated both a significant reduction in HF hospitalization (35.8% vs. 67.9%, $p < 0.001$) and all-cause mortality (29.1% vs. 46.1%, $p < 0.001$) at 24-month follow-up with the MitraClip compared with medical therapy alone [31]. While these results seem contradictory at first, it is important to note that MITRA-FR patients, on average, had a more dilated left ventricle, less aggressive medical therapy, and a lower successful clip implantation rate than those in the COAPT study. Importantly, at three years follow-up, the COAPT results have persisted; this study led to the FDA approval of the MitraClip system for treatment of secondary MR [32].

Other transcatheter mitral valve repair systems are currently in various stages of development. The Edwards PASCAL™ Transcatheter Valve Repair System (Edwards Lifesciences LLC, Irvine, CA, USA; Fig. 5) is another TEER system that has also demonstrated efficacy in treating MR and has recently received FDA approval [33]. In addition to these, many other devices are undergoing investigation, including the Edwards Cardioband Mitral Valve Reconstruction System (Edwards Lifesciences LLC, Irvine, CA, USA), which mimics a surgical annuloplasty ring. Given the challenges that the mitral valve anatomy presents, the demonstrated effectiveness and safety of the MitraClip™ system, and a large number of prior failed transcatheter mitral valve repair devices, we await the results of randomized clinical trials to determine whether any of these devices offer similar or improved transcatheter outcomes.

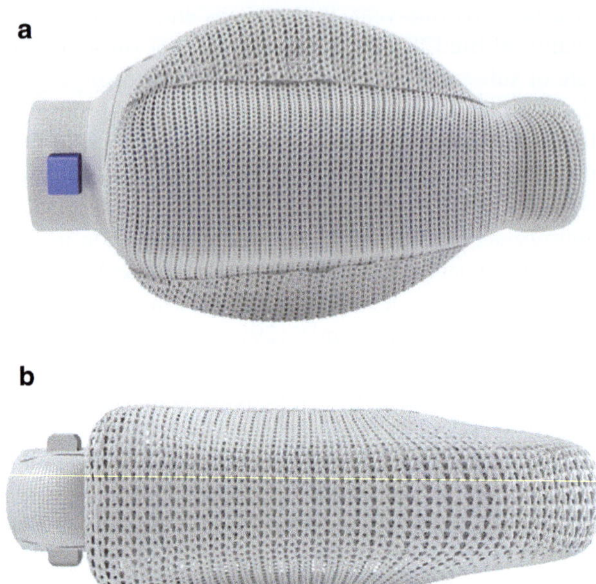

Fig. 5 The Edwards PASCAL™ (**a**) and PASCAL Ace™ (**b**) Transcatheter Valve Repair Systems. Images provided courtesy of Edwards Lifesciences LLC, Irvine, CA. Edwards, the stylized E logo, PASCAL Transcatheter Valve Repair System, and PASCAL Ace Transcatheter Valve Repair System are trademarks of Edwards Lifesciences Corporation

3.2 Transcatheter Mitral Valve Replacement

Transcatheter mitral valve replacement (TMVR) is a developing technology currently reserved for patients at high or prohibitive risk for mitral valve surgery, a population that includes many elderly patients with multiple comorbidities. In a similar fashion to TAVR, a collapsible valve is mounted onto a catheter and delivered to and deployed within the existing mitral valve. Depending on the system and the patient's anatomy, these devices are usually delivered via transapical or transseptal routes. There are a large number of devices currently in development and/or used off-label. Furthermore, because of the necessary displacement of the anterior mitral valve leaflet into the LVOT by the TMVR, careful CT analysis is required pre-procedure to evaluate the LVOT and the neo-LVOT (the expected LVOT after TMVR deployment). The most feared complication of TMVR is LVOT obstruction, with a mortality of approximately 34%; fortunately, studies have shown this can be consistently predicted with CT analysis [34]. Unfortunately, it is not uncommon for the anatomy to be prohibitive for TMVR.

The most TMVR experience worldwide has been achieved with the SAPIEN™ balloon-expandable valve for TAVR. It is a circular-shaped device delivered transseptally, but use is limited to failed bioprosthetic valves, prior annuloplasty ring repairs, or significant mitral annular calcification. According to observational data, successful implantation improves symptoms, hospitalization, and survival when used in a failed bioprosthetic valve. Conversely, severe mitral annular calcification defines a high-risk patient population where LVOT obstruction, valve embolization, or at least moderate paravalvular leak can be present in more than 50% of patients with a one-year mortality of 43% [35].

The SAPIEN 3™ system, however, cannot be used in native valves without significant calcium because of a lack of an anchoring mechanism. For native valve disease, the two systems with the most data are the Intrepid™ (Medtronic, Minneapolis, Minnesota) dual-stent design system and the Tendyne™ (Abbott, Abbott Park, IL). The Intrepid has an outer stent to engage the saddle-shaped annulus and the inner stent that holds the valve. Early experience with the Tendyne™ and the Intrepid™ has demonstrated 96% successful deployment through a transapical approach [36, 37]. Although the early feasibility of transseptal deployment has been demonstrated, that delivery method is not yet available for widespread use. Furthermore, little is known about the durability of these valves in the mitral position. For now, TMVR for native mitral valve disease remains in the realm of research.

4   Mitral Stenosis

The vast majority of mitral stenosis (MS) historically was due to rheumatic heart disease, but over the past two decades has increased due to calcification of the mitral apparatus in developed countries. However, rheumatic MS is still the most common cause of MS worldwide. It is characterized by commissural fusion, thickening at the leaflet tips, chordal shortening, and restricted mobility of the mitral valve leaflets. Patients usually present at a younger age compared with degenerative MS [38]. Conversely, degenerative (calcific) MS is a disease of the elderly resulting from mitral annular calcification, which is a chronic degenerative condition of the mitral annulus that results in progressive calcification that extends to involve the base of the mitral valve leaflets. In the United States, the prevalence of mitral annular calcification was 9% in the Multi-Ethnic Study of Atherosclerosis (MESA; participants age 45–85) [39] and was 42% among individuals ≥65 years of age in the Cardiovascular Health Study [40]. In comparison, the prevalence of rheumatic heart disease ranges from <50 cases per 100,000 in developed countries compared with >500 cases per 100,000 in developing nations [41]. Currently, calcific MS is more common in developed countries, while rheumatic MS dominates in developing countries.

4.1   Balloon Mitral Valvotomy

The differences in the underlying pathophysiology of rheumatic and calcific MS affect the approach to treatment. Percutaneous balloon mitral valvotomy is the mainstay of treatment for rheumatic MS and was first described by Inoue and colleagues [42]. This procedure involves femoral venous access for transseptal puncture and sequential balloon dilation of the mitral valve to split the mitral commissures, typically using the Inoue balloon. In contrast to aortic valvuloplasty, balloon mitral valvotomy has good long-term outcomes, with some variability between different reports. In 5–10 year follow-up, 60–80% of patients appear to be alive without requiring repeat intervention (repeat balloon valvotomy or surgery) and with NYHA Class I-II symptoms [43, 44]. Follow-up over 20 years has shown up to 50% survival without requiring re-intervention [45–47].

Percutaneous balloon mitral valvotomy is recommended if the mitral valve anatomy is favorable, which is defined as mobile, relatively thin valve leaflets that are free of calcium in the absence of significant valvular fusion. A commonly used echocardiographic score that is associated with outcomes is the Wilkins score which grades leaflet mobility, thickening, calcification, and subvalvular thickening, each on a scale of 1–4 [48]. The scoring system effectively evaluates degenerative MS, which has a high risk of disruption of the mitral apparatus if treated with balloon valvotomy and poorer long-term outcomes [45]. Other contraindications to balloon valvotomy in rheumatic MS are more than mild mitral regurgitation and another indication for surgical intervention (e.g. severe coronary artery disease, other valvular abnormalities requiring correction).

4.2 *Transcatheter Mitral Valve Replacement*

There are limited options for transcatheter valve replacement for calcific MS. As discussed earlier, the Edwards system can be used, despite high one-year mortality [35]. An alternative is enrollment in the APOLLO trial for the Intrepid™ valve, but patients require at least moderate mitral regurgitation in combination with calcific mitral stenosis. It is hoped that developing transcatheter therapies for mitral regurgitation may also be applied to calcific mitral stenosis; however, the narrowing of the annulus by mitral annular calcification is a major barrier to the use of transcatheter valves without a good solution presently.

5 Tricuspid Regurgitation

The tricuspid valve has seen a recent explosion of investigation in transcatheter technologies. However, it is a complex apparatus with three leaflets with associated chordae tendineae and papillary muscles, and accordingly, intervention is typically complex. In comparison to the mitral valve, the tricuspid leaflets are thinner, more fragile, and have a larger valve orifice. In addition, the right-sided structures are thin-walled, the right atrium is often smaller, and the angulation from the inferior vena cava into the right atrium and tricuspid valve adds further difficulty. The most common cause of significant tricuspid regurgitation is secondary to annular dilation and leaflet tethering and is associated with increased mortality [49, 50].

Despite these challenges, both transcatheter tricuspid repair and tricuspid valve replacement have been attempted. However, the only device with significant real-world use and availability to use outside of clinical studies is the off-label use of the MitraClip™ system for the tricuspid valve. Edge-to-edge repair requires careful evaluation of the transesophageal echocardiogram to obtain suitable working views and determine valve coaptation, leaflet length, and the approximate location of the primary tricuspid regurgitation jet. Patient selection requires evaluation for possible contraindications, including secondary non-reversible life-limiting conditions, severe pulmonary hypertension, severe right ventricular dysfunction, severe left ventricular dysfunction, and untreated other severe valvular diseases. The multi-center TriValve registry of 249 patients who had undergone tricuspid repair with the MitraClip™ system demonstrated a 77% success rate (defined as at least a two-grade reduction in tricuspid reduction) with a one-year all-cause mortality of 20%. A failed procedure was associated with a higher risk of all-cause mortality or unplanned hospitalization [51]. A modified MitraClip™ delivery system for the tricuspid valve is under investigation in the Evaluation of Treatment with Abbott Transcatheter Clip Repair System in Patients with Moderate or Greater Tricuspid Regurgitation (TRILUMINATE, Clinical) Trial NCT03227757 [52]. Furthermore, the above-mentioned PASCAL™ Transcatheter Valve Repair System (Edwards Lifesciences LLC, Irvine, CA) used for MR has also been shown to be successfully used in tricuspid regurgitation [53, 54]. Several other device systems, including tricuspid valve replacement, are in earlier stages of development and are beyond the scope of this chapter.

6 Paravalvular Leak

Paravalvular leak refers to abnormal communication between two chambers around a prosthetic (mechanical or bioprosthetic) valve and can affect up to 17% of all surgically implanted prosthetic valves [55]. This frequently occurs to a minimal or mild degree after TAVR, but it is not clinically relevant in most cases [56]. However, significant paravalvular leak can be acute or chronic, resulting in heart failure, hemolysis, and/or anemia. Although surgical reoperation is historically the preferred treatment, it is associated with significant short-term (7–8%) and long-term mortality (15% at one year) [57], and many of these patients are at high surgical risk. Therefore, percutaneous paravalvular leak closure in appropriately selected patients offers an alternative, less-invasive option. However, percutaneous closure is not without risk, with approximately a 5.6% risk of death, emergency surgery, or stroke within 30-days. However, outcomes are worse with untreated or incomplete paravalvular leak closure [58].

The first step in evaluation is transesophageal echocardiography to evaluate the one or more locations of the leak and their anatomical suitability for percutaneous closure. Anatomical considerations include the risk of obstructing normal leaflet motion, the ability to provide complete paravalvular leak closure (i.e., size and shape of the defect), and the risk of impingement of surrounding structures (e.g., coronary ostia for the aortic valve). Paravalvular leaks due to active infection or valve dehiscence should not be closed percutaneously. Notably, there are no FDA-approved devices for paravalvular leak closure. Typically, a variety of vascular plugs are used off-label for this purpose.

7 Left Atrial Appendage Closure for Atrial Fibrillation

The left atrial appendage (LAA) is the major source of thromboembolism in atrial fibrillation and accounts for more than 90% of thrombi in cases of AF-related stroke when thrombus was found [59, 60]. Although anticoagulation is the first-line treatment for the prevention of AF-related thromboembolism, even among insured patients, approximately 47% of patients at moderate to high risk of a stroke are not anticoagulated [61]. It is also important to note that patients at higher risk of stroke often have a higher risk of bleeding [62]. For patients who are unable to take oral anticoagulation, mechanical left atrial appendage occlusion reduces the risk of stroke and provides an alternative treatment.

The most commonly used device is the Watchman LAA closure device (Boston Scientific, Marlborough, MA; Fig. 6), the latest iteration of which is the Watchman FLX™. It is a parachute-shaped, self-expanding device that is placed in the ostium of the LAA (Fig. 7). CT and transesophageal echocardiogram imaging are important modalities for anatomical evaluation for the suitability, sizing, and delivery of the system. The two major randomized controlled trials evaluating the Watchman™ device were PROTECT-AF (Watchman™ Left Atrial Appendage System for Embolic Protection in Patients with Atrial Fibrillation) and PREVAIL (Prospective Randomized Evaluation of the Watchman™ Left Atrial Appendage Closure Device in Patients with Atrial Fibrillation Versus Long-Term Warfarin Therapy); both randomized patients to either anticoagulation with warfarin or Watchman™ closure. After Watchman™ implantation, patients received six weeks of warfarin and then aspirin and clopidogrel for six months, followed by aspirin monotherapy after LAA sealing

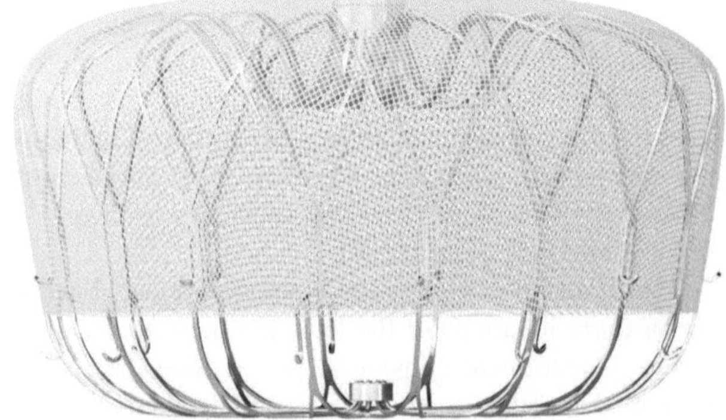

Fig. 6 The Watchman FLX™ device. Image provided courtesy of Boston Scientific, Marlborough, MA. Copyright Boston Scientific Corporation or its affiliates. All rights reserved. Watchman FLX is a trademark of Boston Scientific Corporation

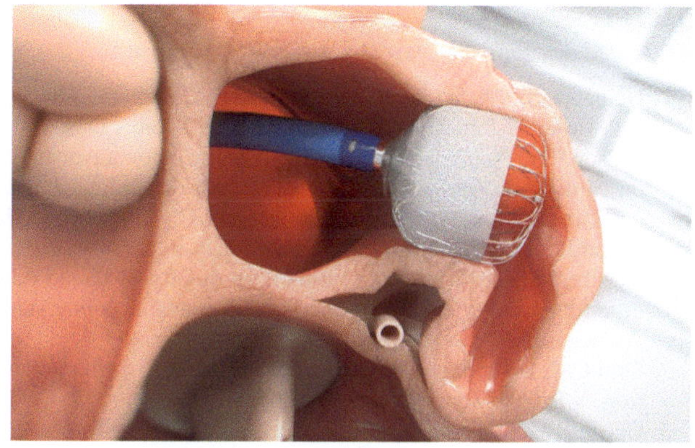

Fig. 7 Illustration of the Watchman FLX device during deployment in the ostium of the left atrial appendage. Image provided courtesy of Boston Scientific, Marlborough, MA. Copyright Boston Scientific Corporation or its affiliates. All rights reserved

was confirmed by TEE. In the PROTECT-AF trial where patients had a $CHADS_2$ score of ≥ 1, the Watchman™ device was shown to be non-inferior to warfarin [63]. Adverse events at a mean follow-up of 3.8 years were similar, although, as would be expected, the initial risk of adverse events is higher with the Watchman™ device because of procedural complications. Although the smaller PREVAIL trial did not confirm noninferiority [64], subsequent meta-analyses have demonstrated the efficacy of the Watchman device [65]. The Lariat™ (SentreHeart, Redwood City, CA) is another device that has FDA approval but with limited evidence for its efficacy and is typically limited to use in patients who are not anticoagulation or Watchman™ candidates but have a high risk of thromboembolism related to atrial fibrillation [66]. In comparison to the Watchman device, the Lariat uses a sutured-based system that requires both venous and epicardial access. The Amplatzer Amulet™ (Abbott, Abbott Park, IL) device is another LAA occlusion device which has recently received FDA approval in the US, in addition to approval for use in Europe.

8 Conclusion

The field of Structural Interventional Cardiology has exploded in the last decade largely due to the advent of TAVR, which revolutionized the treatment of aortic valve disease in the twenty-first century across the surgical risk spectrum. With the addition of transcatheter mitral valve repair, we now have an alternative to surgery to treat many patients with both primary and secondary mitral regurgitation. However, many patients with mitral valve disease are unsuitable for transcatheter repair, and few options are available for the repair or replacement of regurgitant native tricuspid valves. There are currently dozens of devices under investigation to address these gaps, and with time we expect that some of these devices will prove to be effective, less-invasive treatment options. The future of Structural Cardiology is likely to continue its rapid growth and expansion in the coming years, with particular benefits to elderly patients who are often less ideal candidates for cardiac surgery.

References

1. Heidenreich PA, Trogdon JG, Khavjou OA, Butler J, Dracup K, Ezekowitz MD, Finkelstein EA, Hong Y, Johnston SC, Khera A, Lloyd-Jones DM, Nelson SA, Nichol G, Orenstein D, Wilson PW, Woo YJ. American Heart Association advocacy coordinating C, stroke C, council on cardiovascular R, intervention, council on clinical C, council on E, prevention, council on a, thrombosis, vascular B, council on C, critical C, perioperative, resuscitation, council on cardiovascular N, council on the kidney in cardiovascular D, council on cardiovascular S, anesthesia, interdisciplinary council on quality of C and outcomes R. forecasting the future of cardiovascular disease in the United States: a policy statement from the American Heart Association. Circulation. 2011;123:933–44.
2. Otto CM, Prendergast B. Aortic-valve stenosis--from patients at risk to severe valve obstruction. N Engl J Med. 2014;371:744–56.
3. Carita P, Coppola G, Novo G, Caccamo G, Guglielmo M, Balasus F, Novo S, Castrovinci S, Moscarelli M, Fattouch K, Corrado E. Aortic stenosis: insights on pathogenesis and clinical implications. J Geriatr Cardiol. 2016;13:489–98.
4. Ross J Jr, Braunwald E. Aortic stenosis. Circulation. 1968;38:61–7.
5. Litvack F, Jakubowski AT, Buchbinder NA, Eigler N. Lack of sustained clinical improvement in an elderly population after percutaneous aortic valvuloplasty. Am J Cardiol. 1988;62:270–5.
6. Otto CM, Mickel MC, Kennedy JW, Alderman EL, Bashore TM, Block PC, Brinker JA, Diver D, Ferguson J, Holmes DR Jr, et al. Three-year outcome after balloon aortic valvuloplasty. Insights into prognosis of valvular aortic stenosis. Circulation. 1994;89:642–50.
7. Lieberman EB, Bashore TM, Hermiller JB, Wilson JS, Pieper KS, Keeler GP, Pierce CH, Kisslo KB, Harrison JK, Davidson CJ. Balloon aortic valvuloplasty in adults: failure of procedure to improve long-term survival. J Am Coll Cardiol. 1995;26:1522–8.
8. Cribier A, Savin T, Saoudi N, Rocha P, Berland J, Letac B. Percutaneous transluminal valvuloplasty of acquired aortic stenosis in elderly patients: an alternative to valve replacement? Lancet. 1986;1:63–7.
9. Alkhouli M, Zack CJ, Sarraf M, Bashir R, Nishimura RA, Eleid MF, Nkomo VT, Sandhu GS, Gulati R, Greason KL, Holmes DR, Rihal CS. Morbidity and mortality associated with balloon aortic valvuloplasty: a national perspective. Circ Cardiovasc Interv. 2017;10(5):e004481.
10. Writing Committee M, Otto CM, Nishimura RA, Bonow RO, Carabello BA, Erwin JP 3rd, Gentile F, Jneid H, Krieger EV, Mack M, McLeod C, O'Gara PT, Rigolin VH, Sundt TM 3rd, Thompson A, Toly C. 2020 ACC/AHA Guideline for the Management of Patients With Valvular Heart Disease: Executive Summary: A Report of the American College of Cardiology/American Heart Association Joint Committee on Clinical Practice Guidelines. J Am Coll Cardiol. 2021;143(5):e35–71.
11. Carroll JD, Mack MJ, Vemulapalli S, Herrmann HC, Gleason TG, Hanzel G, Deeb GM, Thourani VH, Cohen DJ, Desai N, Kirtane AJ, Fitzgerald S, Michaels J, Krohn C, Masoudi FA, Brindis RG, Bavaria JE. STS-ACC TVT registry of transcatheter aortic valve replacement. J Am Coll Cardiol. 2020;76:2492–516.
12. Leon MB, Smith CR, Mack M, Miller DC, Moses JW, Svensson LG, Tuzcu EM, Webb JG, Fontana GP, Makkar RR, Brown DL, Block PC, Guyton RA, Pichard AD, Bavaria JE, Herrmann HC, Douglas PS, Petersen JL, Akin JJ, Anderson WN, Wang D, Pocock S, Investigators PT. Transcatheter aortic-valve implantation for aortic stenosis in patients who cannot undergo surgery. N Engl J Med. 2010;363:1597–607.
13. Makkar RR, Fontana GP, Jilaihawi H, Kapadia S, Pichard AD, Douglas PS, Thourani VH, Babaliaros VC, Webb JG, Herrmann HC, Bavaria JE, Kodali S, Brown DL, Bowers B, Dewey TM, Svensson LG, Tuzcu M, Moses JW, Williams MR, Siegel RJ, Akin JJ, Anderson WN, Pocock S, Smith CR, Leon MB, Investigators PT. Transcatheter aortic-valve replacement for inoperable severe aortic stenosis. N Engl J Med. 2012;366:1696–704.
14. Popma JJ, Adams DH, Reardon MJ, Yakubov SJ, Kleiman NS, Heimansohn D, Hermiller J Jr, Hughes GC, Harrison JK, Coselli J, Diez J, Kafi A, Schreiber T, Gleason TG, Conte J,

Buchbinder M, Deeb GM, Carabello B, Serruys PW, Chenoweth S, Oh JK, and CoreValve United States Clinical I. transcatheter aortic valve replacement using a self-expanding bioprosthesis in patients with severe aortic stenosis at extreme risk for surgery. J Am Coll Cardiol. 2014;63:1972–81.

15. Smith CR, Leon MB, Mack MJ, Miller DC, Moses JW, Svensson LG, Tuzcu EM, Webb JG, Fontana GP, Makkar RR, Williams M, Dewey T, Kapadia S, Babaliaros V, Thourani VH, Corso P, Pichard AD, Bavaria JE, Herrmann HC, Akin JJ, Anderson WN, Wang D, Pocock SJ, Investigators PT. Transcatheter versus surgical aortic-valve replacement in high-risk patients. N Engl J Med. 2011;364:2187–98.

16. Adams DH, Popma JJ, Reardon MJ, Yakubov SJ, Coselli JS, Deeb GM, Gleason TG, Buchbinder M, Hermiller J Jr, Kleiman NS, Chetcuti S, Heiser J, Merhi W, Zorn G, Tadros P, Robinson N, Petrossian G, Hughes GC, Harrison JK, Conte J, Maini B, Mumtaz M, Chenoweth S, Oh JK, Investigators USCC. Transcatheter aortic-valve replacement with a self-expanding prosthesis. N Engl J Med. 2014;370:1790–8.

17. Leon MB, Smith CR, Mack MJ, Makkar RR, Svensson LG, Kodali SK, Thourani VH, Tuzcu EM, Miller DC, Herrmann HC, Doshi D, Cohen DJ, Pichard AD, Kapadia S, Dewey T, Babaliaros V, Szeto WY, Williams MR, Kereiakes D, Zajarias A, Greason KL, Whisenant BK, Hodson RW, Moses JW, Trento A, Brown DL, Fearon WF, Pibarot P, Hahn RT, Jaber WA, Anderson WN, Alu MC, Webb JG, Investigators P. Transcatheter or surgical aortic-valve replacement in intermediate-risk patients. N Engl J Med. 2016;374:1609–20.

18. Reardon MJ, Van Mieghem NM, Popma JJ, Kleiman NS, Sondergaard L, Mumtaz M, Adams DH, Deeb GM, Maini B, Gada H, Chetcuti S, Gleason T, Heiser J, Lange R, Merhi W, Oh JK, Olsen PS, Piazza N, Williams M, Windecker S, Yakubov SJ, Grube E, Makkar R, Lee JS, Conte J, Vang E, Nguyen H, Chang Y, Mugglin AS, Serruys PW, Kappetein AP, Investigators S. Surgical or transcatheter aortic-valve replacement in intermediate-risk patients. N Engl J Med. 2017;376:1321–31.

19. Thyregod HG, Steinbruchel DA, Ihlemann N, Nissen H, Kjeldsen BJ, Petursson P, Chang Y, Franzen OW, Engstrom T, Clemmensen P, Hansen PB, Andersen LW, Olsen PS, Sondergaard L. Transcatheter versus surgical aortic valve replacement in patients with severe aortic valve stenosis: 1-year results from the all-comers NOTION randomized clinical trial. J Am Coll Cardiol. 2015;65:2184–94.

20. Popma JJ, Deeb GM, Yakubov SJ, Mumtaz M, Gada H, O'Hair D, Bajwa T, Heiser JC, Merhi W, Kleiman NS, Askew J, Sorajja P, Rovin J, Chetcuti SJ, Adams DH, Teirstein PS, Zorn GL 3rd, Forrest JK, Tchetche D, Resar J, Walton A, Piazza N, Ramlawi B, Robinson N, Petrossian G, Gleason TG, Oh JK, Boulware MJ, Qiao H, Mugglin AS, Reardon MJ, and Evolut Low Risk Trial I. Transcatheter aortic-valve replacement with a self-expanding valve in low-risk patients. N Engl J Med. 2019;380:1706–15.

21. Mack MJ, Leon MB, Thourani VH, Makkar R, Kodali SK, Russo M, Kapadia SR, Malaisrie SC, Cohen DJ, Pibarot P, Leipsic J, Hahn RT, Blanke P, Williams MR, McCabe JM, Brown DL, Babaliaros V, Goldman S, Szeto WY, Genereux P, Pershad A, Pocock SJ, Alu MC, Webb JG, Smith CR, Investigators P. Transcatheter aortic-valve replacement with a balloon-expandable valve in low-risk patients. N Engl J Med. 2019;380:1695–705.

22. Khan SU, Lone AN, Saleem MA, Kaluski E. Transcatheter vs surgical aortic-valve replacement in low- to intermediate-surgical-risk candidates: a meta-analysis and systematic review. Clin Cardiol. 2017;40:974–81.

23. Mack MJ, Leon MB, Smith CR, Miller DC, Moses JW, Tuzcu EM, Webb JG, Douglas PS, Anderson WN, Blackstone EH, Kodali SK, Makkar RR, Fontana GP, Kapadia S, Bavaria J, Hahn RT, Thourani VH, Babaliaros V, Pichard A, Herrmann HC, Brown DL, Williams M, Akin J, Davidson MJ, Svensson LG, investigators Pt. 5-year outcomes of transcatheter aortic valve replacement or surgical aortic valve replacement for high surgical risk patients with aortic stenosis (PARTNER 1): a randomised controlled trial. Lancet. 2015;385:2477–84.

24. Makkar RR, Thourani VH, Mack MJ, Kodali SK, Kapadia S, Webb JG, Yoon SH, Trento A, Svensson LG, Herrmann HC, Szeto WY, Miller DC, Satler L, Cohen DJ, Dewey TM,

Babaliaros V, Williams MR, Kereiakes DJ, Zajarias A, Greason KL, Whisenant BK, Hodson RW, Brown DL, Fearon WF, Russo MJ, Pibarot P, Hahn RT, Jaber WA, Rogers E, Xu K, Wheeler J, Alu MC, Smith CR, Leon MB, Investigators P. Five-year outcomes of transcatheter or surgical aortic-valve replacement. N Engl J Med. 2020;382:799–809.

25. Sondergaard L, Ihlemann N, Capodanno D, Jorgensen TH, Nissen H, Kjeldsen BJ, Chang Y, Steinbruchel DA, Olsen PS, Petronio AS, Thyregod HGH. Durability of transcatheter and surgical bioprosthetic aortic valves in patients at lower surgical risk. J Am Coll Cardiol. 2019;73:546–53.

26. Herrmann HC, Daneshvar SA, Fonarow GC, Stebbins A, Vemulapalli S, Desai ND, Malenka DJ, Thourani VH, Rymer J, Kosinski AS. Prosthesis-patient mismatch in patients undergoing transcatheter aortic valve replacement: from the STS/ACC TVT registry. J Am Coll Cardiol. 2018;72:2701–11.

27. Nkomo VT, Gardin JM, Skelton TN, Gottdiener JS, Scott CG, Enriquez-Sarano M. Burden of valvular heart diseases: a population-based study. Lancet. 2006;368:1005–11.

28. Feldman T, Foster E, Glower DD, Kar S, Rinaldi MJ, Fail PS, Smalling RW, Siegel R, Rose GA, Engeron E, Loghin C, Trento A, Skipper ER, Fudge T, Letsou GV, Massaro JM, Mauri L, Investigators EI. Percutaneous repair or surgery for mitral regurgitation. N Engl J Med. 2011;364:1395–406.

29. Glower DD, Kar S, Trento A, Lim DS, Bajwa T, Quesada R, Whitlow PL, Rinaldi MJ, Grayburn P, Mack MJ, Mauri L, McCarthy PM, Feldman T. Percutaneous mitral valve repair for mitral regurgitation in high-risk patients: results of the EVEREST II study. J Am Coll Cardiol. 2014;64:172–81.

30. Obadia JF, Messika-Zeitoun D, Leurent G, Iung B, Bonnet G, Piriou N, Lefevre T, Piot C, Rouleau F, Carrie D, Nejjari M, Ohlmann P, Leclercq F, Saint Etienne C, Teiger E, Leroux L, Karam N, Michel N, Gilard M, Donal E, Trochu JN, Cormier B, Armoiry X, Boutitie F, Maucort-Boulch D, Barnel C, Samson G, Guerin P, Vahanian A, Mewton N, Investigators M-F. Percutaneous repair or medical treatment for secondary mitral regurgitation. N Engl J Med. 2018;379:2297–306.

31. Stone GW, Lindenfeld J, Abraham WT, Kar S, Lim DS, Mishell JM, Whisenant B, Grayburn PA, Rinaldi M, Kapadia SR, Rajagopal V, Sarembock IJ, Brieke A, Marx SO, Cohen DJ, Weissman NJ, Mack MJ, Investigators C. Transcatheter mitral-valve repair in patients with heart failure. N Engl J Med. 2018;379:2307–18.

32. Mack MJ, Lindenfeld J, Abraham WT, Kar S, Lim DS, Mishell JM, Whisenant BK, Grayburn PA, Rinaldi MJ, Kapadia SR, Rajagopal V, Sarembock IJ, Brieke A, Rogers JH, Marx SO, Cohen DJ, Weissman NJ, Stone GW, Investigators C. 3-year outcomes of transcatheter mitral valve repair in patients with heart failure. J Am Coll Cardiol. 2021;77:1029–40.

33. Webb JG, Hensey M, Szerlip M, Schafer U, Cohen GN, Kar S, Makkar R, Kipperman RM, Spargias K, O'Neill WW, Ng MKC, Fam NP, Rinaldi MJ, Smith RL, Walters DL, Raffel CO, Levisay J, Latib A, Montorfano M, Marcoff L, Shrivastava M, Boone R, Gilmore S, Feldman TE, Lim DS. 1-year outcomes for transcatheter repair in patients with mitral regurgitation from the CLASP study. JACC Cardiovasc Interv. 2020;13:2344–57.

34. Yoon SH, Bleiziffer S, Latib A, Eschenbach L, Ancona M, Vincent F, Kim WK, Unbehaum A, Asami M, Dhoble A, Silaschi M, Frangieh AH, Veulemans V, Tang GHL, Kuwata S, Rampat R, Schmidt T, Patel AJ, Nicz PFG, Nombela-Franco L, Kini A, Kitamura M, Sharma R, Chakravarty T, Hildick-Smith D, Arnold M, de Brito FS Jr, Jensen C, Jung C, Jilaihawi H, Smalling RW, Maisano F, Kasel AM, Treede H, Kempfert J, Pilgrim T, Kar S, Bapat V, Whisenant BK, Van Belle E, Delgado V, Modine T, Bax JJ, Makkar RR. Predictors of left ventricular outflow tract obstruction after transcatheter mitral valve replacement. JACC Cardiovasc Interv. 2019;12:182–93.

35. Yoon S-H, Whisenant BK, Bleiziffer S, Delgado V, Dhoble A, Schofer N, Eschenbach L, Bansal E, Murdoch DJ, Ancona M. Outcomes of transcatheter mitral valve replacement for degenerated bioprostheses, failed annuloplasty rings, and mitral annular calcification. Eur Heart J. 2019;40:441–51.

36. Bapat V, Rajagopal V, Meduri C, Farivar RS, Walton A, Duffy SJ, Gooley R, Almeida A, Reardon MJ, Kleiman NS, Spargias K, Pattakos S, Ng MK, Wilson M, Adams DH, Leon M, Mack MJ, Chenoweth S, Sorajja P, and Intrepid Global Pilot Study I. Early experience with new transcatheter mitral valve replacement. J Am Coll Cardiol. 2018;71:12–21.
37. Sorajja P, Moat N, Badhwar V, Walters D, Paone G, Bethea B, Bae R, Dahle G, Mumtaz M, Grayburn P, Kapadia S, Babaliaros V, Guerrero M, Satler L, Thourani V, Bedogni F, Rizik D, Denti P, Dumonteil N, Modine T, Sinhal A, Chuang ML, Popma JJ, Blanke P, Leipsic J, Muller D. Initial feasibility study of a new transcatheter mitral prosthesis: the first 100 patients. J Am Coll Cardiol. 2019;73:1250–60.
38. Akram MR, Chan T, McAuliffe S, Chenzbraun A. Non-rheumatic annular mitral stenosis: prevalence and characteristics. Eur J Echocardiogr. 2009;10:103–5.
39. Kanjanauthai S, Nasir K, Katz R, Rivera JJ, Takasu J, Blumenthal RS, Eng J, Budoff MJ. Relationships of mitral annular calcification to cardiovascular risk factors: the Multi-Ethnic Study of Atherosclerosis (MESA). Atherosclerosis. 2010;213:558–62.
40. Barasch E, Gottdiener JS, Larsen EK, Chaves PH, Newman AB, Manolio TA. Clinical significance of calcification of the fibrous skeleton of the heart and aortosclerosis in community dwelling elderly. The Cardiovascular Health Study (CHS). Am Heart J. 2006;151:39–47.
41. Kumar RK, Antunes MJ, Beaton A, Mirabel M, Nkomo VT, Okello E, Regmi PR, Remenyi B, Sliwa-Hahnle K, Zuhlke LJ, Sable C. American Heart Association Council on Lifelong Congenital Heart D, Heart Health in the Y, Council on C, Stroke N and Council on Clinical C. Contemporary Diagnosis and Management of Rheumatic Heart Disease: Implications for Closing the Gap: A Scientific Statement From the American Heart Association. Circulation. 2020;142:e337–57.
42. Inoue K, Owaki T, Nakamura T, Kitamura F, Miyamoto N. Clinical application of transvenous mitral commissurotomy by a new balloon catheter. J Thorac Cardiovasc Surg. 1984;87:394–402.
43. Hernandez R, Banuelos C, Alfonso F, Goicolea J, Fernandez-Ortiz A, Escaned J, Azcona L, Almeria C, Macaya C. Long-term clinical and echocardiographic follow-up after percutaneous mitral valvuloplasty with the Inoue balloon. Circulation. 1999;99:1580–6.
44. Meneveau N, Schiele F, Seronde MF, Breton V, Gupta S, Bernard Y, Bassand JP. Predictors of event-free survival after percutaneous mitral commissurotomy. Heart. 1998;80:359–64.
45. Bouleti C, Iung B, Himbert D, Messika-Zeitoun D, Brochet E, Garbarz E, Cormier B, Vahanian A. Relationship between valve calcification and long-term results of percutaneous mitral commissurotomy for rheumatic mitral stenosis. Circ Cardiovasc Interv. 2014;7:381–9.
46. Meneguz-Moreno RA, Costa JR Jr, Gomes NL, Braga SLN, Ramos AIO, Meneghelo Z, Maldonado M, Ferreira-Neto AN, Franca JID, Siqueira D, Esteves C, Sousa A, Sousa JE, Abizaid A. Very long term follow-up after percutaneous balloon mitral valvuloplasty. JACC Cardiovasc Interv. 2018;11:1945–52.
47. Ben-Farhat M, Betbout F, Gamra H, Maatouk F, Ben-Hamda K, Abdellaoui M, Hammami S, Jarrar M, Addad F, Dridi Z. Predictors of long-term event-free survival and of freedom from restenosis after percutaneous balloon mitral commissurotomy. Am Heart J. 2001;142:1072–9.
48. Wilkins GT, Weyman AE, Abascal VM, Block PC, Palacios IF. Percutaneous balloon dilatation of the mitral valve: an analysis of echocardiographic variables related to outcome and the mechanism of dilatation. Br Heart J. 1988;60:299–308.
49. Mutlak D, Lessick J, Reisner SA, Aronson D, Dabbah S, Agmon Y. Echocardiography-based spectrum of severe tricuspid regurgitation: the frequency of apparently idiopathic tricuspid regurgitation. J Am Soc Echocardiogr. 2007;20:405–8.
50. Benfari G, Antoine C, Miller WL, Thapa P, Topilsky Y, Rossi A, Michelena HI, Pislaru S, Enriquez-Sarano M. Excess mortality associated with functional tricuspid regurgitation complicating heart failure with reduced ejection fraction. Circulation. 2019;140:196–206.
51. Mehr M, Taramasso M, Besler C, Ruf T, Connelly KA, Weber M, Yzeiraj E, Schiavi D, Mangieri A, Vaskelyte L, Alessandrini H, Deuschl F, Brugger N, Ahmad H, Biasco L, Orban M, Deseive S, Braun D, Rommel KP, Pozzoli A, Frerker C, Nabauer M, Massberg S, Pedrazzini G, Tang

GHL, Windecker S, Schafer U, Kuck KH, Sievert H, Denti P, Latib A, Schofer J, Nickenig G, Fam N, von Bardeleben S, Lurz P, Maisano F, Hausleiter J. 1-year outcomes after edge-to-edge valve repair for symptomatic tricuspid regurgitation: results from the TriValve registry. JACC Cardiovasc Interv. 2019;12:1451–61.

52. Nickenig G, Weber M, Lurz P, von Bardeleben RS, Sitges M, Sorajja P, Hausleiter J, Denti P, Trochu JN, Nabauer M, Dahou A, Hahn RT. Transcatheter edge-to-edge repair for reduction of tricuspid regurgitation: 6-month outcomes of the TRILUMINATE single-arm study. Lancet. 2019;394:2002–11.

53. Fam NP, Braun D, von Bardeleben RS, Nabauer M, Ruf T, Connelly KA, Ho E, Thiele H, Lurz P, Weber M, Nickenig G, Narang A, Davidson CJ, Hausleiter J. Compassionate use of the PASCAL transcatheter valve repair system for severe tricuspid regurgitation: a multicenter, observational, first-in-human experience. JACC Cardiovasc Interv. 2019;12:2488–95.

54. Kitamura M, Fam NP, Braun D, Ruf T, Sugiura A, Narang A, Connelly KA, Ho E, Nabauer M, Hausleiter J, Weber M, Nickenig G, Davidson CJ, Thiele H, von Bardeleben RS, Lurz P. 12-Month outcomes of transcatheter tricuspid valve repair with the PASCAL system for severe tricuspid regurgitation. Catheter Cardiovasc Interv. 2021;97(6):1281–9.

55. Hammermeister K, Sethi GK, Henderson WG, Grover FL, Oprian C, Rahimtoola SH. Outcomes 15 years after valve replacement with a mechanical versus a bioprosthetic valve: final report of the veterans affairs randomized trial. J Am Coll Cardiol. 2000;36:1152–8.

56. Saia F, Martinez C, Gafoor S, Singh V, Ciuca C, Hofmann I, Marrozzini C, Tan J, Webb J, Sievert H, Marzocchi A, O'Neill WW. Long-term outcomes of percutaneous paravalvular regurgitation closure after transcatheter aortic valve replacement: a multicenter experience. JACC Cardiovasc Interv. 2015;8:681–8.

57. Bouhout I, Mazine A, Ghoneim A, Millan X, El-Hamamsy I, Pellerin M, Cartier R, Demers P, Lamarche Y, Bouchard D. Long-term results after surgical treatment of paravalvular leak in the aortic and mitral position. J Thorac Cardiovasc Surg. 2016;151(1260–6):e1.

58. Garcia E, Arzamendi D, Jimenez-Quevedo P, Sarnago F, Marti G, Sanchez-Recalde A, Lasa-Larraya G, Sancho M, Iniguez A, Goicolea J, Garcia-San Roman K, Alonso-Briales JH, Molina E, Calabuig J, Freixa X, Berenguer A, Valdes-Chavarri M, Vazquez N, Diaz JF, Cruz-Gonzalez I. Outcomes and predictors of success and complications for paravalvular leak closure: an analysis of the SpanisH real-wOrld paravalvular LEaks closure (HOLE) registry. EuroIntervention. 2017;12:1962–8.

59. Price MJ. Left atrial appendage occlusion: data update. Interv Cardiol Clin. 2018;7:159–68.

60. Blackshear JL, Odell JA. Appendage obliteration to reduce stroke in cardiac surgical patients with atrial fibrillation. Ann Thorac Surg. 1996;61:755–9.

61. Casciano JP, Dotiwala ZJ, Martin BC, Kwong WJ. The costs of warfarin underuse and non-adherence in patients with atrial fibrillation: a commercial insurer perspective. J Manag Care Pharm. 2013;19:302–16.

62. Hindricks G, Potpara T, Dagres N, Arbelo E, Bax JJ, Blomstrom-Lundqvist C, Boriani G, Castella M, Dan GA, Dilaveris PE, Fauchier L, Filippatos G, Kalman JM, La Meir M, Lane DA, Lebeau JP, Lettino M, GYH L, Pinto FJ, Thomas GN, Valgimigli M, Van Gelder IC, Van Putte BP, Watkins CL and Group ESCSD. ESC guidelines for the diagnosis and management of atrial fibrillation developed in collaboration with the European Association for Cardio-Thoracic Surgery (EACTS). Eur Heart J. 2020;2021(42):373–498.

63. Reddy VY, Sievert H, Halperin J, Doshi SK, Buchbinder M, Neuzil P, Huber K, Whisenant B, Kar S, Swarup V, Gordon N, Holmes D. Committee PAS and Investigators. Percutaneous left atrial appendage closure vs warfarin for atrial fibrillation: a randomized clinical trial. JAMA. 2014;312:1988–98.

64. Holmes DR Jr, Kar S, Price MJ, Whisenant B, Sievert H, Doshi SK, Huber K, Reddy VY. Prospective randomized evaluation of the Watchman left atrial appendage closure device in patients with atrial fibrillation versus long-term warfarin therapy: the PREVAIL trial. J Am Coll Cardiol. 2014;64:1–12.

65. Price MJ, Reddy VY, Valderrabano M, Halperin JL, Gibson DN, Gordon N, Huber KC, Holmes DR Jr. Bleeding outcomes after left atrial appendage closure compared with long-term warfarin: a pooled, patient-level analysis of the WATCHMAN randomized trial experience. JACC Cardiovasc Interv. 2015;8:1925–32.
66. Miller MA, Gangireddy SR, Doshi SK, Aryana A, Koruth JS, Sennhauser S, d'Avila A, Dukkipati SR, Neuzil P, Reddy VY. Multicenter study on acute and long-term safety and efficacy of percutaneous left atrial appendage closure using an epicardial suture snaring device. Heart Rhythm. 2014;11:1853–9.

Cardiovascular Surgery in the Elderly

David Blitzer and David D. Yuh

1 Background

The elderly represent a prominent, with improving life expectancies, rapidly expanding sector of the US population, with currently over 13 million people, and estimates that this number will quadruple in the next 50 years. [1, 2]. In large part, these demographic trends are attributable to improved modalities for preventing and managing cardiovascular disease (CVD) in young and middle-aged adults, which improved survival and delayed the onset of CVD until later in life. These improvements have resulted in an increase in the prevalence of CVD in the population and the incidence of CVD in older adults [3, 4]. CVD remains the leading cause of morbidity and mortality in the elderly, despite advances in medical therapies [5–8]. Elderly patients are thus undergoing more procedures to treat CVD, and the demographics of patients undergoing cardiac surgery, a validated means of increasing survival and improving quality of life, reflect this trend [9]. Compared to a younger cohort, the elderly population generally has higher rates of comorbid disease with lower functional reserve, ultimately predisposing them to a higher risk of complications and death. This increased risk, paired with the institutional and societal emphasis on procedural outcomes, has led many cardiologists and cardiac surgeons to only reluctantly recommend cardiac operations for elderly patients. With the advancement and proliferation of percutaneous technologies, many cardiac surgeons are nonetheless operating on older, sicker patients compared to their training and initial practice. For example, elderly patients comprise an increasingly prominent

D. Blitzer
Division of Cardiac, Thoracic, and Vascular Surgery, Columbia University Vagelos College of Physicians and Surgeons, New York, NY, USA

D. D. Yuh (✉)
Department of Surgery, Division of Cardiac Surgery, Stamford Health, Stamford, CT, USA
e-mail: dyuh@stamhealth.org

© The Author(s), under exclusive license to Springer Nature Switzerland AG 2023
T. M. Leucker, G. Gerstenblith (eds.), *Cardiovascular Disease in the Elderly*, Contemporary Cardiology, https://doi.org/10.1007/978-3-031-16594-8_8

proportion of the population undergoing coronary artery bypass grafting (CABG), and the number of octogenarians undergoing CABG in the United States increased by 67% from 1987 to 1990 [10–12]. There has been a corresponding increase in the literature investigating the CABG outcomes for septuagenarians, octogenarians, and nonagenarians with varied conclusions due to small sample sizes and divergent institutional experiences [3, 5, 6, 10, 11, 13–16]. Regardless of this variance, most of the literature demonstrates that, despite increased costs and longer lengths of stay, cardiac operations can be performed with acceptable hospital mortality rates in carefully selected elderly patients.

2 Evaluation of the Elderly Patient for Cardiac Surgery

2.1 Operation Complexity

Outcomes in the elderly, across several major cardiac operative classifications, have been associated with overall higher mortality and morbidity rates than those observed in younger patients.[16] Among octogenarians without significant comorbidities, operative series have revealed mortality rates of 4.2% with CABG alone and 7% with CABG with aortic valve replacement (AVR), which are comparable to the rates for younger patients. However, while the addition of an AVR increases mortality equally across age categories, the addition of a mitral valve replacement (MVR) adds increasingly to operative mortality risk with advancing age, with mortality rates as high as 18.2% in this population. This finding may result from the impaired left ventricular (LV) function that often results from mitral valve dysfunction and which compounds the diminished physiological reserve of elderly patients. Furthermore, the duration of cardiopulmonary bypass is usually longer for an MVR than for an AVR. Kolh and associates showed that octogenarians experience increased in-hospital mortality directly related to the duration of cardiopulmonary bypass support [23]. Overall, these data suggest that as operative complexity increases, elderly patients experience disproportionately higher mortality and morbidity rates than younger patients. Consequently, surgeons and patients must be pragmatic and balance this heightened operative risk with the projected benefits of any intervention under consideration.

The selection of a valve prosthesis is an area that deserves particular attention with all patients, including the elderly. In general, a bioprosthetic valve (i.e., porcine or bovine pericardial) is preferable to a mechanical valve for most replacement procedures in the elderly, primarily because these devices do not require long-term anticoagulation. In the elderly, the potential for bleeding complications stemming from long-term anticoagulation is magnified by increased rates of falling and pathological bone fractures. Conversely, rates of thrombotic complications are also increased by the greater incidence of inadequate anticoagulation dosing (e.g., confusion, forgetfulness) in this population. Simultaneously, the durability and hemodynamics of bioprosthetic valves continue to improve [17]. With the current selection of mitral valve bioprostheses, an average of 70% will be free of structural valve deterioration at 10 years. Rates of deterioration accelerate over the next five years, with actuarial freedom from primary tissue valve failure ranging from 35–71% at 15 years [18]. In the aortic position, large series have demonstrated greater than 95% and 90% freedom from structural valve deterioration at five and 10 years, respectively. However, at 15 years, this decreases to <70% [19]. In light of these findings, several valve repair techniques have been developed to obviate the need for valve replacement. Such valve-sparing procedures often introduce greater complexity than a standard valve replacement, often requiring greater operative and cardiopulmonary bypass times with the accompanying risks for elderly patients, as previously discussed.

As with cardiac valve pathology, elderly patients have benefited from novel surgical techniques for the management of coronary artery disease. For example, "off-pump" techniques enable CABG to be performed without cardiopulmonary bypass support, which is postulated to be particularly beneficial for the elderly. The appropriate application of such off-pump techniques is controversial compared to a traditional CABG; however, these techniques have been shown to reduce blood loss, fluid overload, early transient renal dysfunction, and myocardial enzyme leak. Such physiological advantages have not consistently translated into improved clinical outcomes such as reduced hospitalization, wound complication rates, and postoperative pain. Similarly, the current evidence has not demonstrated improved neurocognitive outcomes with off-pump CABG in any patient age group. Perhaps most concerning is that several large, well-designed reviews of off-pump CABG indicate that intermediate- to long-term graft patency, completeness of myocardial revascularization, and freedom from coronary reintervention are all compromised with these techniques [20–22]. Nevertheless, off-pump techniques are an important consideration for specific clinical scenarios, particularly the patient with severe calcification of the ascending aorta. Mechanical manipulation or clamping of aortic plaque or calcification is widely considered the most substantial risk factor for embolic stroke, which can be avoided using off-pump techniques. The use of anastomotic stapling devices is another strategy for limiting aortic manipulation in this patient subset. Off-pump CABG is also potentially beneficial for elderly patients with poor left ventricular function by avoiding the need for cardioplegic arrest and thus the potential for global myocardial ischemia or "stunning." This, in turn, can reduce the incidence of post-cardiotomy shock and the need for mechanical circulatory support, which can carry significant risks among the elderly.

3 Suitability for Operation

As will be discussed later, it is well demonstrated that judicious selection of cardiac surgical candidates, particularly among elderly patients, is critical to maintaining acceptable outcomes and avoiding unnecessary risk. The same factors that are predictive of poor operative outcomes in the general population have an even greater influence on operative mortality and morbidity rates for the elderly. Consequently, these factors should be considered even more seriously when evaluating an elderly surgical candidate. These considerations, and their potential impact on postoperative outcomes, should represent an important part of the preoperative discussion between surgeon, patient, and family.

3.1 Emergency Operation

The need for emergent operative intervention is strongly associated with in-hospital mortality. Ko and associates compared outcomes among octogenarians undergoing CABG in emergent, urgent, and elective cases and reported mortality rates of 33.3%, 13.5%, and 2.8%, respectively [8]. They identified emergent status as one of two independent risk factors for mortality, with the other being depressed ejection fraction. Emergent status was also associated with increased morbidity in octogenarians, with 67% experiencing complications in the emergent group compared to 14% in the elective group. Kolh et al. performed a multivariate analysis of 182 octogenarians and noted that urgent procedure status significantly increased the risk for in-hospital mortality [23]. Similarly, Alexander et al. identified preoperative shock, preoperative mechanical circulatory support, and emergent status as factors predictive of in-hospital mortality after CABG in octogenarians [16]. Given the preponderance of the evidence, referring physicians, surgeons and patients alike should have realistic expectations in these scenarios. In the direst of circumstances, those patients who do manage to survive are often relegated to protracted hospitalizations only to be followed by institutional death or disability. A particularly illustrative example of the prohibitively high risk of morbidity or mortality is that of ascending aortic, or Stanford Type A, dissection repair in the very elderly. In a review of 24 consecutive octogenarians who underwent acute type A dissection repair from 1985 to 1999, Neri and colleagues reported overall hospital mortality of 83% [24]. Of the four patients who survived hospital discharge, none were capable of independent function, and all eventually died within 6 months. Although such data should not be used to suggest that all life-saving operations be denied to octogenarians as a matter of policy, they do demonstrate the heightened risks associated with emergent cardiac surgery in the elderly.

3.2 Severe Respiratory Insufficiency

Protracted ventilatory dependence is common among elderly patients, and those suffering from severe chronic obstructive pulmonary disease (COPD) should be excluded from cardiac surgery. All patients with significant pulmonary risk factors should undergo pulmonary function testing prior to any operative intervention. A forced expiratory volume at 1 min (FEV1) less than 65% of the vital capacity or an FEV1 of less than 1 L is indicative of prohibitive risk for postoperative pulmonary failure, and these patients should not be considered for operative intervention.

3.3   Renal Failure

Patients undergoing cardiac surgery are particularly prone to large fluid shifts and electrolyte alterations as a consequence of cardiopulmonary bypass, and these are associated with elevated mortality rates. Given these realities, preoperative renal failure should be considered a strong relative contraindication to cardiac surgery. In a retrospective analysis, Engoren et al. found elevated mortality rates among patients with new dialysis requirements postoperatively, with 70% and 43% rates among octogenarians and septuagenarians, respectively [10].

3.4   Neurological/Physical Disability

In most cases of physical disability among the elderly, the underlying cause is not cardiac in nature. A myriad of pathophysiologic causes, such as osteoarthritis, Alzheimer's disease, cerebrovascular disease, or peripheral vascular disease, may be responsible, none of which would be ameliorated by cardiac surgery. Furthermore, elderly patients who are nonambulatory or otherwise physically disabled as a result of such noncardiac etiologies will be unlikely to meet the substantial physical and occupational rehabilitation requirements necessary to maximize the benefit of cardiac surgery. These cases should be considered as relative contraindications to cardiac surgery.

4   Perioperative Considerations

4.1   Preoperative Evaluation

A thorough preoperative evaluation is a vital component of any cardiac operation. Such an evaluation can identify underlying conditions that may preclude or alter the conduct of the operation. A detailed history and physical examination is the first step and should be obtained from every patient, with particular care taken with elderly patients who may have more complex medical and surgical histories and a prevalence of polypharmacy. Medical conditions that increase morbidity and mortality in elderly cardiac surgical patients include COPD or restrictive pulmonary disease, diabetes, renal insufficiency, and peripheral vascular disease. The presence and severity of these conditions must be well characterized, and treatment should be optimized. Prior surgical history, particularly any history of thoracic surgical procedures (e.g., cardiac, lung, or esophageal resection), peripheral vascular surgery, and saphenous vein stripping, can directly impact the conduct of any planned cardiac operation. A history of mediastinal radiation is important to elicit as it may not only complicate initial entry through a median sternotomy but can also adversely affect sternal healing and internal mammary artery graft patency postoperatively. The physical exam should be guided to assess the patient's preoperative functional status and confirm the underlying cardiac diagnosis, such as a heart murmur on auscultation to confirm valvular stenosis or regurgitation. After the history and physical, a complete blood count, electrolyte panel, urinalysis, and coagulation profile should be obtained to identify undiagnosed blood dyscrasias, electrolyte disturbances, renal insufficiency, active or chronic infections, and coagulopathy. Any such conditions that are discovered should be corrected or ameliorated preoperatively to decrease the attendant risks of postoperative complications. A chest radiograph is routinely obtained to detect underlying pulmonary pathology or malignancy (i.e., pleural effusion, new pulmonary nodule) and aortic pathology (e.g., aneurysmal disease, heavy calcifications). Finally, a 12-lead electrocardiogram should be routinely obtained to detect the presence of arrhythmias and nonviable myocardial territories. Other components of the preoperative evaluation are optional, and their use should be guided by the patient history. These components include pulmonary function tests in the setting of significant pulmonary insufficiency, duplex venous ultrasonography in the setting of varicosities or questionable saphenous vein quality, dental examination to identify and treat caries in valve replacement candidates, and duplex carotid ultrasonography in the setting of prior cerebrovascular events and a carotid bruit, particularly in the elderly [25]. The presence of significant carotid stenosis, defined as luminal narrowing >70%, has been identified as a risk factor for perioperative stroke in CABG patients [26]. In such cases, concomitant or staged carotid endarterectomy and CABG procedures are often performed to reduce the incidence of perioperative stroke or myocardial infarction, depending on the clinical scenario.

4.2   Intraoperative Considerations

In terms of technical considerations, there are few, if any, differences between a cardiac procedure performed on an elderly patient and the same procedure performed on a younger patient. Nevertheless, there are several considerations that the surgeon should bear in mind when operating on elderly patients. First, elderly patients may be more prone to orthopedic and neurological injuries associated with poor positioning, and so particular care should be taken with such patients. This should also be taken into consideration during routine manipulations such as leg abduction to facilitate bladder catheter placement and saphenectomy, cervical extension during intubation, and arm abduction when obtaining vascular access (e.g., radial arterial line, peripheral intravenous line). Transesophageal echocardiography is a critical supplement in elderly patients as a tool to identify high-grade atherosclerotic disease in the ascending aorta, as palpation of the aorta by the surgeon is insensitive. However, placement of the transesophageal ultrasound probe should be performed with care. Higher perfusion pressures are often used in elderly patients to improve end-organ perfusion during cardiopulmonary bypass. A randomized trial comparing a mean arterial pressure (MAP) of 80–100 vs. 50–60 maintained during CABG revealed a significantly lower incidence of cardiac and neurological complications in the higher-pressure group [27]. There is also evidence indicating a pathophysiologic role of relative anemia for postoperative stroke rates in geriatric patients and that optimizing oxygen-carrying capacity by avoiding anemia in geriatric patients undergoing cardiac surgery may play a beneficial role. Floyd et al. reported that such anemia combined with advancing age leads to relative hyperemia or increased cerebral blood flow after cardiac surgery. This may play an important role in the incidence of perioperative stroke and cognitive dysfunction in elderly patients [28]. Furthermore, in a retrospective review of patients with acute myocardial infarctions, Wu et al. reported that maintaining a hematocrit >30% with a more liberal blood transfusion protocol was associated with decreased short-term mortality rates among elderly patients [29]. Finally, as mentioned previously, a key difference between cardiac surgery and other types of surgery is the application of cardiopulmonary bypass, during which blood is exposed to extracorporeal nonendothelial cell surfaces and continuously recirculated throughout the body. The contact between the synthetic surfaces and hematologic, humoral cell lines produces a massive inflammatory cascade, which in turn activates thrombotic, vasoactive, and cytotoxic pathways affecting virtually every organ system. Elderly patients are less capable of tolerating these events, which likely contributes substantially to the heightened morbidity and mortality rates experienced by this age group. Consequently, minimizing the duration of cardiopulmonary bypass, while always considered, is of paramount importance for elderly patients.

4.3 Postoperative Considerations

Postoperatively, elderly patients are treated just like younger cardiac surgery patients, with a few key differences. Special emphasis should be placed on early mobilization, physical and occupational therapy, and pulmonary toilet, all to reduce the incidence of bedsores, deep venous thrombosis/pulmonary embolism, and pneumonia, all of which are particularly detrimental in this population. Furthermore, elderly patients are more prone to "sundowning" or postoperative delirium. Institutional protocols and environmental measures are key to preventing this in the elderly. These measures should include measures to facilitate normal sleep-wake cycles such as single rooms, signposts for time and location (e.g., clock, calendar, and window), and the judicious use of opioid narcotics. Additional emphasis should be placed on preventing patient disorientation by utilizing consistency in care staff, liberalized family visitation, and correcting any pre-existing sensory impairments (e.g., hearing aids, eyeglasses) that may be present.

5   Postoperative Complications

With an appropriate patient selection, cardiac surgery can be performed on elderly patients with acceptable mortality rates; however, hospital morbidity remains a significant concern. Special care must be taken with this population in the postoperative setting. In a review of the literature for octogenarian patients, Bacchetta et al. reported rates of postoperative morbidity ranging from 20 to 68% and 30-day mortality rates of 6–29% [30]. They also reported a series of nonagenarian surgical patients with an overall morbidity rate of 67%, which included arrhythmias, respiratory (e.g., pneumonia, respiratory failure), infectious (e.g., wound, sepsis), and hemorrhagic or embolic (e.g., postoperative bleeding, cerebrovascular accident) complications. While such complications can occur in all patients undergoing cardiac surgery, some are particularly prevalent and devastating among the elderly.

5.1   Delirium

Postoperative delirium and agitation, a neuropsychiatric complication of cardiac surgery, can significantly increase the incidence of other postoperative complications such as mechanical falls, infections, pressure sores, and mortality. It is also associated with prolonged hospital lengths of stay, increased costs, and increased rates of postdischarge institutionalization [31]. Geriatric patients are disproportionately prone to experiencing delirium after cardiac surgery, yet due to its variable presentation, delirium is often overlooked, misdiagnosed, and mistreated in this population. This is reflected in published incidence rates of 3–47% in the literature. Van der Mast and colleagues conducted a prospective study investigating the incidence of and preoperative predictors for delirium after cardiac surgery [32]. They reported postoperative delirium at a rate of 13.5% and identified age over 65 years and plasma albumin concentrations less than 40 g/L as strong predictors for postoperative delirium. Other studies have identified similar risk factors, which include patient age, cerebral disease, and poor preoperative medical status [33–35]. Postoperative delirium is commonly precipitated by infection, hypoxia, myocardial ischemia, metabolic derangements, and anticholinergics. Taken together, these observations suggest that postoperative delirium in geriatric patients is multifactorial, but an underlying medical cause should be investigated when postoperative delirium is identified.

While septuagenarians and octogenarians may undergo cardiac surgery with good in-hospital and late functional outcomes, they also pose a risk to hospitals by incurring greater costs and increased lengths of stay [10]. Postoperative neuropsychiatric dysfunction is a significant cause of these longer lengths of stay and hospital costs. Unfortunately, there are many hurdles to adequately studying this phenomenon, which include methodological hurdles, a lack of consensus on definitions, and a tacit acceptance that it is a natural manifestation of reduced physiological reserve in the geriatric population, to name a few.

One promising therapeutic strategy involves a scheduled regimen of neuroleptics and benzodiazepines for the management of delirium. Neuroleptics are a cornerstone of pharmacological treatment for delirium because they can ameliorate a range of symptoms and are effective both in hyperactive and hypoactive clinical profiles [36]. Benzodiazepines can be useful adjuncts to neuroleptics, particularly when alcohol or sedative withdrawal is a contributing factor. We postulate that a scheduled administration protocol of these agents during acute states of delirium can reduce the total duration of delirium compared to standard "prn" (as needed) administration of high-dose opioids, neuroleptics, and/or benzodiazepines. Some evidence suggests that serotoninergic receptor overstimulation plays a prominent role in delirium after cardiac surgery, leading some researchers to target this pathway. Bayindir et al. demonstrated that the 5-HT3 receptor antagonist, ondansetron, could safely and effectively reduce the severity of delirium in postcardiotomy patients [37].

5.2 Neurological Injury

As patient age increases, so does the incidence of postoperative neurological complications. In a review of patients undergoing CABG, Tuman and coauthors reported an incidence of postoperative neurological events to be 8.9% for patients 75 years of age and older, 3.6% for ages 65–74 years, and 0.9% for ages less than 65 years [38]. Similarly, Alexander and colleagues demonstrated that the incidence of postoperative neurological events increases in parallel with age, with the steepest rise occurring in patients over 75 years old [16]. Octogenarians experienced neurological complications twice as frequently as their younger counterparts. Increasing procedural complexity also plays a role, with 3.9% of octogenarians experiencing a postoperative stroke, compared to 4.9% after combined CABG/AVR and 8.8% after combined CABG/MVR. As mentioned previously, a thorough preoperative evaluation is critical for this population, particularly to identify ascending aortic atherosclerotic disease, which is widely recognized as the most prominent source of embolic stroke in cardiac operations. The frequency and extent of ascending aortic disease increases with advancing age, resulting in higher stroke rates. Furthermore, the increasing prevalence of carotid and intracranial cerebrovascular disease as patients age also contributes to the increased rates of perioperative neurological injury in the elderly. Additionally, increasing procedural complexity also contributes to increased rates of neurological injury. While the precise mechanism by which a valve replacement, when combined with CABG, increases the rates of postoperative stroke, a leading hypothesis suggests that aortic and/or mitral valve debridement generates potential emboli and that the introduction of intracardiac air during valve replacement contributes factors [39].

5.3 Renal Failure

Alexander and associates noted that, as with neurological injury, rates of renal complications increased with increasing patient age, and octogenarians were twice as likely to experience such complications when compared to younger patients. Once again, increasing procedural complexity also plays a role with octogenarians experiencing rates of postoperative renal failure of 6.9%, 12.1%, and 25% after CABG, CABG/AVR, and CABG/MVR, respectively.

5.4 Late Neurocognitive and Physical Functional Impairment

The long-term outcomes in regards to neurocognitive and functional status for the elderly after cardiac surgery remain an area in need of further investigation. Engoren and colleagues reported that while octogenarians generally experienced decreased functional status and overall health, both octogenarians and septuagenarians reported "acceptable" functional outcomes in late follow-up [10]. However, there is a paucity of literature investigating which preoperative factors and patient characteristics predict superior postoperative outcomes among these metrics for the elderly. The ultimate functional and discharge status of these patients has not yet been fully elucidated, though some evidence would suggest the quality of life improvements for the first 12 months postoperatively [40]. Certainly, future efforts should be directed toward answering these questions and would ultimately be of tremendous benefit for appropriate surgical patient selection.

6 Future Directions

6.1 The Relationship Between Frailty and Cardiac Surgery

Current recommendations for appropriate patient selection are largely based on the results of clinical trials performed in younger patients with few comorbidities. Thus, the ability to extrapolate these results to patients that are older and have a greater prevalence of underlying comorbidities is limited. The underlying vulnerability of older patients with altered physiology is generally referred to as "frailty," and this metric is used to differentiate physiological status from chronologic age [41]. In the clinical setting, a subset of older patients who are frailer tends to tolerate cardiovascular procedures poorly [11, 42]. In fact, short- and long-term cardiovascular outcomes appear to be substantially poorer in frailer patients [15, 43–45]. Therefore, more refined approaches to decision-making regarding cardiac operations in the elderly should be based on frailty and the specific contributors to frailty that most impact operative outcomes [46, 47]. Developing such decision-making algorithms is predicated on defining and validating the concept of frailty as it applies to these procedures; however, a standardized definition for frailty remains elusive. Early on, the concept of frailty was equated with a disability, comorbidity, or advanced age in general [48–52]. More recently, the definition of frailty has been further refined as a distinct biological syndrome characterized by a decreased reserve to respond to stressors resulting from an accumulation of decrements across multiple physiological systems, ultimately leading to a predisposition toward adverse outcomes [48, 51, 53, 54]. There is increasing consensus that frailty is characterized by age-associated declines in lean body mass, strength, endurance, balance, walking performance, and low activity, with multiple such components being necessary to establish a clinical diagnosis of frailty. Fried et al. have postulated that many of these components are interrelated and can be characterized by a "cycle of frailty" associated with declining energetics and reserve and with multiple components of the cycle being necessary to identify the presence of frailty [55]. They were then able to develop a standardized definition for frailty in older adults based on this cycle and to validate this definition in community-dwelling older adults, establishing an intermediate stage identifying those at high risk of frailty. Using this definition, they also demonstrated that frailty is not merely synonymous with either co-morbidity or disability but rather that co-morbidity is an etiological risk factor, and disability is an outcome of frailty [55]. Such a standardized definition is critical in clinical decision-making, as it creates a means to (a) identify frail patients at high risk for morbidity or mortality from cardiac surgery and (b) identify potentially treatable physiologic deficiencies in the preoperative setting to improve patient outcomes. To better understand the distinct pathological processes leading to frailty and develop objective screening tests to identify frail patients, several studies have attempted to identify the physiologic and metabolic markers of frailty [56–58]. While a complete understanding remains a goal for the future, there are several physiological and metabolic markers that have been correlated with the state of frailty. After identifying a subset of frail patients in the Cardiovascular Health Study using the aforementioned definition, Newman and Fried demonstrated that, as hypothesized, frailty was associated with older age and a propensity toward clinical cardiovascular disease, particularly congestive heart failure [43]. Inflammatory markers appear to be the most promising metabolic markers of frailty, which is consistent with the hypothesis that the chronic inflammatory changes typical of frail individuals result from subclinical chronic disease processes. Walston and Fried demonstrated that frail individuals had higher serum levels of several inflammatory markers, including C-reactive protein, factor VIII, and D-dimer, when compared to non-frail individuals and that these differences were present independent of the presence of CVD [56]. Similarly, Ershler and Keller demonstrated that elevated levels of interleukin-6 were associated with the development of disability and early mortality in healthy older adults [58]. Frailty is more than a purely physiologic process, as its presence has also been associated with lower education and income, poorer health, comorbid disease and disability (e.g., malignancy, chronic disease, anemia, thyroid disease, and diabetes mellitus), psychological impairment (e.g., depression, senile dementia), and lack of social or financial support. Although advanced age and physical disability are associated with frailty, this evidence suggests that neither old age nor disability alone accurately and predictively identify which elderly patients are at the highest risk of adverse outcomes after cardiac surgery. More importantly, there is some evidence indicating that cardiac surgical interventions can reduce frailty, implicating the role of cardiac pathophysiology in physiologic pathways leading to frailty and emphasizing the need to consider this physiology in individual patients when making evaluations for operative intervention [59, 60].

6.2   *Minimally Invasive Cardiac Surgery*

Recently, the focus in cardiac surgical evolution has been aimed toward minimally invasive techniques, which aim not only to minimize trauma but also the physiologic insult associated with cardiac surgery and cardiopulmonary bypass. This has led to the widespread adoption of robot-assisted, endoscopic, and endovascular techniques, all hoping to reduce the inherent morbidity of cardiovascular operations. The proposed benefits are particularly alluring for elderly patients and include reduced postoperative pain, wound-healing complications, and sequelae of the systemic inflammatory response seen as mentioned previously [61]. Evidence suggests that minimally invasive procedures such as transcatheter aortic valve replacement can be performed safely in nonagenarians and that transcatheter aortic valve replacement is associated with a decrease in postoperative delirium [62, 63]. Other studies evaluating the impact of frailty on patients undergoing surgical or transcatheter aortic valve replacement indicate there is no difference between groups, further emphasizing the need for further study of this phenomenon and its impact on cardiac surgery outcomes [64].

7   Summary

As the population continues to age, the proportion of elderly patients being considered for cardiac surgery will continue to increase. These patients present cardiac surgeons with a unique set of operative risk factors that require careful consideration and perioperative planning. Reviewing the outcomes for this population suggests that cardiac surgery can be safely performed in carefully selected elderly patients with acceptable results. Refined surgical techniques, particularly minimally invasive procedures, combined with accumulating clinical experience, will hopefully continue to improve outcomes for these patients. Nevertheless, the elderly patient warrants careful consideration between cardiologists, cardiac surgeons, patients, and their families, to maintain realistic expectations in regard to the risk and benefits to be derived from surgery. Disregarding such considerations can only result in poor clinical outcomes that will translate to unanticipated anguish and deprivation of dignity for patients and their families. Over time, well-designed clinical research will continue to identify the preoperative factors and physiologic markers to identify patients with extremely elevated operative risk profiles and facilitate interventions that can ameliorate these risks and discussions about when such interventions are best avoided.

References

1. U.S. Census Bureau. Population projections program. Washington, DC: U.S. Census Bureau; 2000.
2. U.S. Census Bureau. Statistical abstract of the United States: 2000. Washington, DC: U.S. Bureau of the Census; 2000. p. 85.
3. Roberts WC, Shirani J. Comparison of cardiac findings at necropsy in octogenarians, nonagenarians, and centenarians. Am J Cardiol. 1998;82:627–31.
4. Foot DK, et al. Demography and cardiology, 1950–2050. J Am Coll Cardiol. 2000;35(4):1076–81.
5. Craver JM, et al. 601 octogenarians undergoing cardiac surgery: outcome and comparison with younger age groups. Ann Thorac Surg. 1999;67:1104–10.
6. Tsai TP, et al. Aortocoronary bypass surgery in septuagenarians and octogenarians. J Cardiovasc Surg. 1989;30:364–8.
7. Weintraub WS, et al. Influence of age on results of coronary artery surgery. Circulation. 1991;84(Suppl 3):226–35.
8. Ko W, et al. Isolated coronary artery bypass grafting in one hundred consecutive octogenarian patients: a multivariate analysis. J Thorac Cardiovasc Surg. 1991;102:532–8.
9. Kumar P, et al. Quality of life in octogenarians after open heart surgery. Chest. 1995;108:919–26.
10. Engoren M, et al. Cost, outcome, and functional status in octogenarians and septuagenarians after cardiac surgery. Chest. 2002;122:1309–15.
11. Peterson ED, Cowper PA, Jollis JG. Outcomes of coronary artery bypass surgery in 24461 patients aged 80 years or older. Circulation. 1995;92(Suppl II):II-85–95.
12. Peterson ED, et al. Changing mortality following myocardial revascularization in the elderly: the national Medicare experience. Ann Int Med. 1994;1212:919–27.
13. Smith KM, et al. Outcomes and costs of coronary artery bypass grafting: comparison between octogenarians and septuagenarians at a tertiary care center. CMAJ. 2001;165(6):759–64.
14. Mullaney CJ, et al. Early and late results after isolated coronary artery bypass surgery in 159 patients aged 80 years and older. Circulation. 1991;82(Suppl IV):IV229–36.
15. Glower DD, Christopher TD, Milano CA. Performance status and outcome after coronary artery bypass grafting in persons 80 to 93 years. Am J Cardiol. 1992;70:567–71.
16. Alexander KP, et al. Outcomes of cardiac surgery in patients age > 80 years: results from the National Cardiovascular Network. J Am Coll Cardiol. 2000;35:731–8.
17. Tseng EE, et al. Aortic valve replacement in the elderly. Ann Surgery. 1997;225(6):793–804.
18. Gudbjartsson T, Aranki S, Cohn LH. Mechanical/bioprosthetic mitral valve replacement. In: Edmunds Jr HL, editor. Cardiac surgery in the adult. New York: McGraw-Hill; 2003. p. 951–86.

19. Desai ND, Christakis GT. Stented mechanical/bioprosthetic aortic valve replacement. In: Edmunds Jr HL, editor. Cardiac surgery in the adult. New York: McGraw-Hill; 2003. p. 825–55.
20. Khan NE, et al. A randomized comparison of off-pump and on-pump multivessel coronary artery bypass surgery. N Engl J Med. 2004;350(1):21–8.
21. Legare JF, et al. Coronary bypass surgery performed off pump does not result in lower in-hospital morbidity than coronary artery bypass grafting performed on pump. Circulation. 2004;109(7):810–2.
22. Racz MJ, Hannan EL, Isom OW. A comparison of short- and long-term outcomes after off-pump and on-pump coronary artery bypass surgery with sternotomy. J Am Coll Cardiol. 2004;43(4):557–64.
23. Kolh P, et al. Cardiac surgery in octogenarians: perioperative outcome and longterm results. Eur Heart J. 2001;22:1235–43.
24. Neri E, et al. Operation for acute type a aortic dissection in octogenarians: is it justified? J Thorac Cardiovasc Surg. 2001;121:259–67.
25. Durand DJ, et al. Mandatory versus selective preoperative carotid screening: a retrospective analysis. Ann Thorac Surg. 2004;77:TBD.
26. Naylor AR, et al. Carotid artery disease and stroke during coronary artery bypass: a critical review of the literature. Eur J Vasc Endovasc Surg. 2002;23(4):283–94.
27. Gold JP, et al. Improvement of outcomes after coronary artery bypass: a randomized trial comparing intraoperative high versus low mean arterial pressure. J Thorac Cardiovasc Surg. 1995;110(5):1302–11.
28. Floyd TF, et al. Perioperative changes in cerebral blood flow after cardiac surgery: influence of anemia and aging. Ann Thorac Surg. 2003;76(6):2037–42.
29. Wu WC, et al. Blood transfusion in elderly patients with acute myocardial infarction. N Engl J Med. 2001;345(17):1230–6.
30. Bacchetta MD, et al. Outcomes of cardiac surgery in nonagenarians: a 10-year experience. Ann Thorac Surg. 2002;75:1215–20.
31. Van der Mast RC. Delirium after cardiac surgery. PhD Dissertation 1994.
32. Van der Mast RC, et al. Incidence of and preoperative predictors for delirium after cardiac surgery. J Psychosom Res. 1998;46(5):479–83.
33. Rolfson DB, et al. Incidence and risk factors for delirium and other adverse outcomes in older adults after coronary artery bypass graft surgery. Can J Cardiol. 1999;15(7):771–6.
34. Bitondo Dyer C, Ashton CM, Teasdale TA. Postoperative delirium: a review of 80 primary data-collection studies. Arch Intern Med. 1995;155:461–5.
35. Gokgoz L, et al. Psychiatric complications of cardiac surgery: postoperative delirium syndrome. Scand Cardiovasc J. 1997;31:217–22.
36. Meagher DJ. Delirium: optimising management. BMJ. 2001;322:144–9.
37. Bayindir O, et al. The use of the 5-HT3-receptor antagonist ondansetron for the treatment of postcardiotomy delirium. J Cardiothorac Vasc Anesth. 2000;14(3):288–92.
38. Taylor HL, et al. A questionnaire for the assessment of leisure-time physical activities. J Chronic Dis. 1978;31:745–55.
39. Salazar JD, et al. Stroke after cardiac surgery: short and long-term outcomes. Ann Thorac Surg. 2001;72:1195–202.
40. Coelho PNMP, Miranda LMRPC, Barros PMP, Fragata JIG. Quality of life after elective cardiac surgery in elderly patients. Interact Cardiovasc Thorac Surg. 2019;28(2):199–205. https://doi.org/10.1093/icvts/ivy235.
41. Krumholz HM, Herrin J. Quality improvement studies: the need is there but so are the challenges. Am J Med. 2000;109:501–3.
42. Gersh BJ, Kronmal RA, Frye RL. Coronary arteriography and coronary artery bypass surgery; morbidity and mortality in patients aged 65 years or older: a report from the coronary artery surgery study. Circulation. 1983;67:483–91.
43. Newman AB, et al. Associations of subclinical cardiovascular disease with frailty. J Gerontol A Biol Scie Med Sci. 2001;56(3):M158–66.

44. Fried LP, et al. Risk factors for 5-year mortality in older adults: the cardiovascular health study. JAMA. 1998;279(8):585–92.
45. Pendergast DR, Fisher NM, Calkins E. Cardiovascular, neuromuscular, and metabolic alterations with age leading to frailty. J Gerontol. 1993;48:61–7.
46. Fried LP, et al. Physical disability in older adults: a physiologic approach. Cardiovascular health study research group. Clin Epidemiol. 1994;47(7):747–60.
47. Bild DE, et al. Age-related trends in cardiovascular morbidity and physical functioning in the elderly: the cardiovascular health study. J Am Geriatr Soc. 1993;41(10):1047–56.
48. Fried LP, Walston J. Frailty and failure to thrive. In: Hazzard WR, et al., editors. Principles of geriatric medicine and gerontology. New York: McGraw-Hill; 1998. p. 1387–402.
49. Rockwood K, et al. A brief clinical instrument to classify frailty in elderly people. Lancet. 1999;353:205–6.
50. Winograd CH, et al. Screening for frailty: criteria and predictors of outcomes. J Am Geriatr Soc. 1991;39:778–84.
51. Campbell AJ, Buchner DM. Unstable disability and the fluctuations of frailty. Age Aging. 1997;26:315–8.
52. Winograd CH. Targeting strategies: an overview of criteria and outcomes. J Am Geriatr Soc. 1991;39S:25S–35S.
53. Buchner DM, Wagner EH. Preventing frail health. Clin Geriatr Med. 1992;8:1–17.
54. Bortz WM II. A conceptual framework of frailty: a review. J Gerontol A Biol Sci Med Sci. 2002;57(5):M283–8.
55. Fried LP, et al. Frailty in older adults: evidence for a phenotype. J Gerontol A Biol Scie Med Sci. 2001;56(3):M146–56.
56. Walston J, et al. Frailty and activation of the inflammation and coagulation systems with and without clinical comorbidities: results from the cardiovascular health study. Arch Intern Med. 2002;162(20):2333–41.
57. Zieman SJ, et al. Upregulation of the nitric oxide-cGMP pathway in aged myocardium: physiological response to L-arginine. Circ Res. 2001;88:97–102.
58. Ershler WB, Keller ET. Age-associated increased interleukin-6 gene expression, late-life diseases, and frailty. Annu Rev Med. 2000;51:245–70.
59. Miguelena-Hycka J, Lopez-Menendez J, Prada PC, García MM, Vigil-Escalera C, Harmand MG, Pérez RM, Rodriguez-Roda J. Changes in frailty status after cardiac surgery. A prospective cohort study Arch Gerontol Geriatr. 2022;98:104568. https://doi.org/10.1016/j.archger.2021.104568. Epub 2021 Nov 9
60. Jha SR, Hannu MK, Newton PJ, Wilhelm K, Hayward CS, Jabbour A, et al. Reversibility of frailty after bridge-to-transplant ventricular assist device implantation or heart transplantation. Transplant Direct. 2017;3(7):E167.
61. Plomondon ME, et al. Off-pump coronary artery bypass is associated with improved risk-adjusted outcomes. Ann Thorac Surg. 2001;72(1):114–9.
62. Habertheuer A, Aranda-Michel E, Schindler J, Gleason TG, Kilic A, Kliner D, Bianco V, Toma C, Sultan I. Longitudinal outcomes of nonagenarians undergoing transcatheter aortic valve replacement. Ann Thorac Surg. 2021;111(5):1520–8.
63. Hoogma DF, Venmans E, Al Tmimi L, Tournoy J, Verbrugghe P, Jacobs S, Fieuws S, Milisen K, Adriaenssens T, Dubois C, Rex S. Postoperative delirium and quality of life after transcatheter and surgical aortic valve replacement: a prospective observational study. J Thorac Cardiovasc Surg. 2021; https://doi.org/10.1016/j.jtcvs.2021.11.023. Epub ahead of print
64. Strom JB, Xu J, Orkaby AR, Shen C, Song Y, Charest BR, Kim DH, Cohen DJ, Kramer DB, Spertus JA, Gerszten RE, Yeh RW. The role of frailty in identifying benefit from transcatheter versus surgical aortic valve replacement. Circ Cardiovasc Qual Outcomes. 2021;14(12):e008566. https://doi.org/10.1161/CIRCOUTCOMES.121.008566. Epub ahead of print

Valvular Heart Disease in the Elderly: Clinical and Multi-Modality Imaging Perspectives

Tom Kai Ming Wang and Milind Y. Desai

1 Aortic Stenosis

1.1 Etiologies and Epidemiology

Aortic stenosis (AS) is an exemplary age-related valve disease with a prevalence of 12.4% (and severe AS of 3.4%) in a recent meta-analysis, and also important as the most common indication for valve surgery and interventions [7, 8]. In those with severe symptomatic AS on medical therapy alone, the prognosis is poor at a median of two years in those with dyspnea and heart failure, three years in those with syncope, and five years in those with angina [9]. The main etiologies by valvular heart disease lesion are listed in Table 1. The most common etiology for AS is age-related degenerative sclerosis and calcifications of the aortic valve leading to leaflet restriction, with the two other important causes more common in younger patients being bicuspid aortic valve and rheumatic heart disease [10]. Studies have shown that conventional cardiovascular risk factors beyond age, such as male gender, hypertension, dyslipidemia, obesity, diabetes, smoking, and renal dysfunction, are also associated with a higher risk of developing AS [11]. AS leads to pressure loading of the left ventricle during systole, leading to concentric hypertrophy, and later impaired systolic function and sometimes demand myocardial ischemia.

T. K. M. Wang · M. Y. Desai (✉)
Section of Cardiovascular Imaging, Heart, Vascular and Thoracic Institute, Cleveland Clinic, Cleveland, OH, USA
e-mail: desaim2@ccf.org

T. M. Leucker, G. Gerstenblith (eds.), *Cardiovascular Disease in the Elderly*, Contemporary Cardiology, https://doi.org/10.1007/978-3-031-16594-8_9

Table 1 Common etiologies of valvular heart disease by lesion

Aortic stenosis	Aortic regurgitation	Mitral regurgitation	Tricuspid regurgitation
Primary causes			
Degenerative/calcific	Degenerative/prolapse	Degenerative/prolapse	Degenerative/prolapse
	Infective endocarditis	Infective endocarditis	Infective endocarditis
Rheumatic heart disease	Rheumatic heart disease	Rheumatic heart disease	Rheumatic heart disease
	Connective tissue disorders	Connective tissue disorders	Carcinoid syndrome
	Acute aortic syndrome (aortic dissection)	Acute myocardial infarction (papillary muscle rupture)	Trauma
Prosthetic degeneration, pannus, and thrombosis	Prosthetic degeneration and paravalvular leak	Prosthetic degeneration and paravalvular leak	Prosthetic degeneration and paravalvular leak
			Cardiac implantable device lead
Bicuspid aortic valve	Bicuspid aortic valve		Ebstein's anomaly/dysplastic
Secondary causes			
Not applicable	Dilated thoracic aorta/root	Ischemic cardiomyopathy	Left heart disease
		Nonischemic cardiomyopathy	Pulmonary disease
		Atrial functional	Atrial functional
		Left-to-right shunt lesions	Primary right heart disease

1.2 Clinical Presentation

Current guidelines use the four stages A–D framework for characterizing the clinical status for all valvular heart diseases, including AS—A: at risk (risk factors for valve disease), B: progressive (asymptomatic with mild-moderate valve severity), C: asymptomatic severe (C1 and C2 if there is no or presence of left or right ventricle decompensation), and D: symptomatic severe [4]. Heart failure symptoms can also be graded based on the New York Heart Association classification for dyspnea severity. The majority of AS patients are asymptomatic with a long latent period before progressing into the C2 or D phases. Common symptoms of severe symptomatic AS are dyspnea (on exertion, orthopnea, at rest or overt pulmonary edema from systolic and/or diastolic dysfunction), angina (demand ischemia from the increased left ventricular systolic pressure required in the setting of aortic stenosis, left ventricle hypertrophy, and/or concomitant coronary heart disease), and dizziness or syncope (related to hypotension from fixed obstruction, arrhythmia, and/ or abnormal baroreceptor response). A small minority of patients have gastrointestinal bleeding from angiodysplasia or Heyde's syndrome, which is associated with von Willebrand syndrome [12, 13]. The history needs to be actively sought in the elderly patient with at least moderate AS, because, AS is progressive and severe symptomatic AS is associated with a dismal prognosis warranting assessment towards aortic valve intervention [9].

AS often has a loud, harsh ejection systolic murmur at the right upper sternal edge, which radiates to both carotid arteries and is louder on expiration but softens when progressing to critical AS. Signs of severe AS include slow-rising plateau pulse, narrow pulse pressure, aortic stenosis thrill on palpitation, paradoxical splitting of S2, presence of S4, and signs of left ventricular failure. Elevated B-type natriuretic peptide is associated with adverse outcomes in AS, and along with other biomarkers, such as renal function, are important in the risk stratification for aortic valve surgeries and interventions [8, 14, 15].

1.3   Echocardiography

The strengths and limitations of the various imaging modalities for evaluating valvular heart disease are shown in Table 2. Transthoracic echocardiography (TTE) remains the first-line imaging modality for evaluating all valvular heart diseases including AS. The main TTE views and modalities for AS include the parasternal long axis, parasternal short axis at aortic valve level, apical five- and three-chamber

Table 2 Strengths and limitations of imaging modalities for evaluating valvular heart diseases

	Echocardiography	CT	MRI
Strengths	High availability, low cost	High availability, low cost	
	High temporal resolution	High spatial resolution	High spatial resolution
	First-line valve assessment		Gold standard chamber quantification
	Doppler evaluation		Direct flow quantification
		Extracardiac structures	Extracardiac structures
			Tissue characterization
	Intraprocedural guidance	Procedural planning	Procedural planning
Limitations	Operator dependent	Radiation	Lower availability, high cost
	Body habitus	Iodinated contrast	Gadolinium contrast
	Lower spatial resolution	Lower temporal resolution	Lower temporal resolution
	Right heart quantification	No flow quantification	Non-compatible device/ prosthesis
	Extracardiac structures limited	Not portable for sick patients	Breath-hold instructions, claustrophobia
	Tissue characterization limited		Not portable for sick patients

views, and all two-dimensional, color, continuous and pulsed wave Doppler techniques [16]. The Pedoff probe is often used in the apical, suprasternal, and right parasternal areas to try and detect the maximal aortic valve systolic velocities, with one study showing that 61% of severe AS patients did not have the highest velocity detected on apical windows [17]. The main quantitative parameters for AS assessment are peak systolic velocity, mean gradient, valve area, and dimensionless index, with mild AS being 2.6–2.9 m/s, <20 mmHg, >1.5 cm^2, and >0.50; moderate AS being 3.0–4.0 m/s, 20–40 mmHg, 1.0–1.5 cm^2, and 0.25–0.50 cm; and severe AS being ≥4.0 m/s, ≥40 mmHg, ≤1.0 cm^2, and ≤0.25, respectively [5]. The aortic valve area is often determined using the continuity equation from the left ventricular outflow tract (LVOT) diameter (to calculate area), LVOT velocity time integral (VTI), and aortic valve VTI. It should be noted that the LVOT diameter measurement needs to be accurate as it can lead to the widest margin of error in area calculation. Multiple methods of determining left ventricular stroke volume can be used, which are divide by aortic valve VTI to obtain the valve area. The dimensionless index is also useful and can be determined by either the ratio of peak velocities or VTIs of the LVOT divided by the aortic valve VTI.

Not uncommonly, there are challenges in grading AS severity from the discrepancies between aortic valve peak velocity, mean gradient, and valve area [5]. It is important to check for measurement errors that underestimate the gradient, flow, and valve area under-estimation, along with quantifying flow status, ejection fraction (<50% warrants dobutamine stress echocardiography), and flow reserve (by dobutamine stress echocardiography, if present to help distinguish true severe or pseudosevere AS). Parameters that increase the chance of severe AS in those with an area <1.0 cm^2 but gradient <40 mmHg (low gradient AS) include left ventricular hypertrophy, mean aortic valve gradient 30–40 mmHg, valve area ≤0.8 cm^2, dimensionless index ≤0.25, low flow stroke volume index <35 mL/m^2 and left ventricular ejection fraction<50%, and high aortic valve calcium scores by CT, with specific criteria discussed in the next section. Separate guidelines exist for the evaluation of prosthetic AS, which is beyond the scope of this chapter [18]. In addition to the aortic valve, a complete TTE examination should be performed, including chamber quantification, left ventricle mass, systolic and diastolic function, and assessment for other valvular heart diseases, as they may influence surgical decision-making [4, 6, 16]. Exercise stress ECG or echocardiography may be helpful to identify exercise intolerance and symptoms in reportedly asymptomatic patients with severe AS with potential surgical implications; however, it is contraindicated in those with known symptomatic severe AS [19]. Several studies have also demonstrated the prognostic utility of left ventricular global longitudinal strain (LVGLS) in aortic stenosis that should be part of the comprehensive TTE study [20].

Transesophageal echocardiography (TEE) can also be used to assess aortic valve stenosis severity, with aortic valve morphology and motion assessment in midesophageal aortic valve long and short axis views, Doppler interrogation of the aortic valve occurs in the transgastric long axis view, whereas the LVOT and aortic annulus are measured using three-dimensional (3D) echocardiography, although these are usually underestimated compared with cross-sectional imaging techniques. Therefore, TEE is no longer the first-line test to assess aortic valve stenosis severity [21, 22]. In the intraprocedural setting for aortic valve surgery (TEE) or transcatheter intervention (TTE or TEE), echocardiography can assess the prosthetic valve placement, presence of prosthetic valve stenosis or regurgitation, aortic complications, pericardial effusion, cardiac chamber size and function, LVOT obstruction, and other valvular diseases [23].

1.4   Cardiac Computed Tomography

Cardiac computed tomography (CT) has important clinical utility in both aortic valve stenosis evaluation as well as being the preferred modality in the preprocedural evaluation prior to transcatheter aortic valve replacement (TAVR) [5, 24]. Aortic valve morphology, thickening, calcifications, and leaflet motion can be assessed, using retrospective-gated four-dimensional (4D) imaging that spans the entire cardiac cycle and valve planimetry can be performed if image quality is sufficient. The Agatston calcium score of the aortic valve has been incorporated into the guidelines for grading AS, especially when echocardiography parameters are conflicting, such as in low gradient AS. The diagnosis of severe AS is likely in men with a calcium score $\geq$2000 units and women $\geq$1200 units and unlikely in men <1600 units, women <800 units, and higher calcium scores portends worse survival [5, 25]. As part of TAVR workup, multiplanar reconstruction (MPR) assessment on contrast-enhanced CT (Fig. 1) includes the aortic annulus diameter, area, and perimeter to inform TAVR prosthesis sizing, annulus to left and right coronary artery heights (to prevent coronary obstruction), left ventricular outflow tract, aortic root, thoracoabdominal aorta and peripheral arterial anatomy, tortuosity, dimensions and calcifications (as part of vascular access evaluation, including iliofemoral and aortic arch branch vessels), coronary artery evaluation (to determine the need for revascularization), and chamber size, mass, and function quantification [24, 26]. Additionally, 4D-CT is also valuable in assessing prosthetic aortic valve stenosis and related reduced leaflet motion, hypoattenuating leaflet thickening (also known as HALT), pannus, and thrombosis [27]. CT with or without contrast can be useful in the preoperative evaluation for all valvular heart surgeries. The assessment should include relations between the sternum, especially in redo cardiac surgery, key vascular structures such as the brachiocephalic vein, ascending aorta, bypass grafts, and right ventricle, assessment of thoracic aorta dimensions, calcifications, lung assessment, and any other acute pathologies.

1.5   Magnetic Resonance Imaging

Cardiac magnetic resonance imaging (MRI) has some unique roles in the evaluation of AS, although it is not the first line imaging modality for diagnosing AS severity. Phase contrast sequences performed at the aortic valve, sinotubular junction, and ascending aorta levels can quantitatively assess peak systolic velocity, as long as the

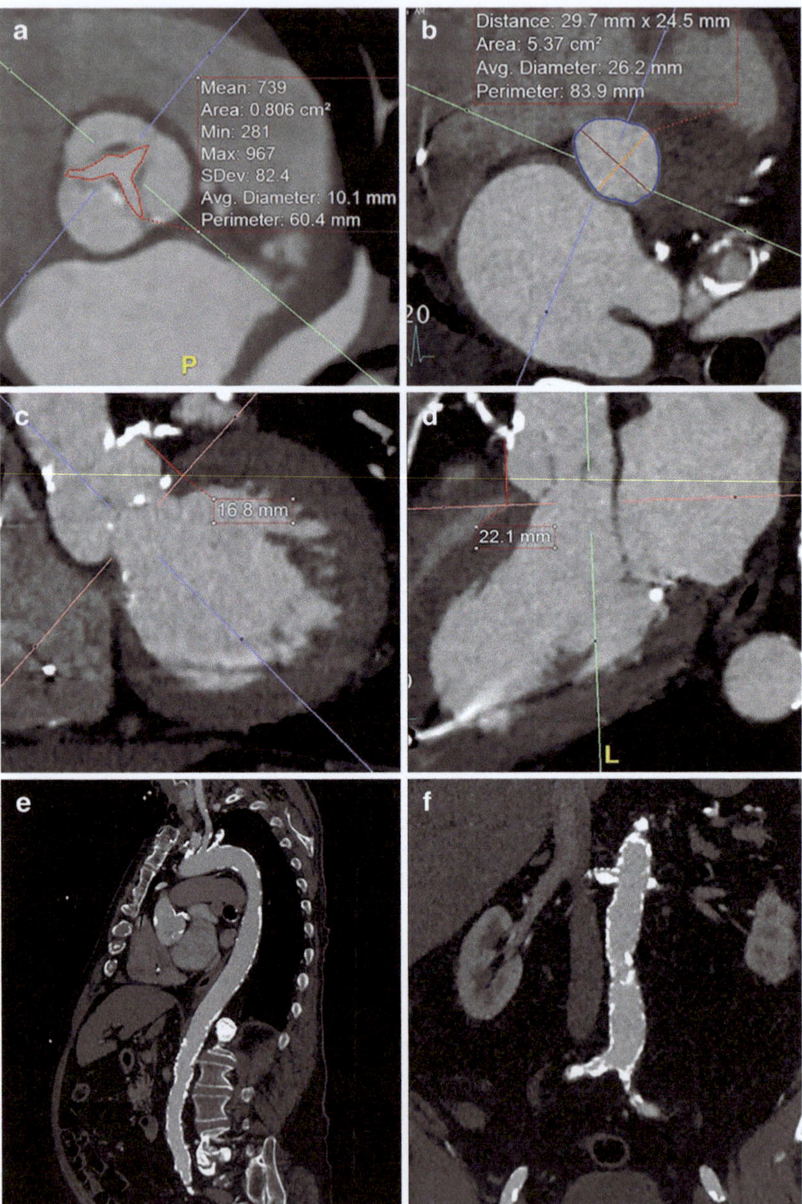

Fig. 1 CT evaluation of aortic stenosis in an 83-year-old man prior to transcatheter aortic valve replacement, including retrospective 4D-gating and multiplanar reconstruction (**a**) aortic valve planimetry showing severe aortic stenosis, (**b**) aortic annulus sizing, (**c**) annulus to left coronary artery height (note sinotubular junction and coronary calcifications), (**d**) annulus to the right coronary artery height, (**e**) significant thoracoabdominal aortic and arch branch vessel calcifications, prohibiting subclavian artery access, and (**f**) severe common iliac artery calcifications prohibiting transfemoral access (note right renal artery stenting)

velocity encoding is set high enough to not have aliasing, along with concurrent regurgitant volume and fraction [28]. Only a few studies have compared TTE and MRI grading of AS severity, with varrying correlations from modest to strong, highlighting MRI's limitations for valve stenosis evaluation for velocities and gradients. Compared to TTE, MRI is superior in assessing left ventricular outflow tract area [29]. Furthermore, bright blood gradient echo cine sequences are used to allow for visual assessment of aortic valve morphology, thickening of the valve, calcification (signal void), flow acceleration, and to determine whether the level of obstruction is below, at, or above, the aortic valve [28]. MRI is the gold standard for quantification of chamber size, mass, especially if TTE imaging is suboptimal [30]. Perhaps one of the most important utilities of MRI is its 3D whole heart sequence, which provides a noncontrast imaging alternative to CT in the preprocedural evaluation of TAVR in those patients with significant renal impairment [26]. Noncontrast CT is still preferred for evaluating peripheral vascular access for TAVR. Lastly, MRI uniquely has the capabilities of myocardial tissue characterization, such as late gadolinium enhancement imaging, native T1-mapping, and extracellular volume fraction analysis, and all of these as binary and/or continuous parameters have been demonstrated in recent studies to be prognostic of survival in aortic stenosis with or without intervention [31–33].

2   Aortic Regurgitation

2.1   Etiologies and Epidemiology

Approximately 11% of the general population have at least mild AR and 0.5% have at least moderate aortic regurgitation (AR) [2, 34]. One classification commonly used to, assess aortic valve cusp mobility in AR is type 1 normal cusp motion with aortic dilation (functional) or perforation, type 2 cusp prolapse (excessive motion), and type 3 cusp restriction [3]. There are a wide range of different AR etiologies (Table 1) including limpaired eaflet morphology (bicuspid, unicuspid, or quadricuspid), dilated thoracic aorta causing a "functional" AR (includes idiopathic, aortopathies from connective tissues diseases such as Marfan syndrome, Ehlers-Danlos and Loeys-Dietz, autoimmune diseases such as lupus and ankylosing spondylitis, and acute aortic syndromes including dissection), structural valve degeneration (such as calcification and prolapse, sometimes with concurrent AS), and other acquired leaflet abnormalities (including infective endocarditis, rheumatic heart disease, connective tissue diseases, radiotherapy, and toxins). Unlike AS, AR has etiologies that can affect patients over the entire age spectrum and not just the elderly. Chronic AR leads to left ventricular volume overload, eccentric hypertrophy remodeling, and eventually left heart failure, while acute AR, when there is insufficient time for the left ventricle to compensate, can result in acute pulmonary edema and cardiogenic shock.

2.2 Clinical Evaluation

The aforementioned four stages A–D framework for characterizing the clinical status of AS also apply to AR [4]. Acute AR can develop in patients with infective endocarditis, acute aortic syndromes, and trauma; otherwise, most cases are chronic and asymptomatic until stage D. Dyspnea and left heart failure symptoms eventually develop, while chest pains and palpitations are less common and usually related to mechanical interaction between the dilated heart and chest wall, or concurrent coronary heart disease.

On clinical examination, the AR murmur is typically described as early diastolic, loudest at the left lower sternal edge, louder with expiration and handgrip, and better appreciated with the patient sitting up and leaning forward. Additional physical exam findings of severe AR include a collapsing higher volume pulse, wide pulse pressure, longer duration of diastolic murmur, soft A2, presence of S3, Austin-Flint murmur (mid to late diastolic apical rumble from turbulence between regurgitant AR flow and antegrade mitral valve inflow during diastole) and other signs of left heart failure. Other less utilized signs of severe AR from a widened pulse pressure and increased stroke volume include Corrigan's pulse, deMusset's sign, Traube's sign, Duroziez's sign, Quincke's sign, and Mueller's sign [35]. Acute AR can also exhibit the following exam findings: tachycardia, hypotension, pulmonary edema, and at times cardiogenic shock. The B-type natriuretic peptide is a useful biomarker to monitor disease progression in asymptomatic chronic AR and elevated levels are associated with adverse clinical outcomes [36].

2.3 Echocardiography

A multi-parametric approach is necessary for the echocardiography evaluation of AR [3]. The aortic valve is evaluated on the same aforementioned views and using the same techniques in AR as in AS [16]. To evaluate the AR mechanism it is important to examine the aortic valve morphology, thickening, prolapse or flail leaflets, vegetations, regurgitation jet location, direction, and number. Qualitative features suggestive of significant AR include coaptation defect, flow convergence, increased jet density on continuous wave Doppler, flow reversal in the descending and abdominal aorta (holodiastolic), and a dilated left ventricle [3]. Semiquantitative and quantitative TTE parameters in AR and thresholds according to the guidelines are shown in Table 3, including vena contracta width, jet width or area, pressure half-time, effective regurgitant orifice area, regurgitant volume, and regurgitant fraction. A high-frequency diastolic fluttering of the anterior mitral valve leaflet may occasionally be present. Separate guidelines also exist for the evaluation of prosthetic AR, which share some common criteria for its severity grading [18]. A complete TTE examination including left ventricular and other chamber dimensions and function (left ventricle size being part of the criteria for aortic valve

Table 3 Quantitative and semi-quantitative echocardiographic grading of valvular regurgitation by lesion (modified from ASE guidelines)

Parameter	Aortic regurgitation				Mitral regurgitation				Tricuspid regurgitation			
Severity	Mild	Moderate		Severe	Mild	Moderate		Severe	Mild	Moderate		Severe
Color Doppler jet area (cm^2 for AR/TR, % of left atrium for MR)	<5	5–20	21–59	>60	Small	Variable		>50%	N/A			>10
Flow in proximal descending aorta (AR), pulmonary vein (MR) or hepatic vein (TR)	Brief early diastolic reversal	Intermediate		Holo-diastolic reversal	Systolic dominance	Systolic blunting		Systolic flow reversal	Systolic dominance	Systolic blunting		Systolic flow reversal
Pressure half-time (ms)	>500	200–500		≤200	N/A				N/A			
Valve inflow E-wave (m/s)	N/A				A-wave dominant	Variable		>1.2	A-wave dominant	Variable		>1.0
Vena contracta width (cm)	<0.3	0.3–0.6		≥0.6	<0.3	0.3–0.7		≥0.7	<0.3	0.3–0.7		≥0.7
Effective regurgitant orifice area (cm^2)	<0.10	0.10–0.19	0.20–0.29	≥0.30	<0.20	0.20–0.29	0.30–0.39	≥0.40	<0.20	0.20–0.29	0.30–0.39	≥0.40
Regurgitant volume (mL)	<30	30–44	45–59	≥60	<30	30–44	45–59	≥60	<30	30–44		≥45
Regurgitant fraction (%)	<30	30–39	40–49	≥50	<30	30–39	40–49	≥50	N/A			

surgery), other valvular heart diseases, and thoracic aorta measurements (if visible), including the aortic root and ascending aorta should be performed [16]. Additionally, LVGLS has been shown to provide incremental prognostic utility in asymptomatic severe AR before and after aortic valve surgery and should also be measured during the TTE examination [37]. TEE can be used in selected patients to further assess the AR mechanism and should include an evaluation for acute pathologies such as aortic dissection, evidence of endocarditis complications like root abscess, and prosthetic AR. Furthermore, TEE imaging can be helpful in the intraoperative setting to guide the surgeon [3].

2.4 Magnetic Resonance Imaging

The key components of MRI evaluation in AR are shown in Fig. 2. AR is arguably the valve lesion most often evaluated with cardiac MRI to quantify aortic regurgitation volume and fraction, left ventricle volumes and function, and for concurrent evaluation of the thoracic aorta, especially as TTE assessment is sometimes challenging [3]. Phase contrast sequence imaging performed at the aortic valve, sinotubular junction, and/or ascending aorta level can directly quantify regurgitant volume and fraction [28]. In addition, measurements of the flow over time at the descending aorta by this sequence can demonstrate holodiastolic flow reversal, a specific sign of severe AR [38]. Chamber quantification especially left ventricle end-diastolic volume, end-systolic volume, and ejection fraction are traced and calculated on bright blood gradient echo sequences, along with visualization of aortic valve morphology (aortic valve short axis view), regurgitant flow, and forward flow acceleration (3-chamber and oblique coronal views), and finally, the thoracic aorta dimensions can be measured on whole-heart without contrast or magnetic resonance angiography sequences [28]. There is a modest correlation between TTE and MRI assessment of AR regurgitant volume and fraction, and lower values are typically seen by MRI, especially if measured further along the ascending aorta compared to at the aortic valve/sinotubular junction [39]. Guidelines have not established AR severity thresholds by MRI, although one study proposed <8%, 8–19%, 20–29%, and 30 + % as the MRI thresholds for 0–1+, 2+ (moderate), 3+ (moderate to severe), and 4+ (severe) AR. Finally, increasing AR severity and holodiastolic flow reversal by MRI are associated with an adverse prognosis, and have potential implications for the timing of aortic valve procedures [40].

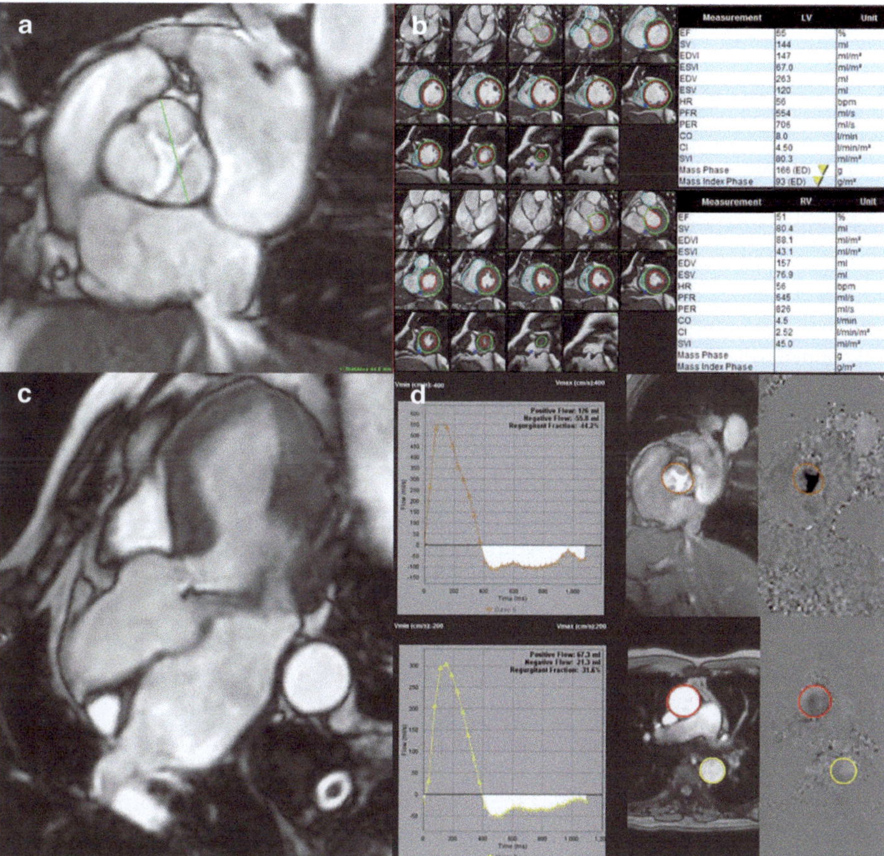

Fig. 2 MRI evaluation of aortic regurgitation in a 78-year-old man (**a**) trileaflet aortic valve morphology and dilated aortic root (4.4 cm), (**b**) left and right ventricle chamber quantification using bright blood gradient echo images, (**c**) cine 3-chamber view showing significant posteriorly directed eccentric jet of aortic regurgitation impeding anterior mitral valve leaflet opening in diastole, and (**d**) phase contrast sequence to quantify aortic regurgitation at the valve level (regurgitant volume 56 mL, fraction 44%) in the upper panel, and holodiastolic flow reversal at the descending thoracic aorta (yellow circle) in the lower panel. (Note the mitral regurgitant volume would be left ventricular stroke volume—aortic valve forward flow = 144–126 = 18 mL, and regurgitant fraction 18/144 = 12.5%)

3 Mitral Regurgitation

3.1 *Etiologies and Epidemiology*

Mitral regurgitation (MR) occurs in up to 19% of patients 65-years old (at least mild severity) and is the second commonest valve lesion treated by both cardiac surgery and transcatheter interventions [8, 41]. The Carpentier classification divides MR etiologies based on leaflet motion: type 1 has normal leaflet motion including annular dilation and perforation, type 2 has excessive leaflet motion including prolapse and flail, and type 3 has restricted leaflet motion including thickening/fusion and left ventricular/atrial dilation [3, 42]. Clinically, however, the distinction between primary and secondary MR is perhaps more critical in guiding the direction of subsequent procedural management [8, 41] and medical therapies for heart failure [43, 44]. Primary MR refers to pathology directly affecting the mitral valve leaflets. The most common cause is degenerative MR with mitral valve prolapse, associated with fibroelastic deficiency with typically one to two segment prolapse, and less commonly Barlow's disease (often with bileaflet prolapse). Mitral valve prolapse is present in 0.6–2.4% of the general population, and a subset of these patients are increasingly recognized to be associated with ventricular arrhythmias and sudden cardiac death, including those with bileaflet prolapse, prior syncope, higher premature ventricular complex burden, mitral annular dysfunction, and late gadolinium enhancement on MRI [45–47]. Other important primary MR causes are endocarditis, rheumatic (often with concurrent mitral stenosis), and connective tissue diseases (such as rheumatoid arthritis).

Secondary MR (also known as functional MR) refers to abnormal left ventricular and/or atrial remodeling with and without dysfunction leading to malcoaptation of the otherwise structurally normal leaflets. Some patients have mixed MR etiologies and this is much more common in the elderly [48]. Secondary MR causes include ischemic cardiomyopathy (which may be regional or global left ventricular dysfunction), nonischemic cardiomyopathy, and atrial functional MR (from the dilated left atrium and mitral annulus, which can be associated with atrial fibrillation) [8, 41, 48]. Most of these patients have central MR jets, except for ischemic MR with regional dysfunction, such as posteromedial papillary muscle restriction from right coronary artery territory infarction, which usually yields a posteriorly directed MR jet [3, 48]. Of note, there are a heterogeneous range of factors at play in leading to secondary MR, including left ventricular, atrial, and mitral annular dilation, leaflet tethering and restriction, reduced left ventricular systolic function, elevated left ventricular filling and left atrial pressures, leaflet thickening, annular contraction, and dyssynchrony. Secondary MR has consistently been shown to be associated with a poor prognosis in heart failure and cardiomyopathy patients [48, 49].

3.2   Clinical Evaluation

The majority of MR patients are asymptomatic in stages A–C [4]. Acute MR is uncommon but rapidly leads to pulmonary edema and cardiogenic shock. Symptomatic chronic MR leads to exercise intolerance, fatigue, and weakness, before progressing to heart failure symptoms of dyspnea, orthopnea, paroxysmal nocturnal dyspnea, and edema. Rarely, symptoms like chest pain, palpitations, thromboembolism, and hemoptysis are encountered; more commonly these symptoms are associated with concomittant atrial fibrillation.

The MR murmur is generally described as pan-systolic at the apex of the heart, louder on expiration, and with hand grip. In mitral valve prolapse, there may be a mid-systolic click, and the murmur can radiate posteriorly for anterior leaflet prolapse and to the base of the heart anteriorly for posterior leaflet prolapse, corresponding to jet direction. Clinical signs of severe MR include soft S2, presence of S3, small volume pulse, displaced apical impulse early diastolic rumble, and signs of left ventricular failure and/or pulmonary hypertension. Again, B-type natriuretic peptides also demonstrate prognostic utility in MR, especially for primary etiology and medically managed patients [50].

3.3   Echocardiography

MR assessment begins with TTE, using parasternal long and short axis and apical 4-, 2-, and 3-chamber views [16]. The mitral valve apparatus including the leaflets, annulus, chordae, and papillary muscles are assessed for thickness, calcifications, motion (including prolapse, flail, rupture papillary muscle, perforation, tenting, coaptation defect, and systolic anterior motion), and vegetations. Additionally, the TTE examination should include color Doppler to interrogate the regurgitant jet number, origin, direction, and size, keeping the range of possible MR etiologies in mind [3]. Qualitative features that suggest severe MR include a large central or eccentric wall-impinging MR jet, dense triangular MR jet by continuous wave Doppler, dilated left ventricle and left atrium, large flow convergence, pan-systolic regurgitant jet, E-wave dominant mitral inflow (>1.2 m/s), and systolic flow reversal within the pulmonary veins. Quantitative TTE parameters and thresholds for mild, moderate, and severe MR are shown in Table 3, including vena contracta width, effective regurgitant orifice area, regurgitant volume, and regurgitant fraction. Notably, some guidelines and studies have suggested lower thresholds for these quantitative parameters in secondary MR, given the impaired systolic function in these patients [4, 6, 51], while others suggest the same thresholds [3]. Chamber quantification for the left ventricle, left atrium and right atrium, right ventricular systolic pressure estimate and other concurrent valve diseases must be evaluated, given their important implications for both prognosis and subsequent management [4, 6]. Left ventricle ejection fraction is considered abnormal when below 60%, given MR's volume loading and reduced afterload on the left ventricle. LVGLS should also be measured, because impaired strain is associated with worse survival in both primary and secondary MR [52–54]. Finally, the proportionate versus disproportionate MR hypothesis was recently proposed to reconcile the conflicting findings between the two Mitraclip randomized trials (COAPT strongly positive, Mitra-FR neutral), and this ratio between a quantitative estimate of MR severity and left ventricle volume can be assessed by TTE (or MRI) [55–57].

TEE has arguably the most important role in MR amongst all valvular heart diseases, including advanced techniques with biplane, 3D, and MPR to accurately diagnose the structure and pathology (both primary and secondary) in most patients with MR [4, 6]. The main two-dimensional views are mid-esophageal 4-, bicomissural, two-chamber, long-axis, left and right pulmonary veins (assess pulmonary vein flow), left atrial appendage (to exclude thrombus), and transgastric long axis and mitral valve short axis views, and 3D views which can add complementary information [21]. TEE can help determine if the MR is amenable to surgical and percutaneous repair and can provide intraprocedural guidance and postoperative evaluation for these procedures such as transseptal puncture, prosthesis positioning or grasp of leaflets, mitral valve gradient measurements for stenosis, valvular and paravalvular leak, cardiac chamber size and function, LVOT obstruction and any evidence of pericardial effusion [21, 58, 59]. Figure 3 provides an example of an intraprocedural TEE for a Mitraclip procedure using 3D-MPR. Furthermore, stress echocardiography may also be helpful for evaluating functional capacity, changes in ejection fraction, MR severity, right ventricular systolic pressure, arrhythmias, and heart rate recovery. Many of these findings are associated with reduced survival in MR and greater need to undergo mitral procedures [54, 60].

3.4   *Magnetic Resonance Imaging*

Similar to AR, MRI may be considered for evaluating MR when there is evidence of significant MR and a discrepancy between TTE parameters and the clinical status. Additionally, MRI can be useful to determine the etiology of MR, and a viability assessment of any associated cardiomyopathy (secondary MR), and assessment of MR related to systolic anterior motion in hypertrophic cardiomyopathy [3]. The mitral valve is visualized on the 4-, 2-, and 3-chamber along with short axis views on bright blood gradient sequence images for leaflet structure (morphology, thickening, calcification represented by signal void), abnormal motion (both prolapse and

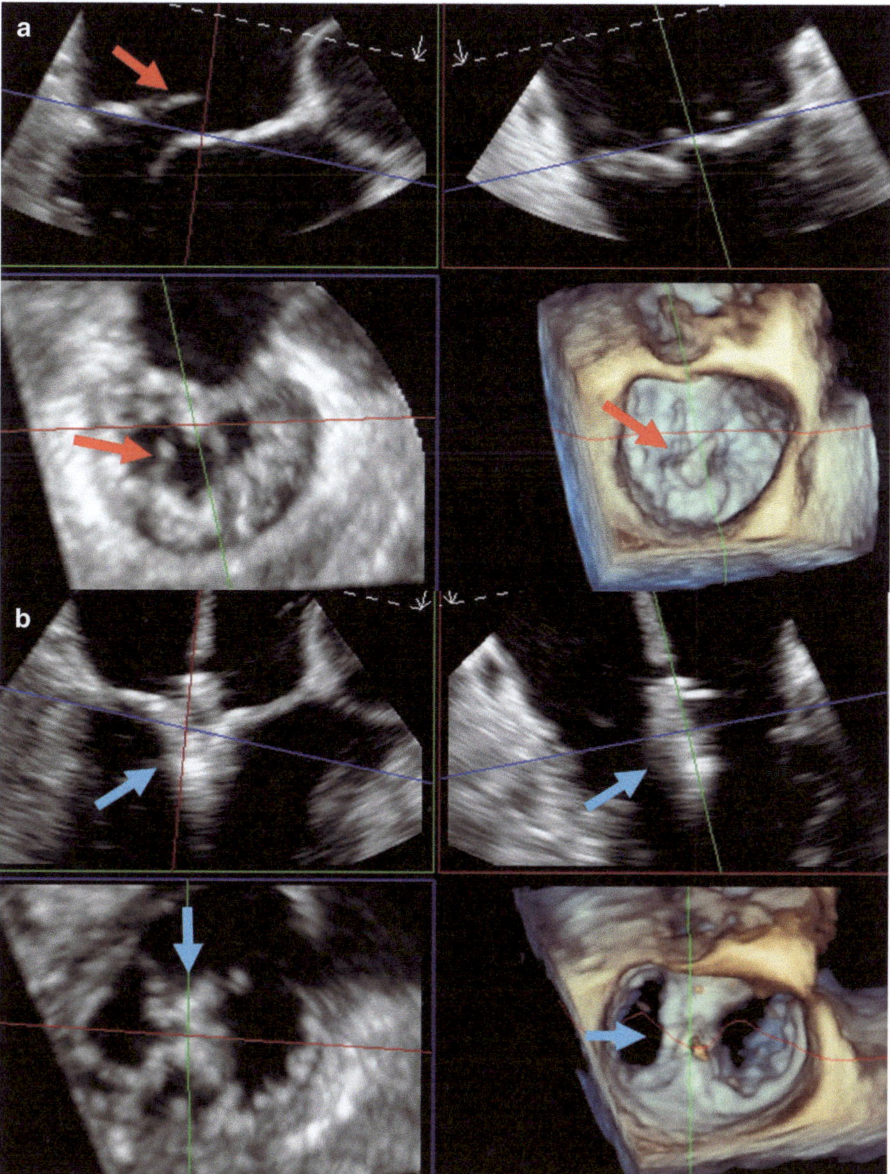

Fig. 3 Three-dimensional transesophageal echocardiography evaluation of mitral regurgitation in an 87-year-old woman with live multiplanar reconstruction software (**a**) P2 mitral valve prolapse with flail (red arrows) pre-procedure and (**b**) guidance for Mitraclip (blue arrows) deployment grasping the mitral valve leaflets during the procedure

restriction can be seen), regurgitant jet, and mitral annular disjunction [28, 44]. Unlike the aortic valve, phase contrast sequences in MRI are not usually directly applied at the mitral and tricuspid valves to assess flow because of the marked through-plane motion of the atrioventricular valves during the cardiac cycle [28]. Mitral regurgitant volume is generally calculated by subtracting the aortic valve forward flow (by phase contrast sequence) from the left ventricle stroke volume (on cine images) and this can then be divided by the stroke volume to calculate the mitral regurgitant fraction. The remaining chamber quantifications of both the left and right ventricles on bright blood gradient echo sequences are also important. Studies comparing TTE and MRI have found a modest correlation with a tendency for TTE to over-estimate MR severity (approximately 16 mL higher regurgitant volume in one prospective study). MRI had a better association with predicting post-surgical left ventricle remodeling and improvement compared to TTE [61]. Optimal thresholds of MRI-derived MR are not well established, with one study defining regurgitant fraction of 40+ % as severe and associated with a worse prognosis. This MRI derived threshold is lower than the TTE threshold [62]. Late gadolinium enhancement sequences are valuable in MR evaluation for both primary and secondary MR, along with helping diagnose cardiomyopathy in secondary MR [28, 44, 63]. Other features that can be evaluated on MRI in MR patients include mitral annular disjunction, papillary muscles, and systolic anterior motion especially related to hypertrophic cardiomyopathy.

3.5 Computed Tomography

Although CT has the least role in the diagnosis of MR, it can provide some important additional information. CT is the best modality to visualize and semi-quantitate mitral annular calcifications, which is not only associated with cardiovascular events but also reduces the chance for successful surgical and percutaneous repair [64]. Similar to its role in TAVR patients, CT is useful in the pre-procedural evaluation for transcatheter mitral valve repair or replacement using ECG-gating contrast-enhanced acquisition [65]. Key parts of this assessment include mitral annulus sizing (at various phases of the cardiac cycle if possible), characterization of the landing zone dependent on device planned, neo-LVOT dimensions and obstruction risk, localization of interatrial septum and apex, predicting angulations for fluoroscopy and determining the anatomic relations between the coronary arteries especially the left circumflex vessel with the mitral annulus. Furthermore, CT is an adjunctive modality to TTE and TEE in the diagnosis of infective endocarditis findings, including vegetation, pseudoaneurysm/abscess, and fistula, especially with retrospective 4D-protocols, which also have prognostic implications [43, 47, 66]. Finally, CT can be useful in the evaluation prior to cardiac surgery to evaluate thoracic anatomy and its relations to the sternum, aortic calcifications, and dilation.

4   Tricuspid Regurgitation

4.1   Etiologies and Epidemiology

The tricuspid valve has often been termed the forgotten valve, given the traditional focus and effective treatment options for left-sided heart valve disease. However, there is renewed interest because of the rising prevalence and adverse outcomes of tricuspid valve associated pathologies, and tricuspid valve interventions are the next frontier in structural heart imaging and procedures [3, 67, 68]. Although trivial to mild TR is common in the general population, significant TR is present in approximately 1.2–1.5% of the general population and 16% of patients referred for transthoracic echocardiography [1, 2, 67]. Similar to MR, tricuspid regurgitation (TR) etiologies are classified as primary, with pathology directly affecting the valve leaflets, and secondary, where right ventricular and/or atrial remodeling and dysfunction lead to malcoaptation of the valve leaflets. The, distinction between primary and secondary TR is important for the appropriate treatment (see Table 1) [4, 6]. Recent epidemiological studies demonstrate that the vast majority (85–95%) of TR is secondary TR [69–71], and this is more common in the elderly. However, among the patients undergoing tricuspid valve surgery for TR, about half have a primary and half have a secondary cause [72].

The most common secondary etiology of TR is related to left heart disease, in approximately 54–70% of cases [69–71]. These range from mitral and/or aortic valve disease to any cause of left ventricle systolic and/or diastolic dysfunction that directly or indirectly via secondary pulmonary hypertension leads to right ventricle remodeling, tricuspid annular dilation, and resulting TR. The second class of secondary TR etiologies is that related to chronic lung diseases, including chronic obstructive lung disease, bronchiectasis, interstitial lung disease, and pulmonary thromboembolic disease, with associated pulmonary hypertension and cor pulmonale; however, with reduced smoking and treatments, it currently makes up only 2.3–17% of secondary TR [69–71]. Another class of increasingly recognized causes is atrial functional TR, often in patients with atrial fibrillation, reported in 17–40% of secondary TR cases [71, 73]. These patients usually have an enlarged right atrium leading to dilatation of the tricuspid valve annulus without significant right ventricular remodeling. Other less frequent causes of secondary TR are associated with primary right ventricular cardiomyopathy (such as arrhythmogenic or myocardial infarction) and congenital left-to-right shunting lesions such as septal defects and anomalous pulmonary venous drainage that cause right ventricle volume overload [74, 75]. Secondary TR severity may improve with treatment of the right ventricular pathology.

Primary TR causes are well-known despite being less common. Degenerative TR related to prolapse is less common than in MR, accounting for 9–34% of primary TR cases [69–71]. Cardiac implantable electronic device lead-associated TR is another common cause of primary TR in 17–67% of cases; however, it is important to carefully image these patients to be certain that the lead is indead affecting valve leaflet motion to cause the TR [69–71]. Other causes of primary TR include infective endocarditis (especially in intravenous drug users), prosthetic valve degeneration, rheumatic heart disease, carcinoid syndrome, trauma, and congenital heart disease (especially Ebstein's anomaly and tricuspid valve dysplasia) [4, 6, 66, 75].

4.2 Clinical Evaluation

Patients with significant TR have some unique clinical characteristics compared to those with left heart valve disease, with a higher prevalence of women (over 50%), heart failure, atrial fibrillation, prior cardiac surgery, chronic lung disease, and chronic kidney disease [70, 72, 76–79], and several of these are related to secondary TR etiologies. It is, therefore, important to einquire about these characteristics and other potential etiologies of TR in the patient's history. Many patients with TR are asymptomatic, even for those with moderate to severe TR, as volume overload of the right heart is generally well-tolerated until late in the disease course. The TR disease course is often chronic except in primary TR scenarios such as from acute infective endocarditis and trauma. Early clinical symptoms are nonspecific, including fatigue, impaired exercise capacity, and peripheral edema, and therefore the diagnosis is often missed as these symptoms are common with advanced age [80]. Symptoms of advanced TR associated with developing right heart failure include abdominal bloating, ascites, hepatomegaly, pleural effusion, chronic kidney and liver disease, coagulopathy, cachexia, low cardiac output, and absolute or relative hypotension.

A thorough history and clinical examination of the elderly patient and obtaining collateral history are critical in identifying the above mentioned clinical manifestations. Characteristic examination findings that may be present include a pan-systolic but often soft murmur at the left lower sternal edge louder on inspiration, right ventricular heave, prominent v-waves of the jugular venous pressure, pulsatile and at times a larg and tender liver, ascites, and peripheral edema. Many clinical factors associated with an adverse prognosis have been identified in TR patients, such as older age, heart failure, cardiogenic shock, chronic kidney disease, liver cirrhosis, malnutrition, decubitus ulcer, endocarditis, carcinoid syndrome, and emergency surgery [67, 76, 77, 81]. Laboratory tests that should be performed in patients with TR include a complete blood count (especially platelet count), metabolic panel (especially renal function), coagulation screen, liver function (including albumin), and B-type natriuretic peptide.

4.3   Echocardiography

The standard TTE examination is mandatory in the initial imaging assessment of TR. The key views to visualize the tricuspid valve include the parasternal right ventricle inflow view, parasternal short axis view at the aortic and mitral valve leaflet levels, apical 4-chamber and right ventricle focused views, apical reverse 3-chamber view, subcostal 4-chamber view, and subcostal long axis inferior vena cava and hepatic vein views [16]. The tricuspid valve is inspected with two-dimensional imaging for thickness, motion, vegetations, and any other clues to suggest etiology of TR, then with color, continuous wave, and pulsed wave Doppler interrogation. Qualitative observations of TR include valve malcoaptation, color jet area, flow convergence, continuous wave Doppler jet (dense and triangular suggestive of severe TR), and systolic flow reversal in the hepatic veins by pulsed wave Doppler [3]. The conventional quantitative and semiquantitative parameters for grading TR severity are listed in Table 3. Some authors have recently proposed expanding the severe TR grade to add "massive" and "torrential" TR to fully capture the range of severe TR encountered clinically, with "massive" TR corresponding to a vena contracta of 14–20 and 21+ mm, and "torrential" TR to a vena contracta of 0.60–0.79 and 0.80+ mm^2 [82]. Multiple studies have demonstrated that increasing TR severity is associated with a worse prognosis [67, 81].

TR evaluation is not complete without evaluating the cardiac chambers, starting with the right ventricle, as its dimensions and function are also potential indications for valve surgery [4, 6]. The right ventricle is visualized on the same aforementioned views of the tricuspid valve [16]. The right ventricle dimensions to measure with normal reference ranges available are right ventricular basal, mid, longitudinal, and outflow tract proximal and distal diameters, end-diastolic and end-systolic areas, and volumes and wall thickness [30]. Right ventricle systolic function is assessed using a combination of visual evaluation, tricuspid annular plane systolic excursion, tissue Doppler lateral annular S wave, pulsed wave or tissue Doppler index of myocardial performance, fractional area change, ejection fraction, and longitudinal strain (free-wall). Diastolic and systolic interventricular septal deviation to the left ventricle can be observed with right ventricle volume and pressure overload, respectively, and may co-exist. The right heart assessment also includes right atrial dimensions (indexed right atrial volume is preferred), right ventricular systolic pressure with TR peak systolic velocity and modified Bernoulli's equations, and right atrial pressure estimated by inferior vena cava size and collapsibility. Finally, dedicated assessments of left heart size, systolic and diastolic function, mitral, aortic, pulmonic valves, pericardium, and congenital heart lesions are all potentially relevant to the full TTE examination [16, 30, 82]. 3D echocardiography and TEE can further evaluate the tricuspid valve, the tricuspid valve annulus other aspects of right heart anatomy, TR etiology, and severity. TEE is also useful for real-time guidance during tricuspid valve interventions [21, 83].

4.4 Magnetic Resonance Imaging

Examples of MRI indications in TR patients include cases when the TR severity is indeterminant because of discrepancies between TTE parameters and clinical assessment, or TTE views are suboptimal, and to accurately quantify right heart size and function [3]. The bright-blood gradient echo, most commonly SSFP, is the sequence used to quantify right ventricle size (end-diastolic volume, end-systolic volume) and function (ejection fraction, cardiac output, and strain using feature tracking) [28, 84]. Phase contrast imaging placed at the main pulmonic artery quantifies pulmonic forward and regurgitant flows, and volumes, and subtracting the former from the right ventricle stroke volume gives the TR regurgitant volume, and then the regurgitant fraction after dividing by the stroke volume [3]. Unlike TTE, guidelines have not officially established thresholds for MRI-derived TR severity by regurgitant volume or fraction. A recent study found 65–68% agreement between TTE and MRI grading of TR, with effective regurgitant orifice area above $0.4cm^2$ being the most sensitive, and triangular and dense jet contour and density by continuous wave Doppler being the most specific at predicting severe TR by MRI [85]. Another functional TR study confirmed increasing MRI-grading of TR severity (moderate 30–44 mL or 30–49% and severe 45+ mL or 50+ % for regurgitant volume and fraction, respectively) to be associated with worse survival in unadjusted and adjusted analyses [86]. However, because lower regurgitant volumes and fractions are typically quantified by MRI than TTE, another MRI study identified 35+ mL or 30+ % respectively as the optimal thresholds for severe TR associated with worse prognosis [87]. MRI is the gold standard for chamber quantification and accuracy for regurgitant volume and fraction quantification.

4.5 Computed Tomography

Cardiac CT has had relatively limited roles in TR assessment, however, it can be additive to echocardiography and MRI assessment. Right heart imaging by CT can be challenging with contrast timing to interrogate the tricuspid valve, requiring dedicated protocols with electrocardiogram gating [88]. Retrospective-gated 4D CT can assess right heart size and function [84]. In the era of rapidly evolving transcatheter tricuspid interventions, however, CT can provide a means to visualize and directly measure the tricuspid annulus, identify the course of the right coronary artery relative to the annulus for suitability of annuloplasty devices, along with trajectories of the superior and inferior vena cavae connecting with the right atrium for caval valve implantation [89]. CT also allows extracardiac thoracic anatomy assessment, often as part of redo cardiac surgery, which is prevalent in TR patients, along with assessing for pulmonary, congenital heart, and pericardial diseases that are other potential etiologies for TR.

5   Conclusion

The elderly population with valvular heart disease continues to grow worldwide and places a heavy mortality and morbidity burden on society. Aortic stenosis and regurgitation, mitral regurgitation, and tricuspid regurgitation are the most frequently encountered in the elderly. Each valve lesion has unique and also common etiologies, pathophysiology, epidemiology, and clinical features that clinicians should be alert to. The rapidly evolving landscape and technologies in advanced cardiac imaging for diagnosis and risk stratification, along with surgical and transcatheter treatments, have extended boundaries in the management of the range of valvular heart disease in the elderly with a multi-disciplinary approach. Following both contemporary valve guidelines along with the flexibility of adapting novel imaging and therapeutic technologies have enabled the ongoing optimization of clinical outcomes in valvular heart disease. This chapter provides guidance on the clinical and imaging approaches for this often complex group of elderly patients.

References

1. Iung B, Baron G, Butchart EG, Delahaye F, Gohlke-Bärwolf C, Levang OW, et al. A prospective survey of patients with valvular heart disease in Europe: The Euro Heart Survey on Valvular Heart Disease. Eur Heart J. 2003;24(13):1231–43.
2. Nkomo VT, Gardin JM, Skelton TN, Gottdiener JS, Scott CG, Enriquez-Sarano M. Burden of valvular heart diseases: a population-based study. Lancet (London, England). 2006;368(9540):1005–11.
3. Zoghbi WA, Adams D, Bonow RO, Enriquez-Sarano M, Foster E, Grayburn PA, et al. Recommendations for Noninvasive Evaluation of Native Valvular Regurgitation: A Report from the American Society of Echocardiography Developed in Collaboration with the Society for Cardiovascular Magnetic Resonance. J Am Soc Echocardiogr. 2017;30(4):303–71.
4. Otto CM, Nishimura RA, Bonow RO, Carabello BA, Erwin JP 3rd, Gentile F, et al. 2020 ACC/AHA Guideline for the Management of Patients With Valvular Heart Disease: A Report of the American College of Cardiology/American Heart Association Joint Committee on Clinical Practice Guidelines. J Am Coll Cardiol. 2021;143(5):e35–71.
5. Baumgartner HC, Hung JC-C, Bermejo J, Chambers JB, Edvardsen T, Goldstein S, et al. Recommendations on the echocardiographic assessment of aortic valve stenosis: a focused update from the European Association of Cardiovascular Imaging and the American Society of Echocardiography. Eur Heart J Cardiovasc Imaging. 2017;18(3):254–75.
6. Baumgartner H, Falk V, Bax JJ, De Bonis M, Hamm C, Holm PJ, et al. 2017 ESC/EACTS guidelines for the management of valvular heart disease. Eur Heart J. 2017;38(36):2739–91.
7. Osnabrugge RL, Mylotte D, Head SJ, Van Mieghem NM, Nkomo VT, LeReun CM, et al. Aortic stenosis in the elderly: disease prevalence and number of candidates for transcatheter aortic valve replacement: a meta-analysis and modeling study. J Am Coll Cardiol. 2013;62(11):1002–12.
8. O'Brien SM, Feng L, He X, Xian Y, Jacobs JP, Badhwar V, et al. The Society of Thoracic Surgeons 2018 adult cardiac surgery risk models: part 2-statistical methods and results. Ann Thorac Surg. 2018;105(5):1419–28.

9. Varadarajan P, Kapoor N, Bansal RC, Pai RG. Survival in elderly patients with severe aortic stenosis is dramatically improved by aortic valve replacement: results from a cohort of 277 patients aged > or =80 years. Eur J Cardiothorac Surg. 2006;30(5):722–7.

10. Roberts WC, Ko JM. Frequency by decades of unicuspid, bicuspid, and tricuspid aortic valves in adults having isolated aortic valve replacement for aortic stenosis, with or without associated aortic regurgitation. Circulation. 2005;111(7):920–5.

11. Stewart BF, Siscovick D, Lind BK, Gardin JM, Gottdiener JS, Smith VE, et al. Clinical factors associated with calcific aortic valve disease. Cardiovascular health study. J Am Coll Cardiol. 1997;29(3):630–4.

12. King RM, Pluth JR, Giuliani ER. The association of unexplained gastrointestinal bleeding with calcific aortic stenosis. Ann Thorac Surg. 1987;44(5):514–6.

13. Vincentelli A, Susen S, Le Tourneau T, Six I, Fabre O, Juthier F, et al. Acquired von Willebrand syndrome in aortic stenosis. N Engl J Med. 2003;349(4):343–9.

14. Chen S, Redfors B, O'Neill BP, Clavel MA, Pibarot P, Elmariah S, et al. Low and elevated B-type natriuretic peptide levels are associated with increased mortality in patients with preserved ejection fraction undergoing transcatheter aortic valve replacement: an analysis of the PARTNER II trial and registry. Eur Heart J. 2020;41(8):958–69.

15. Nakatsuma K, Taniguchi T, Morimoto T, Shiomi H, Ando K, Kanamori N, et al. B-type natriuretic peptide in patients with asymptomatic severe aortic stenosis. Heart. 2019;105(5):384–90.

16. Mitchell C, Rahko PS, Blauwet LA, Canaday B, Finstuen JA, Foster MC, et al. Guidelines for performing a comprehensive transthoracic echocardiographic examination in adults: recommendations from the American Society of Echocardiography. J Am Soc Echocardiogr. 2019;32(1):1–64.

17. Thaden JJ, Nkomo VT, Lee KJ, Oh JK. Doppler imaging in aortic stenosis: the importance of the nonapical imaging windows to determine severity in a contemporary cohort. J Am Soc Echocardiogr. 2015;28(7):780–5.

18. Zoghbi WA, Chambers JB, Dumesnil JG, Foster E, Gottdiener JS, Grayburn PA, et al. Recommendations for evaluation of prosthetic valves with echocardiography and doppler ultrasound: a report From the American Society of Echocardiography's Guidelines and Standards Committee and the Task Force on Prosthetic Valves, developed in conjunction with the American College of Cardiology Cardiovascular Imaging Committee, Cardiac Imaging Committee of the American Heart Association, the European Association of Echocardiography, a registered branch of the European Society of Cardiology, the Japanese Society of Echocardiography and the Canadian Society of Echocardiography, endorsed by the American College of Cardiology Foundation, American Heart Association, European Association of Echocardiography, a registered branch of the European Society of Cardiology, the Japanese Society of Echocardiography, and Canadian Society of Echocardiography. J Am Soc Echocardiogr. 2009;22(9):975–1014. quiz 82–4

19. Saeed S, Rajani R, Seifert R, Parkin D, Chambers JB. Exercise testing in patients with asymptomatic moderate or severe aortic stenosis. Heart. 2018;104(22):1836–42.

20. Magne J, Cosyns B, Popescu BA, Carstensen HG, Dahl J, Desai MY, et al. Distribution and prognostic significance of left ventricular global longitudinal strain in asymptomatic significant aortic stenosis: an individual participant data meta-analysis. J Am Coll Cardiol Img. 2019;12(1):84–92.

21. Hahn RT, Abraham T, Adams MS, Bruce CJ, Glas KE, Lang RM, et al. Guidelines for performing a comprehensive transesophageal echocardiographic examination: recommendations from the American Society of Echocardiography and the Society of Cardiovascular Anesthesiologists. J Am Soc Echocardiogr. 2013;26(9):921–64.

22. Vaquerizo B, Spaziano M, Alali J, Mylote D, Theriault-Lauzier P, Alfagih R, et al. Three-dimensional echocardiography vs. computed tomography for transcatheter aortic valve replacement sizing. Eur Heart J Cardiovasc Imaging. 2016;17(1):15–23.

23. Nicoara A, Skubas N, Ad N, Finley A, Hahn RT, Mahmood F, et al. Guidelines for the Use of Transesophageal Echocardiography to Assist with Surgical Decision-Making in the Operating

Room: A Surgery-Based Approach: From the American Society of Echocardiography in Collaboration with the Society of Cardiovascular Anesthesiologists and the Society of Thoracic Surgeons. J Am Soc Echocardiogr. 2020;33(6):692–734.

24. Blanke P, Weir-McCall JR, Achenbach S, Delgado V, Hausleiter J, Jilaihawi H, et al. Computed tomography imaging in the context of transcatheter aortic valve implantation (TAVI)/transcatheter aortic valve replacement (TAVR): an expert consensus document of the Society of Cardiovascular Computed Tomography. J Cardiovasc Comput Tomogr. 2019;13(1):1–20.

25. Clavel MA, Pibarot P, Messika-Zeitoun D, Capoulade R, Malouf J, Aggarval S, et al. Impact of aortic valve calcification, as measured by MDCT, on survival in patients with aortic stenosis: results of an international registry study. J Am Coll Cardiol. 2014;64(12):1202–13.

26. Francone M, Budde RPJ, Bremerich J, Dacher JN, Loewe C, Wolf F, et al. CT and MR imaging prior to transcatheter aortic valve implantation: standardisation of scanning protocols, measurements and reporting-a consensus document by the European Society of Cardiovascular Radiology (ESCR). Eur Radiol. 2020;30(5):2627–50.

27. Makkar RR, Fontana G, Jilaihawi H, Chakravarty T, Kofoed KF, De Backer O, et al. Possible subclinical leaflet thrombosis in bioprosthetic aortic valves. N Engl J Med. 2015;373(21):2015–24.

28. Kramer CM, Barkhausen J, Bucciarelli-Ducci C, Flamm SD, Kim RJ, Nagel E. Standardized cardiovascular magnetic resonance imaging (CMR) protocols: 2020 update. J Cardiovasc Magn Resonan. 2020;22(1):17.

29. Pouleur AC, le Polain de Waroux JB, Pasquet A, Vancraeynest D, Vanoverschelde JL, Gerber BL. Planimetric and continuity equation assessment of aortic valve area: Head to head comparison between cardiac magnetic resonance and echocardiography. J Magn Reson Imaging. 2007;26(6):1436–43.

30. Lang RM, Badano LP, Mor-Avi V, Afilalo J, Armstrong A, Ernande L, et al. Recommendations for cardiac chamber quantification by echocardiography in adults: an update from the American Society of Echocardiography and the European Association of Cardiovascular Imaging. Eur Heart J Cardiovasc Imaging. 2015;16(3):233–70.

31. Balciunaite G, Skorniakov V, Rimkus A, Zaremba T, Palionis D, Valeviciene N, et al. Prevalence and prognostic value of late gadolinium enhancement on CMR in aortic stenosis: meta-analysis. Eur Radiol. 2020;30(1):640–51.

32. Lee H, Park JB, Yoon YE, Park EA, Kim HK, Lee W, et al. Noncontrast myocardial T1 mapping by cardiac magnetic resonance predicts outcome in patients with aortic stenosis. J Am Coll Cardiol Img. 2018;11(7):974–83.

33. Everett RJ, Treibel TA, Fukui M, Lee H, Rigolli M, Singh A, et al. Extracellular myocardial volume in patients with aortic stenosis. J Am Coll Cardiol. 2020;75(3):304–16.

34. Coffey S, Cairns BJ, Iung B. The modern epidemiology of heart valve disease. Heart. 2016;102(1):75–85.

35. Babu AN, Kymes SM, Carpenter Fryer SM. Eponyms and the diagnosis of aortic regurgitation: what says the evidence? Ann Intern Med. 2003;138(9):736–42.

36. Pizarro R, Bazzino OO, Oberti PF, Falconi ML, Arias AM, Krauss JG, et al. Prospective validation of the prognostic usefulness of B-type natriuretic peptide in asymptomatic patients with chronic severe aortic regurgitation. J Am Coll Cardiol. 2011;58(16):1705–14.

37. Alashi A, Khullar T, Mentias A, Gillinov AM, Roselli EE, Svensson LG, et al. Long-term outcomes after aortic valve surgery in patients with asymptomatic chronic aortic regurgitation and preserved LVEF: impact of baseline and follow-up global longitudinal strain. J Am Coll Cardiol Img. 2020;13(1 Pt 1):12–21.

38. Bolen MA, Popovic ZB, Rajiah P, Gabriel RS, Zurick AO, Lieber ML, et al. Cardiac MR assessment of aortic regurgitation: holodiastolic flow reversal in the descending aorta helps stratify severity. Radiology. 2011;260(1):98–104.

39. Gabriel RS, Renapurkar R, Bolen MA, Verhaert D, Leiber M, Flamm SD, et al. Comparison of severity of aortic regurgitation by cardiovascular magnetic resonance versus transthoracic echocardiography. Am J Cardiol. 2011;108(7):1014–20.

40. Kammerlander AA, Wiesinger M, Duca F, Aschauer S, Binder C, Zotter Tufaro C, et al. Diagnostic and prognostic utility of cardiac magnetic resonance imaging in aortic regurgitation. J Am Coll Cardiol Img. 2019;12(8 Pt 1):1474–83.
41. Singh JP, Evans JC, Levy D, Larson MG, Freed LA, Fuller DL, et al. Prevalence and clinical determinants of mitral, tricuspid, and aortic regurgitation (the Framingham Heart Study). Am J Cardiol. 1999;83(6):897–902.
42. Carpentier A. Cardiac valve surgery—the "French correction". J Thorac Cardiovasc Surg. 1983;86(3):323–37.
43. Ponikowski P, Voors AA, Anker SD, Bueno H, Cleland JGF, Coats AJS, et al. 2016 ESC Guidelines for the diagnosis and treatment of acute and chronic heart failure: The Task Force for the diagnosis and treatment of acute and chronic heart failure of the European Society of Cardiology (ESC)Developed with the special contribution of the heart failure association (HFA) of the ESC. Eur Heart J. 2016;37(27):2129–200.
44. Yancy CW, Jessup M, Bozkurt B, Butler J, Casey DE Jr, Colvin MM, et al. 2017 ACC/AHA/HFSA Focused Update of the 2013 ACCF/AHA Guideline for the Management of Heart Failure: A Report of the American College of Cardiology/American Heart Association Task Force on Clinical Practice Guidelines and the Heart Failure Society of America. Circulation. 2017;136(6):e137–e61.
45. Dejgaard LA, Skjølsvik ET, Lie ØH, Ribe M, Stokke MK, Hegbom F, et al. The mitral annulus disjunction arrhythmic syndrome. J Am Coll Cardiol. 2018;72(14):1600–9.
46. Essayagh B, Sabbag A, Antoine C, Benfari G, Yang LT, Maalouf J, et al. Presentation and outcome of arrhythmic mitral valve prolapse. J Am Coll Cardiol. 2020;76(6):637–49.
47. Nordhues BD, Siontis KC, Scott CG, Nkomo VT, Ackerman MJ, Asirvatham SJ, et al. Bileaflet mitral valve prolapse and risk of ventricular dysrhythmias and death. J Cardiovasc Electrophysiol. 2016;27(4):463–8.
48. Chehab O, Roberts-Thomson R, Ng Yin Ling C, Marber M, Prendergast BD, Rajani R, et al. Secondary mitral regurgitation: pathophysiology, proportionality and prognosis. Heart. 2020;106(10):716–23.
49. Sannino A, Smith RL 2nd, Schiattarella GG, Trimarco B, Esposito G, Grayburn PA. Survival and cardiovascular outcomes of patients with secondary mitral regurgitation: a systematic review and meta-analysis. JAMA Cardiol. 2017;2(10):1130–9.
50. Clavel MA, Tribouilloy C, Vanoverschelde JL, Pizarro R, Suri RM, Szymanski C, et al. Association of B-type natriuretic peptide with survival in patients with degenerative mitral regurgitation. J Am Coll Cardiol. 2016;68(12):1297–307.
51. Bartko PE, Arfsten H, Heitzinger G, Pavo N, Toma A, Strunk G, et al. A unifying concept for the quantitative assessment of secondary mitral regurgitation. J Am Coll Cardiol. 2019;73(20):2506–17.
52. Bijvoet GP, Teske AJ, Chamuleau SAJ, Hart EA, Jansen R, Schaap J. Global longitudinal strain to predict left ventricular dysfunction in asymptomatic patients with severe mitral valve regurgitation: literature review. Netherlands Heart J. 2020;28(2):63–72.
53. Namazi F, van der Bij P, Hirasawa K, Kamperidis V, van Wijngaarden S, Mertens B, et al. Prognostic value of left ventricular global longitudinal strain in patients with significant 2 secondary mitral regurgitation. J Am Coll Cardiol. 2019;
54. Mentias A, Naji P, Gillinov AM, Rodriguez LL, Reed G, Mihaljevic T, et al. Strain echocardiography and functional capacity in asymptomatic primary mitral regurgitation with preserved ejection fraction. J Am Coll Cardiol. 2016;68(18):1974–86.
55. Stone GW, Lindenfeld J, Abraham WT, Kar S, Lim DS, Mishell JM, et al. Transcatheter mitral-valve repair in patients with heart failure. N Engl J Med. 2018;379(24):2307–18.
56. Obadia JF, Messika-Zeitoun D, Leurent G, Iung B, Bonnet G, Piriou N, et al. Percutaneous repair or medical treatment for secondary mitral regurgitation. N Engl J Med. 2018;379(24):2297–306.
57. Grayburn PA, Sannino A, Packer M. Proportionate and disproportionate functional mitral regurgitation: A new conceptual framework that reconciles the results of the MITRA-FR and COAPT trials. J Am Coll Cardiol Img. 2019;12(2):353–62.

58. Bushari LI, Reeder GS, Eleid MF, Chandrasekaran K, Eriquez-Sarano M, Rihal CS, et al. Percutaneous transcatheter edge-to-edge MitraClip technique: a practical "step-by-step" 3-dimensional transesophageal echocardiography guide. Mayo Clin Proc. 2019;94(1):89–102.
59. Zoghbi WA, Asch FM, Bruce C, Gillam LD, Grayburn PA, Hahn RT, et al. Guidelines for the Evaluation of Valvular Regurgitation After Percutaneous Valve Repair or Replacement: A Report from the American Society of Echocardiography Developed in Collaboration with the Society for Cardiovascular Angiography and Interventions, Japanese Society of Echocardiography, and Society for Cardiovascular Magnetic Resonance. J Am Soc Echocardiogr. 2019;32(4):431–75.
60. Naji P, Griffin BP, Asfahan F, Barr T, Rodriguez LL, Grimm R, et al. Predictors of long-term outcomes in patients with significant myxomatous mitral regurgitation undergoing exercise echocardiography. Circulation. 2014;129(12):1310–9.
61. Uretsky S, Gillam L, Lang R, Chaudhry FA, Argulian E, Supariwala A, et al. Discordance between echocardiography and MRI in the assessment of mitral regurgitation severity: a prospective multicenter trial. J Am Coll Cardiol. 2015;65(11):1078–88.
62. Myerson SG, d'Arcy J, Christiansen JP, Dobson LE, Mohiaddin R, Francis JM, et al. Determination of clinical outcome in mitral regurgitation with cardiovascular magnetic resonance quantification. Circulation. 2016;133(23):2287–96.
63. Cavalcante JL, Kusunose K, Obuchowski NA, Jellis C, Griffin BP, Flamm SD, et al. Prognostic impact of ischemic mitral regurgitation severity and myocardial infarct quantification by cardiovascular magnetic resonance. J Am Coll Cardiol Img. 2020;13(7):1489–501.
64. Guerrero M, Wang DD, Pursnani A, Eleid M, Khalique O, Urena M, et al. A cardiac computed tomography-based score to categorize mitral annular calcification severity and predict valve embolization. J Am Coll Cardiol Img. 2020;13(9):1945–57.
65. Weir-McCall JR, Blanke P, Naoum C, Delgado V, Bax JJ, Leipsic J. Mitral valve imaging with CT: relationship with transcatheter mitral valve interventions. Radiology. 2018;288(3):638–55.
66. Habib G, Lancellotti P, Antunes MJ, Bongiorni MG, Casalta JP, Del Zotti F, et al. 2015 ESC Guidelines for the management of infective endocarditis: The Task Force for the Management of Infective Endocarditis of the European Society of Cardiology (ESC). Endorsed by: European Association for Cardio-Thoracic Surgery (EACTS), the European Association of Nuclear Medicine (EANM). Eur Heart J. 2015;36(44):3075–128.
67. Nath J, Foster E, Heidenreich PA. Impact of tricuspid regurgitation on long-term survival. J Am Coll Cardiol. 2004;43(3):405–9.
68. Taramasso M, Alessandrini H, Latib A, Asami M, Attinger-Toller A, Biasco L, et al. Outcomes after current transcatheter tricuspid valve intervention: mid-term results from the international TriValve registry. JACC Cardiovasc Interv. 2019;12(2):155–65.
69. Bohbot Y, Chadha G, Delabre J, Landemaine T, Beyls C, Tribouilloy C. Characteristics and prognosis of patients with significant tricuspid regurgitation. Arch Cardiovasc Dis. 2019;112(10):604–14.
70. Vieitez JM, Monteagudo JM, Mahia P, Perez L, Lopez T, Marco I, et al. New insights of tricuspid regurgitation: a large-scale prospective cohort study. Eur Heart J Cardiovasc Imaging. 2021;22(2):196–202.
71. Wang TKM, Akyuz K, Mentias A, Kirincich J, Duran Crane A, Xu S, et al. Contemporary etiologies, outcomes, and novel risk score for isolated tricuspid regurgitation. JACC Cardiovasc Imaging. 2022;15(5):731–44.
72. Dreyfus J, Flagiello M, Bazire B, Eggenspieler F, Viau F, Riant E, et al. Isolated tricuspid valve surgery: impact of aetiology and clinical presentation on outcomes. Eur Heart J. 2020;41(45):4304–17.
73. Muraru D, Guta AC, Ochoa-Jimenez RC, Bartos D, Aruta P, Mihaila S, et al. Functional regurgitation of atrioventricular valves and atrial fibrillation: an elusive pathophysiological link deserving further attention. J Am Soc Echocardiogr. 2020;33(1):42–53.
74. Góngora E, Dearani JA, Orszulak TA, Schaff HV, Li Z, Sundt TM. 3rd. Tricuspid regurgitation in patients undergoing pericardiectomy for constrictive pericarditis. Ann Thorac Surg. 2008;85(1):163–70; discussion 70–1

75. Stout KK, Daniels CJ, Aboulhosn JA, Bozkurt B, Broberg CS, Colman JM, et al. 2018 AHA/ACC Guideline for the Management of Adults With Congenital Heart Disease: A Report of the American College of Cardiology/American Heart Association Task Force on Clinical Practice Guidelines. J Am Coll Cardiol. 2019;73(12):e81–e192.
76. Axtell AL, Bhambhani V, Moonsamy P, Healy EW, Picard MH, Sundt TM, et al. Surgery is not associated with improved survival compared to medical therapy in isolated severe tricuspid regurgitation. J Am Coll Cardiol. 2019;74(6):715–25.
77. Kundi H, Popma JJ, Cohen DJ, Liu DC, Laham RJ, Pinto DS, et al. Prevalence and outcomes of isolated tricuspid valve surgery among Medicare beneficiaries. Am J Cardiol. 2019;123(1):132–8.
78. Vassileva CM, Shabosky J, Boley T, Markwell S, Hazelrigg S. Tricuspid valve surgery: the past 10 years from the Nationwide inpatient sample (NIS) database. J Thorac Cardiovasc Surg. 2012;143(5):1043–9.
79. Zack CJ, Fender EA, Chandrashekar P, Reddy YNV, Bennett CE, Stulak JM, et al. National trends and outcomes in isolated tricuspid valve surgery. J Am Coll Cardiol. 2017;70(24):2953–60.
80. Konstam MA, Kiernan MS, Bernstein D, Bozkurt B, Jacob M, Kapur NK, et al. Evaluation and Management of Right-Sided Heart Failure: A Scientific Statement From the American Heart Association. Circulation. 2018;137(20):e578–622.
81. Chorin E, Rozenbaum Z, Topilsky Y, Konigstein M, Ziv-Baran T, Richert E, et al. Tricuspid regurgitation and long-term clinical outcomes. Eur Heart J Cardiovasc Imaging. 2020;21(2):157–65.
82. Hahn RT, Zamorano JL. The need for a new tricuspid regurgitation grading scheme. Eur Heart J Cardiovasc Imaging. 2017;18(12):1342–3.
83. Muraru D, Hahn RT, Soliman OI, Faletra FF, Basso C, Badano LP. 3-dimensional echocardiography in imaging the tricuspid valve. J Am Coll Cardiol Img. 2019;12(3):500–15.
84. Doherty JU, Kort S, Mehran R, Schoenhagen P, Soman P. ACC/AATS/AHA/ASE/ASNC/HRS/SCAI/SCCT/SCMR/STS 2017 Appropriate Use Criteria for Multimodality Imaging in Valvular Heart Disease: A Report of the American College of Cardiology Appropriate Use Criteria Task Force, American Association for Thoracic Surgery, American Heart Association, American Society of Echocardiography, American Society of Nuclear Cardiology, Heart Rhythm Society, Society for Cardiovascular Angiography and Interventions, Society of Cardiovascular Computed Tomography, Society for Cardiovascular Magnetic Resonance, and Society of Thoracic Surgeons. J Am Coll Cardiol. 2017;70(13):1647–72.
85. Zhan Y, Senapati A, Vejpongsa P, Xu J, Shah DJ, Nagueh SF. Comparison of echocardiographic assessment of tricuspid regurgitation against cardiovascular magnetic resonance. J Am Coll Cardiol Img. 2020;13(7):1461–71.
86. Zhan Y, Debs D, Khan MA, Nguyen DT, Graviss EA, Khalaf S, et al. Natural history of functional tricuspid regurgitation quantified by cardiovascular magnetic resonance. J Am Coll Cardiol. 2020;76(11):1291–301.
87. Wang TKM, Akyuz K, Reyaldeen R, Griffin BP, Popovic ZB, Pettersson GB, et al. Prognostic value of complementary echocardiography and magnetic resonance imaging quantitative evaluation for isolated tricuspid regurgitation. Circ Cardiovasc Imaging. 2021;14(9):e012211.
88. Khalique OK, Cavalcante JL, Shah D, Guta AC, Zhan Y, Piazza N, et al. Multimodality imaging of the tricuspid valve and right heart anatomy. J Am Coll Cardiol Img. 2019;12(3):516–31.
89. van Rosendael PJ, Kamperidis V, Kong WK, van Rosendael AR, van der Kley F, Ajmone Marsan N, et al. Computed tomography for planning transcatheter tricuspid valve therapy. Eur Heart J. 2017;38(9):665–74.

Acute Coronary Syndrome in the Older Adult Populations

Amit Rout, Sheraz Hussain, and Abdulla A. Damluji

1 Introduction

The world population is changing rapidly with a demographic shift towards a large expansion of older adults. Of all the age categories, adults older than 65 years of age are the fastest growing segment of the U.S. population, with recent data indicating that 9% of the population in 2019 was over 65 years old, and this estimate is projected to increase to 16% by 2050. While the population above 80 years of age was around 143 million in 2019, the "oldest old" is projected to increase to 426 million by 2050 [1, 2]. Aging is associated with the risk of developing certain biologic processes collectively known as geriatric syndromes. The intermix of age-related biological factors and concurrent geriatric risks or syndromes leads to a higher likelihood of developing cardiovascular disease (CVD). Similarly, the presence of CVD further worsens preexisting geriatric risks.

Age is an independent risk factor for CVD, which is endemic in the older adult populations, with an estimated prevalence of 89.3% among men and 91.8% among women aged >80 years [2]. According to the 2019 American Heart Association (AHA) annual update on heart disease and stroke statistics, the prevalence of CVD was 70–75% in those aged 60–79 years and 79–86% in adults 80 years and older [1,

A. Rout
University of Louisville School of Medicine, Louisville, KY, USA

S. Hussain
Geriatrics and Palliative Care Medicine, University of Chicago, Chicago, IL, USA

Cardiovascular Disease, Advocate Christ Medical Center, Oak Lawn, IL, USA

A. A. Damluji (✉)
The Inova Center of Outcomes Research, Inova Heart and Vascular Institute, Falls Church, VA, USA
e-mail: Abdulla.Damluji@jhu.edu

T. M. Leucker, G. Gerstenblith (eds.), *Cardiovascular Disease in the Elderly*, Contemporary Cardiology, https://doi.org/10.1007/978-3-031-16594-8_10

2]. As older age could be accompanied by geriatric-specific conditions, older patients with the acute coronary syndrome (ACS) are at higher risk for adverse outcomes, including mortality, rehospitalizations, diminished quality of life, and functional decline [3]. The significance of preventing and managing coronary disease is highlighted by the fact that the lifetime risk of a first coronary event at the age of 70 years is approximately 35% in men and 24% in women [4]. As a group, CVD contributes to 20% of all disability-adjusted life-years (DALY) burden by age 65 years, of which coronary disease is a dominant cause [3].

Coronary disease portends a significant burden on society as it relates to healthcare utilization and costs. The direct medical costs of coronary disease are projected to increase from $89 billion in 2015 to $215 billion in 2035. The indirect costs attributed to coronary disease were $99 billion in 2015 and are projected to increase to $151 billion in 2035 [4, 5]. The rate of hospital admission for ACS is highest among patients older than 65 years, along with the length of hospital stay and mean charges for hospitalization [6, 7]. The increased cost could be attributed to multiple factors, including the complexity associated with caring for older patients because of increased age-associated risks, including multiple comorbidities, frailty, adverse events, and other age-associated risk factors [7]. As such, the cost-benefit analysis of the management of ACS and the health resources utilization among older patients remains an area of active debate among specialists in geriatric cardiology [8, 9]. While observational evidence suggests the benefits of pharmaco- and catheter-based therapies among older patients, large randomized controlled trials have traditionally excluded older adults because of the complexity associated with their care [10, 11]. Geriatric syndromes, including multimorbidity, polypharmacy, cognitive impairment, frailty, disability, and functional decline, usually are age-associated risks that strongly influence the management of ACS. In this chapter, we will discuss the bidirectional association between geriatric syndromes and ACS and highlight an approach to managing coronary syndromes in older adult populations in light of these age-associated risks.

2 The Aging Process and the Pathophysiology of ACS

Atherosclerosis is the hallmark of coronary disease development and progression. Atherosclerosis consists of plaques in the intima, which contain smooth muscle cells, inflammatory cells, calcium, coagulation factors, and lipids. Inflammation develops as early as the second decade of life and continues to progress with aging. The pathophysiology of ACS involves an event that triggers myocardial ischemia or infarction from acute plaque rupture, erosion, or thrombosis resulting in supply-demand mismatch. ACS encompasses ST-segment elevation myocardial infarction (STEMI/STE-ACS), non-ST-segment elevation myocardial infarction (NSTEMI/NSTE-ACS) and unstable angina (UA) [12, 13]. With advancing age, coronary disease complexity increases with calcification, bifurcation lesions, and multivessel or left main involvement. In the Multi-Ethnic Study of Atherosclerosis (MESA) study, coronary artery calcium deposition increased in all age groups, but the highest prevalence was in older adult populations [14]. In the meta-analysis of older patients involving octogenarians, the prevalence of left main coronary artery disease was around 7.3% vs. 5.7%, and three-vessel disease was 29% vs. 20% when compared to patients <80 years old [15]. In another registry, the prevalence of multivessel disease was 39.8% in <60 years old, 50.3% for the 60–80 age group, and 58.7% in >80 years old. The use of multivessel or left main PCI increased with age, with 14.4% in <60 years old, 14.7% in 60–80 years old, and 16.8% in >80 years old [16].

As the individual ages, various physiologic changes affect the cardiovascular system leading to both cellular and functional level changes, which ultimately lead to increased coronary disease risk [17]. These changes impact ventricularsystolic and diastolic function, valvular structures, electrical conduction system, and vasculature, contributing to increased mortality and morbidity in older patients [17, 18]. The presence of multiple coexisting conditions like hypertension, diabetes, and chronic kidney disease also contributes to increased CVD risk with age [18, 19]. Advancing age affects the integrity of the vasculature, causing loss of elasticity, increased stiffness, and arterial thickening in large- to medium-sized arteries [17, 20]. Endothelial dysfunction, smooth muscle cell thickening, collagen deposition, calcification, and atherosclerosis of the vascular wall worsen with age leading to arterial wall stiffness and isolated systolic hypertension. The endothelium plays a major role in vascular homeostasis by regulating vasodilation, vasoconstriction, smooth muscle cell growth, platelet and inflammatory cell migrations and activations. Atherosclerosis begins with endothelial dysfunction and later progresses to decreased bioavailability of the endothelial vasodilators like nitric oxide (NO) and prostacyclin while the level of vasoconstrictors like thromboxane and endothelin are increased [17, 21]. Overall, this leads to decreased vascular dilation, increased vasoconstriction, endothelial dysfunction, and subsequently vascular wall injury and the development of atherosclerosis. These vascular changes also influence target blood pressure goals and end-organ function [21, 22].

3 Epidemiology of ACS in Older Adults

Cardiovascular disease remains the leading cause of death worldwide, and coronary heart disease accounts for 42.1% of all CVD-related deaths. Based on the National Health and Nutrition Examination Survey (NHANES) between 2015 and 2018, the prevalence of CAD in the 60–79 years age group was 22% of males and 13.4% of females, of which 12.6% of males and 4.5% of females in this age group had a prior myocardial infarction (MI) event. In the same survey, the prevalence of CAD in the 80 years and older age group was 33.9% of males and 21.6% of females, of which 15.8% of males and 8.7% of females had a prior MI [23]. In the Atherosclerosis Risk in Communities (ARIC) Study between 1987 and 2002, the prevalence of MI in patients aged 65–74 years old was around 37–39% [24]. In the multicenter EUROHEART ACS study, 53.9% of patients with ACS were >65 years old, while

25% were above 75 years old. The percentage of women with ACS increased with age, similar to men after the age of 75 years [25]. Data from large registries for NSTE-ACS reported a prevalence of around 32–40%, and for STE-ACS, around 25–29% in those above 75 years old [10, 11]. The National Heart, Lung, and Blood Institute (NHLBI) reported data from the ARIC study between 2005 and 2014 that in the 65-to-74-year age group, the incidence of MI was highest in black males, 10.7 per 1000 person-years compared to 7.3 in white males, 7.7 in black females and 3.7 in white females. The incidence of MI increases significantly in those aged 75–84 years group approximating 15.9 vs. 9.4 per 1000 person-years for black and white males, respectively, and 12.0 vs. 8.5 per 1000 person-years for black and white females, respectively [23]. In the Cardiovascular Health Study (CHS), the 10-year incidence rate for MI in patients 65 years or older was 19.3/1000 person-years for male and 9.4/1000 person-years for females [26].

Table 1 Common geriatric syndromes and their interaction with acute coronary syndromes

Geriatric syndrome	Definition	Interaction with ACS
Multimorbidity [27, 30, 32]	Presence of two or more medical disease conditions in the same individual	Prevalence increases with age, lower rates of revascularization, increased hospital stays and mortality
Polypharmacy [34, 38, 40]	Daily use of five or more medications	Increased risk of bleeding and other adverse events
Cognitive impairment [42, 50, 53]	Memory impairment more than expected for age and education level, dementia is the final form	Increased risk of developing cognitive impairment, major barrier in management of ACS
Delirium [57, 58, 60]	Acute disturbance in attention and awareness that fluctuates with time	High incidence in hospitalized patients with ACS, associated with increased stay, bleeding, functional/cognitive decline and mortality
Frailty [61, 62, 64, 78]	Decline in physical reserve associated with increased vulnerability	Less revascularization like PCI and CABG in frail patients, increased risk of mortality, MI, stroke, rehospitalization and bleeding
Disability [87, 89, 93]	Difficulty performing basic or complex activities essential to independent living	Increased risk of CAD in disabled patients, increased adverse events, prolonged recovery
Functional decline [97, 101, 103]	Reduced capacity to perform activities of daily living secondary to worsening physical and cognitive dysfunction	ACS event worsens functional decline, increased risk of adverse events and mortality after ACS

ACS acute coronary syndrome, *CAD* coronary artery disease, *CABG* coronary artery bypass grafting, *PCI* percutaneous coronary intervention

4   Geriatric Syndromes and ACS

Several geriatric syndromes are present in older patients admitted with ACS (Table 1). These age-related risks affect health outcomes because ACS exacerbates the burden of these geriatric syndromes. We aim to define and discuss the most commonly encountered geriatric syndromes among older adults with ACS.

4.1   Multimorbidity

Multimorbidity is the presence of two or more medical conditions in the same individual. While sometimes used interchangeably, comorbidity is defined as the concurrent presence of diseases associated with a primary condition like CAD [27, 28]. The prevalence of multimorbidity increases with age, reaching above 70% in those ≥75 years old [29]. Older CVD patients often live with multimorbidity, which has significant effects on their overall care. Among Medicare beneficiaries ≥65 years old, the three most common comorbidities in patients with CAD are hypertension, hyperlipidemia, and diabetes mellitus, all risk factors for coronary events. Arthritis, anemia, heart failure, chronic kidney disease, atrial fibrillation, and chronic obstructive pulmonary disease (COPD) are among the top 10 comorbidities [30, 31]. The prevalence of multimorbidity in patients with ACS is reported from 25 to 96% and increases with age and is associated with lower rates of revascularization, increased hospital stays, and mortality [32]. The pathophysiological implication of multimorbidity is the complex interaction of each disease at various levels of cardiovascular risk with physiologic risks, hemodynamic response, its impact on multiple organs system, medication interaction and subsequent further increase in atherosclerosis and inflammation [33].

4.2   Polypharmacy and Deprescribing

Polypharmacy is defined as the concomitant use of at least five or more medications daily. Older patients presenting with ACS and with comorbidities are frequently managed with >5 concurrent medications as part of guideline-directed medical therapy, thus fulfilling the definition of polypharmacy [34]. However, multiple therapies may also have a negative effect on the overall well-being of older patients because of frequently encountered medication related adverse events. Interactions between the various drugs can potentiate the risk of adverse effects of one or more medication. In a registry-based Swedish study of older patients, the prevalence of polypharmacy, defined as the use of more than five drugs, was 44%, while almost 12% of older patients were on more than 10 different medications on a daily basis, i.e. hyperpolypharmacy [35]. In another European study, 8% of the population were on nine or more drugs, and 90% of these were from cardiovascular medications [36]. Similarly, in a large US population-based study in patients >65 years old, the prevalence of polypharmacy with five or more drugs was 36.8% [37]. Older patients frequently encountered higher healthcare utilization secondary to adverse drug reactions from polypharmacy [38–40]. Adverse reactions associated with cardiovascular medications include bleeding, hypotension, electrolyte imbalance, and renal injury [38–40]. Polypharmacy is very common in patients with CAD. Current guidelines recommend dual antiplatelet therapy (DAPT), statin, beta blockers, and enin-angiotensin-aldosterone system (RAAS) antagonist for patients with ACS. Furthermore, many of these patients have comorbidities, like diabetes, hypertension, chronic kidney disease, and other chronic conditions for which these patients are already on multiple medications. These adverse drug events can be mitigated by actively evaluating a patient's medication list with a pharmacist trained in managing geriatric patients with the goals of discontinuing non-essential medications, those with little or no benefits, and evaluating for dose reductions of essential medications, a term known as *deprescribing* [41].

4.3 *Cognitive Impairment*

Mild cognitive impairment (MCI) is defined as memory impairment more than expected for a patient's age and educational level [42]. Dementia is the final form of cognitive dysfunction, also known as a major neurocognitive disorder. Patients with MCI have an estimated 10–30% risk of developing dementia [43–45]. Alzheimer's disease is the most common cause of dementia (60–80%), followed by cerebrovascular disease or vascular dementia (5–10%); other causes include Lewy body disease, frontotemporal lobar degeneration, Parkinson's disease, hippocampal sclerosis, and mixed pathologies [46]. The prevalence of dementia increases with age, with approximately 5% of the population at age 65–74 years, 10–14% between ages 75 and 84 years, and 29–35% of age 85 years and older [46]. Similarly, the prevalence of MCI was 19%, 28%, and 38% for those aged 65–74 years, 75–84 years, and ≥85 years old, respectively [47]. In a large US population study, the prevalence of cognitive impairment without dementia was around 22% in those older than 71 years old [48]. Studies have shown not only increased prevalence but also increased risk of developing dementia and cognitive impairment in patients with CAD [49, 50]; cognitive impairment and dementia present major barriers in diagnosis and management in patients with ACS. Events like ACS worsen cognition in older patients, which then affects their future cardiovascular management and outcomes [51–53].

4.4 Delirium

Delirium is defined as an acute disturbance in attention and awareness in one's state of mind that tends to fluctuate with time [54]. It is triggered by the presence of physiological stressors, inflammation, hemodynamic instability, drug therapy, electrolyte imbalances, or the actual underlying condition [55]. Delirium more commonly occurs in older adults when placed in an unfamiliar environment, such as hospitals especially the critical care setting. It is associated with a prolonged hospital stay, more extensive disease work-up, and with overall poor outcomes [56]. The prevalence of delirium in older patients in a nonhospital setting is usually low, around 1–2%, and further increases with age. In the hospital setting, the prevalence of delirium varies with the level of acuity, with 8–17% in the Emergency Department to as high as 50–82% in postoperative and intensive care units [57]. In one study involving ≥65 years old coronary care unit patients, the overall incidence of delirium increased with age and reached 50% in those ≥85 years old. Furthermore, those with delirium were found to have five times increased mortality at 30 days [58]. Another study found an overall prevalence of around 26% in cardiac intensive care units [59]. In a prospective multicenter registry study including NSTE-ACS patients aged 80 years or older, the incidence of delirium during hospitalization was 37% and was associated with prolonged hospitalizations and increased bleeding and mortality at six-month follow-up [60].

4.5 Frailty

Commonly present in the older adult population, frailty is defined as the progressive decline in physical reserve, which is associated with increased vulnerability to acute stressors, adverse health outcomes, increased hospitalizations, and mortality [61, 62]. In a large US population-based study, frailty was present in 15% of those over 65 years old. Frailty was more prevalent among women, racial minorities, lower income groups, and with advanced age (9% in 65–70 years old versus 38% in those ≥90 years old) [63]. In a Medicare-based registry study, frail patients without CVDs had more major cardiovascular events, including MI and mortality, compared to nonfrail patients when followed longitudinally [64]. Frailty is a clinical diagnosis and can be assessed by using various tools and indexes. One of the initial tools is the Fried physical frailty phenotype that consists of five components: slowness (time to walk 15 feet- slowest 20%; cutoff depends on sex and height), weakness (grip strength measured using hand dynamometer, lowest 20%; cut off depends on gender and BMI), low physical activity (expends <270 kcal/week, calculated from activity scale incorporating episodes of walking, household chores, yard work etc.), exhaustion (subjective self-reported of feeling everything being an effort or 'I could not get going'), and weight loss (lost >10 pounds unintentionally in one year) [65]. The FRAIL scale is an interview-based screening tool that includes fatigue, resistance, ambulation, illnesses, and weight loss. This scale is commonly used in acute settings because of its convenience [66]. The Clinical Frailty Scale (CFS) is a commonly used instrument in cardiovascular trials and is based on fitness, active disease, activities of daily living, and cognition [67]. Other frailty tools include the Frailty Index, Reported Edmonton Frail Scale, Tilburg Frailty Indicator, Hospital Frailty Risk Score, and Comprehensive Geriatric Assessment [68–72]. Some frailty scales, like the FRAIL scale, Frailty Index, and CFS, have been used in cardiovascular trials and for prognostication in patients with ACS [73]. Gait speed or walking speed had been used as a surrogate for frailty and was a risk factor for disability, cognitive dysfunction, hospitalization, mortality, and cardiovascular death in older patients [74, 75]. Frailty is also associated with adverse cardiovascular outcomes, and frail patients experience worse functional decline after a cardiovascular event [76].

Multiple studies using various frailty tools had shown an increased risk of mortality and other cardiovascular outcomes in frail compared to nonfrail patients [77–81]. In the TRIOLOGY ACS trial, the medical managements using prasugrel and clopidogrel were compared in NSTE-ACS patients. The Fried scale was used to calculate frailty in patients aged 65 years or older. The authors reported that compared to nonfrail patients, frail patients had an increased risk of the primary outcome of the composite of cardiovascular death, MI, stroke, and all-cause death over a period of 30 months [79]. Large population-based studies using health care databases persistently show the reduced use of PCI and coronary artery bypass grafting (CABG) revascularization procedures in frail compared to nonfrail patients. Furthermore, the incidence of adverse cardiovascular outcomes was significantly higher in frail than in nonfrail patients [80, 81]. In a meta-analysis of 15 studies including older patients with ACS, frailty was associated with a significantly higher risk of mortality, reinfarction, stroke/transient ischemic attack (TIA), major bleeding, and rehospitalization rates [82].

4.6 Disability

Disability is defined as difficulty performing basic or complex activities essential to independent living [83]. Older populations commonly encounter multiple disabilities ranging from hearing, vision, cognition, mobility, self-care, or independent living, which compromises their ability to carry out activities of daily living and instrumental activities of daily living [84]. In the US, almost 42% of the older (≥65 years) population reported the presence of one or more disabilities. Impaired mobility is the most prevalent, with 26.9% reporting this disability [84]. Similarly, the United Nations Department of Economic and Social Affairs Disability estimates that 46% of the 60 years and older population have some form of disability [85]. Disability in older adults is mainly related to the geriatric syndromes discussed earlier pertaining to multimorbidity, polypharmacy, cognitive dysfunction, and frailty. Population studies found multiple causes of disability, including advanced age, overweight, depression, stroke, cardiovascular disease, diabetes, hypertension, cognitive impairment, osteoarthritis, and falls [86–88]. Cardiovascular disease remains an independent risk factor for increasing disability in older patients [89, 90]. Disability is also associated with an increased incidence of CAD and overall cardiovascular adverse events [91–93].

4.7 Functional Decline

Functional decline is defined as a reduced capacity to perform activities of daily living because of worsening physical and/or cognitive function [94]. Functional decline is very common and usually becomes progressive with age. It is associated with deterioration in the quality of life and adverse health outcomes. Risk factors like mobility disability, cognitive impairments, arthritis, depression, and other common geriatrics risks were associated with increased functional decline in older patients [95–98]. In a Japanese study involving older patients admitted to the hospital for heart failure, multiple risk factors leading to functional decline were identified, including age 80 years or older, prior stroke, dementia, mobility impairment, advanced heart failure, hyponatremia, and renal disease [99]. In the same study, patients with functional decline experienced increased cardiovascular adverse events and mortality [99]. In another study, older patients with a history of or a new vascular event, including hospitalization for MI, experienced an increased risk of functional decline [100–102]. Prospective studies in patients with MI have found that older age, longer hospital stays, mobility dysfunction, preadmission physical activity, and depression were important risk factors for functional decline [103].

5 Management Strategy of ACS in Older Adults

5.1 Presentation and Diagnostic Approach

The diagnostic criteria for ACS in older patients are similar to those in the general population. A detailed history and clinical examination become much more important in the older patient given multiple comorbidities and polypharmacy, which can affect the diagnostic approach for ACS. Multimorbidity such as prior atherosclerotic cardiovascular diseases and chronic kidney disease is common in older patients, and many patients are on some pharmacotherapy which includes an antiplatelet or an anticoagulant. A detailed past medical and a review of medication history are important as it often impacts the initial diagnostic approach and further pharmacotherapy. Cognitive impairment and functional decline in older patients are likely to act as barriers to performing a full evaluation, and it is often necessary to obtain medical information from patients' families and caretakers. While classical chest pain remains one of the common presentations of ACS in all populations, including older adults, the frequency of typical ischemic symptoms decreases with age [10]. In the GRACE registry, an atypical presentation was present in 43% of patients older than 75 years [104]. In the National Registry of Myocardial Infarction (NRMI), chest pain was not the initial presentation in more than 40% of patients in the 75–84-year age group and was absent in more than 50% of patients 85 years or older [10]. In a recent prospective observational study SILVER-AMI, which included patients ≥75 years of age, chest pain was absent in 44% [105]; the commonly reported atypical symptoms were dyspnea, diaphoresis, nausea, vomiting, and syncope [10]. It is important to recognize these atypical symptoms and maintain a high degree of suspicion because several studies have reported a poor prognosis in patients with atypical ACS presentation [10, 104, 106].

The 12-lead electrocardiogram (ECG) is one of the first and most readily available diagnostic tests in patients presenting with ACS. While the diagnosis of STE-ACS can be made with ECG in the appropriate setting, ECG in NSTE-ACS may be nonspecific and require serial monitoring. The yield of an ECG in diagnosing ACS decreases in the presence of other ECG abnormalities, especially with left bundle branch block (LBBB). These abnormalities are common in older patients, with studies reporting their presence in almost 70% of patients over the age of 75 years [107–109]. In addition to LBBB, they include right bundle branch blocks, left ventricular hypertrophy, atrial fibrillation, atrial flutter , and a paced ventricular rhythm. The presence of these ECG abnormalities increases with age [107–109].

A cardiac troponin assay is a biomarker that aids in the diagnosis of MI, even among older patients. With the advent of high sensitivity troponin, diagnostic yield is significantly improved and is currently being recommended in clinical practice guidelines [110]. Variations in levels of these troponin assays based on patient factors like age, gender, race, and chronic diseases can occur, and clinicians should be cognizant of these variations while interpreting them [110]. Baseline elevated levels of cardiac troponin levels have been reported in older patients in the community [111, 112]. In a large general population study, the levels of high-sensitivity cardiac troponin T and cardiac troponin I were noted to correlate well for patients younger than 60 years. However mild elevation above the 99th percentile was observed with age and those with muscle mass disorder, particularly high sensitivity troponin T [113]. Similarly, data from large population studies reported possible overdiagnosis of MI in the older adult population with the use of the 14 ng/l cutoffs of high sensitivity cardiac troponin T [114]. With the availability of cardiac troponin, current guidelines do not recommend routine use of creatine kinase myocardial isoenzyme and myoglobin for diagnosis of ACS [113].

6 Pharmacotherapy in ACS

6.1 Antiplatelet Therapy

Aspirin is an irreversible platelet cyclooxygenase-1 inhibitor. Current American and European guidelines recommend the use of a loading dose (325 mg) at the initial presentation of ACS, followed by a daily maintenance dose (81 mg) [13, 115–120]. The role of aspirin in MI was established in the Second International Study of Infarct Survival (ISIS-2); aspirin was associated with a significant reduction in vascular death when used alone or in combination with streptokinase compared to placebo. In the ISIS-2 study of patients treated with aspirin, the reduction in deaths for those ≥70 years old was higher than for those 60–69 years old [121]. In the Antithrombotic Trialists' Collaboration meta-analysis, aspirin was associated with a significant reduction in the risk of MI, and this benefit was higher in the ≥65-year-old age group compared to the younger patients [122]. In an observational study, the role of aspirin in ≥65 years old patients after an MI event was compared with patients discharged without aspirin. Of the 5490 patients included in this study, 24% were discharged without aspirin. At 6 months follow up, mortality in patients discharged on aspirin was significantly lower than in patients discharged without aspirin (8.4% vs. 17%) [123]. While the role of aspirin is well established in secondary prevention, concerns regarding increased bleeding risk remain high, especially in the older population [124–126].

Clopidogrel is recommended as an alternative to aspirin in a patient with aspirin intolerance or allergy [118, 119]. The role of clopidogrel in addition to aspirin was first established in the CURE (Clopidogrel in Unstable angina to Prevent Recurrent ischemic Events) trial. In this trial, NSTEMI patients randomized to clopidogrel experienced a significant reduction in CV death, MI, or stroke at 1 year. Compared to patients <65 years, those ≥65 years had a similar and significant reduction in these outcomes [127]. However, in the PCI Cure trial, the impact of clopidogrel on death or MI was not significant in the ≥65 years old subgroup [128]. While clopidogrel is one of the most widely used P2Y12 receptor inhibitors, there is a substantial population that exhibits clopidogrel resistance or residual high treatment platelet reactivity; thus, this population experiences an increased risk of ischemic events [129].

Potent P2Y12 inhibitors like ticagrelor and prasugrel have a more rapid onset of action and more pronounced platelet inhibition than clopidogrel. In the PLATO trial, vascular death, MI, or stroke was significantly lower in ACS patients randomized to ticagrelor than in those randomized to clopidogrel. In the PLATO trial, 15% ($n = 2878$) of patients were ≥75 years old, though there was a numerical decrease in primary events (16.8% vs. 18.3%) the difference was not significant, while the <75 years old ($n = 15{,}744$) patients had a significant reduction in primary events (8.6% vs. 10.4%) [130]. In a detailed post hoc analysis of PLATO based on age ≥75 or <75 years, the mortality and CV death outcomes were significantly reduced in the ticagrelor group; however, there was no difference in the MI, stent thrombosis, and stroke outcomes. Major bleeding was similar in both the ticagrelor and clopidogrel groups, including those >75 years [131]. The TRITON–TIMI 38 trial reported a significant reduction in the primary endpoint of CV death, MI, or stroke with prasugrel when compared with clopidogrel in ACS patients. In the 1769 (13%) patients ≥75 years old, there was a numerical but nonsignificant reduction in the primary endpoint with prasugrel (17.2% vs. 18.3%). The risk of TIMI major bleeding, fatal and life-threatening bleeding was significantly increased in the prasugrel patients who were ≥75 years old. Furthermore, the ≥75-year-old group experienced no difference in the composite of death, MI, stroke, or TIMI major bleeding with prasugrel when compared to clopidogrel. The recommended doses of prasugrel in ACS are a 60 mg loading dose and a 10 mg maintenance dose [132]. The European Medicines Agency and United States Food and Drug Administration (FDA) recommend a 30 mg loading dose and a 5 mg maintenance dose in patients ≥75 years old because older patients usually have higher concentrations of the active prasugrel metabolite [133]. The Assessment of a Normal versus Tailored Dose of Prasugrel after Stenting in Patients Aged ≥75 years to Reduce the Composite of Bleeding, Stent Thrombosis, and Ischemic Complications (ANTARCTIC) trial that randomized ≥75-year-old patients with PCI for ACS found no extra benefit of a platelet function-based dose adjustment of prasugrel [134]. In the TRIOLOGY-ACS trial, which compared prasugrel and clopidogrel in NSTE-ACS patients and among the elderly subgroup (≥75 years), 5 mg of prasugrel was used rather than 10 mg [135]. Overall, there were no differences in CV death, MI, stroke, or bleeding events among all participants and among those in the older age group [136]. The Elderly ACS 2 trial, which randomized patients >74-year-old with ACS to prasugrel (5 mg) or clopidogrel, reported no difference between the two groups in the composite of mortality, MI, stroke, rehospitalization, or bleeding [137]. The POPular AGE (Ticagrelor or Prasugrel Versus Clopidogrel in Elderly Patients with an Acute Coronary Syndrome and a High Bleeding Risk: Optimization of Antiplatelet Treatment in High-Risk Elderly) trial included those over 70 years old with NSTE-ACS. The use of clopidogrel was associated with less bleeding but a similar risk of ischemic events when compared to ticagrelor or prasugrel [138]. Registry studies provide conflicting results, with the Bremen STEMI registry, including patients ≥75 years old, reported decreased ischemic events with ticagrelor when compared to clopidogrel without any difference in bleeding, while the SWEDEHEART (Swedish Web System for Enhancement and Development of Evidence-Based Care in Heart Disease Evaluated According to Recommended Therapies) including patients ≥80 years old, reported an increased risk of mortality and bleeding with ticagrelor when compared to clopidogrel [139, 140].

Dual-antiplatelet therapy with aspirin and a P2Y12 inhibitor remains the cornerstone of treatment to prevent recurrent ischemic events in patients with ACS undergoing PCI. Despite guideline recommendations for DAPT in all age groups, the use of aspirin and P2Y12 inhibitors is often significantly reduced in older patients [10, 141–143]. Current ACC/AHA DAPT guidelines recommend 12 months of DAPT after an ACS event [13, 120]. Depending on patients' bleeding and ischemic risks, the duration can vary from 6 to 12 months. The guidelines also recommend the use of the more potent P2Y12 inhibitors, prasugrel, and ticagrelor, in patients with ACS rather than clopidogrel, except that the use of prasugrel is contraindicated in patients with a history of stroke or TIA [13]. The FDA highlighted that prasugrel is generally not recommended in patients >75 years of age because of an increased risk of fatal and intracranial bleeding and uncertain benefits, but exceptions are made for high-ischemic risk patients with diabetes and prior acute MI in whom the benefits appear to be greater than the risks. The 2017 European Society of Cardiology (ESC) guidelines similarly recommend 12 months of DAPT in patients with ACS, and six months in patients with ACS and high bleeding risk [119]. Though the recommendations are similar for the older population, they are usually considered at high risk for bleeding with DAPT, and the duration of DAPT should be individualized in this age group [124, 138, 144]. In a meta-analysis of six randomized control trials including both stable CAD and ACS patients, the risk of ischemic events in those with six months of DAPT was similar to the risk in those with 12 months of DAPT, but there was a significant reduction in major bleeding with six months of treatment duration [145].

6.2 Parenteral Anticoagulation Therapy

Parenteral anticoagulation is recommended in the acute setting in patients presenting with ACS [13, 115–119]. Multiple trials have shown the benefits of unfractionated heparin (UFH), and low-molecular-weight heparins (LMWHs) compared to placebo in patients with NSTE-ACS [146–150], although the representation of older patients was minimal in these trials. Multiple randomized controlled trials (RCTs) also compared UFH with LMWH in NSTE-ACS patients, and overall, there was no significant difference between the two [10, 149, 151–153]. In a meta-analysis comparing six trials of enoxaparin versus UFH, there was a significant reduction in death or MI with enoxaparin. Age-based subgroup data available from these trials were limited [154]. However, in a post-hoc age-related analysis of The Superior Yield of the New Strategy of Enoxaparin, Revascularization and Glycoprotein IIb/ IIIa Inhibitors (SYNERGY) trial, involving patients ≥75 years reported increased bleeding with enoxaparin when compared to UFH [155]. LMWHs are eliminated by the kidneys, and this complicates their use in older patients with chronic kidney disease. UFH is not renally cleared and remains a useful option in the older population. However, the dosing of UFH is frequently associated with under or overdosing, leading to increased recurrent ischemic events and bleeding risks with UFH in older adults [156].

The Fifth Organization to Assess Strategies in Acute Ischemic Syndromes (OASIS-5) trial compared fondaparinux, a parenteral factor Xa inhibitor, versus enoxaparin in ACS patients. The primary outcome of death, MI, or refractory ischemia was similar in both groups; however, the risks of major bleeding and death at 1 and 6 months were significantly lower in the fondaparinux group. In patients ≥65 years old, the risks of bleeding (4.1% vs. 8%) and mortality were significantly lower in the fondaparinux group [157, 158]. Similarly, in the OASIS-6 trial, the risks of mortality and MI in STEMI patients were significantly less in those treated with fondaparinux than in those treated with UFH [159]. These benefits were noted in all age groups [157–159]. One caveat of using fondaparinux in ACS that limits its use in this setting is an increased risk of catheter-related thrombosis and requiring a switch to other parenteral anticoagulants [157, 159]. The use of fondaparinux is attractive during PCI because of its relatively short, 17–21-hour half-life. This short half-life allows single fixed daily dosing. However, catheter-related thrombosis remains a major adverse cardiovascular event that increases the risk of MI and stroke. Fondaparinux is primarily used when conservative management of ACS is contemplated.

Bivalirudin was evaluated in ACS in multiple RCTs and offered an alternative to UFH and LMWHs, especially in patients with heparin-induced thrombocytopenia [160]. Trials comparing bivalirudin with heparin plus GP IIb-IIIa inhibitors showed a significant reduction in major bleeding without increasing the risk of ischemic events with bivalirudin; however, when GP IIb-IIIa inhibitors were not used or were optional, the risk of bleeding was similar between bivalirudin and heparin. Age-specific data from RCTs support similar results in the older population [160–165]. The use of bivalirudin is limited because of high cost and some concern for an increased risk of stent thrombosis [160, 166].

6.3   Oral Anticoagulation Therapy

Warfarin is the first and the oldest oral anticoagulant. It is a vitamin K antagonist that exerts anticoagulant activity by interfering with the function of the vitamin K-dependent clotting factors II, VII, IX, X, protein C, and protein S [167]. Initial studies showing a mortality benefit with warfarin post ACS event were published in 1949, with subsequent studies confirming those findings [168]. Later studies revealed that the combination of aspirin and warfarin, as opposed to aspirin alone, significantly reduced cardiovascular death, recurrent myocardial infarction, and thromboembolic strokes after an ACS event. Meta-analysis of such trials demonstrated a reduction in ischemic events; however, these benefits were offset by an increased incidence of major bleeding complications [169, 170]. Direct oral anticoagulants have been evaluated in the setting of recent ACS for secondary prevention with or without DAPT, however, with limited success. Dabigatran was evaluated in ACS patients in the RandomizEd Dabigatran Etexilate Dose Finding Study (RE-DEEM) trial. At the six-months follow-up, major bleeding was significantly increased based on the dose of dabigatran used [171]. A subsequent meta-analysis reported an increased risk of MI event with dabigatran when compared to heparin products or warfarin use in different settings like stroke, venous thromboembolism, and ACS patients [172]. The Apixaban for Prevention of Acute Ischemic and Safety Events (APPRAISE-1) trial compared apixaban with a placebo in a patient with ACS who were on DAPT. The results showed an increased risk of major bleeding and a nonsignificant reduction in CV mortality, MI, and stroke with apixaban [173].

APPRAISE-2 trial was a large-scale (7392) patient trial that compared apixaban 5 mg twice daily with a placebo in ACS patients. There was no reduction in CV mortality, MI, or stroke with apixaban compared to placebo and a significant increase in TIMI major bleeding. Subgroup analysis based on the patients age ≥75-years found no benefit in ischemic events with a significantly increased risk of bleeding, which was five to six times more than in the <75-year-old group [174]. Rivaroxaban is a direct factor Xa inhibitor. It was initially evaluated in the ATLAS ACS TIMI 46 (Aspirin with or without Thienopyridine Therapy in Subjects with Acute Coronary Syndrome Thrombolysis in Myocardial Infarction 46). This trial enrolled only a limited number of ≥75-year-old patients. It reported a dose-dependent increase in major bleeding and a reduction in ischemic events [175]. The ATLAS ACS 2-TIMI 51 (Acute Coronary Syndrome ACS 2–Thrombolysis in Myocardial Infarction 51) trial with 15,526 patients compared twice daily low dose rivaroxaban 2.5 mg or 5 mg dose with placebo in patients with recent ACS and already on DAPT. Both rivaroxaban doses were significantly associated with reductions in CV death, MI, or stroke; however all-cause mortality and CV death were significantly reduced in the 2.5 mg dose but not in the 5 mg dose group. Furthermore, rivaroxaban was associated with an increased risk of TIMI major bleeding, which was lower in the 2.5 mg dose compared to the 5 mg dose group. The trial included 1405 (9%) patients ≥75 years old. While specific primary and safety events for this age group were not reported, those older than 65 years had a significant reduction in ischemic events and an increased risk of bleeding events in the primary trial analysis [176]. Based on this trial, 2.5 mg twice daily rivaroxaban was approved after ACS in Europe but not by the US FDA [177].

6.4 Oral Anticoagulant Therapy in Patients with Atrial Fibrillation and ACS

ACS and concomitant atrial fibrillation (AF) are fairly common in older populations [178]. Patients with AF who present with ACS and undergo PCI are complicated in terms of anticoagulation and antiplatelet therapies. The WOEST (What is the Optimal antiplatelet and anticoagulant therapy in patients with oral anticoagulation and coronary StenTing) trial compared dual therapy with warfarin plus clopidogrel and triple therapy with warfarin, aspirin, and clopidogrel. The trial included both stable CAD and ACS patients, and the average age of study participants was 70 years old. Compared to triple therapy, dual therapy was associated with a significant reduction in bleeding events. Subgroup analysis based on age ≥75 years showed similar benefits as the overall study [179]. Similar trials using DOACs compared dual therapy with DOAC plus a P2Y12 inhibitor versus triple therapy with warfarin plus DAPT. The RE-DUAL PCI (Randomized Evaluation of Dual Therapy with Dabigatran (plus a P2Y12 inhibitor) vs. Triple Therapy with Warfarin (plus a P2Y12 inhibitor and aspirin) in Patients with Atrial Fibrillation That Undergo a Percutaneous

Coronary Intervention with Stenting) trial compared dabigatran (110 mg and 150 mg) based dual therapy with warfarin plus DAPT triple therapy in patients with non-valvular AF who underwent PCI. Compared to triple therapy with warfarin, dual therapy with dabigatran was associated with a significant reduction in bleeding with no increase in thrombotic risk [180]. In a post-hoc analysis in patients $\geq$75 years old, dabigatran 110 mg was associated with a significant reduction in bleeding but with increased risk of thrombotic events, while the 150 mg dabigatran group failed to offer any additional reduction in bleeding events but was non-inferior to warfarin included triple therapy for thrombotic events [181]. The AUGUSTUS (Antithrombotic Therapy after Acute Coronary Syndrome or PCI in Atrial Fibrillation) trial evaluated the use of apixaban versus warfarin and with or without aspirin in patients with AF undergoing coronary revascularization for ACS [182]. Dual therapy with apixaban and a P2Y12 inhibitor was associated with the reduction in bleeding without an increase in ischemic events when compared to double warfarin therapy (plus P2Y12 inhibitor) or triple therapy (aspirin + P2Y12 inhibitor) or apixaban (aspirin + P2Y12 inhibitor) Similar results were noted in the subgroup of $\geq$80-year-old patients [182]. The PIONEER AF-PCI (Prevention of Bleeding in Patients with Atrial Fibrillation Undergoing PCI) compared the safety of rivaroxaban and warfarin in patients with AF who underwent PCI. Dual therapy with rivaroxaban (15 mg) plus a P2Y12 inhibitor was associated with a reduction in bleeding without an increased risk of ischemic events when compared to warfarin-based triple therapy (aspirin plus P2Y12 inhibitor). The results in the $\geq$75-year-old subgroup were associated with reduced bleeding (20.6% vs. 31.4%) and a similar risk of ischemic events (5.6% vs. 6.5%) [183]. The ENTRUST-AF PCI (evaluation of the safety and efficacy of an edoxaban-based antithrombotic regimen in patients with AF following successful percutaneous coronary intervention) trial compared edoxaban-based dual therapy with warfarin-based triple therapy in patients with AF undergoing PCI for stable CAD or ACS. The trial found similar risks of bleeding and ischemic events in the two groups. In the age group $\geq$75 years old, the risk of bleeding was similar in edoxaban dual therapy, and the warfarin-based triple therapy regimens [184]. Based on these results, it is reasonable to consider dual therapy with P2Y12 inhibitor and a DOAC over triple therapy in most older patients undergoing PCI. For those with complex disease or high risk of ischemic events, triple therapy for a month post PCI followed by dual therapy of DOAC plus P2Y12 inhibitor or coumadin plus P2Y12 inhibitor is also a reasonable strategy.

7 Revascularization for STEMI

7.1 *Role of Fibrinolysis*

While PCI is the preferred revascularization technique in STEMI, fibrinolytic therapy still remains an important therapeutic option when timely PCI is not available. The role of fibrinolysis in older adults is mainly available from subgroups of large RCTs and observational studies, as there are no dedicated trials for this population. The GISSI-1 (Gruppo Italiano per lo Studio della Streptochinasi nell'Infarto Miocardico) trial found a non-significant decrease in mortality in patients >75 years old with streptokinase [185]. In the ISIS-2 trial (Second International Study of Infarct Survival), the use of streptokinase was associated with a significant reduction (15.8% vs. 23.8%) in mortality in patients ≥70 years old [121]. The original FTT (Fibrinolytic Therapy Trialists' Collaborative Group) study, which included all ACS patients, found a nonsignificant relative reduction in mortality in the elderly ≥75-year-old, which on further analysis after excluding NSTEMI patients found a significant reduction in mortality (26% vs. 29.4%) [186, 187]. Registry and observational data had reported conflicting results with some showing no additional benefits of fibrinolytic therapy in the elderly, while other showed a significant reduction in mortality especially with long-term follow-up [188–190]. Fibrinolysis increases the risk of bleeding in all age groups, but the elderly are more prone to bleeding. The FTT study reported a higher risk of stroke in the elderly (2.0% vs. 1.2%). The risk of intracranial hemorrhage (ICH) increases with age and is associated with increased mortality in the elderly; however, the overall risk remains low [191–193].

Trials comparing alternative agents for fibrinolysis showed improved benefits in terms of reduction in ICH. In the GUSTO-I trial, tissue plasminogen activator (tPA) was associated with a significant reduction in mortality and stroke in all patients, including elderly 75–84 years of age; however ≥85 years old had benefit from streptokinase [191]. In the ASSENT-2 (Assessment of the Safety of a New Thrombolytic 2) trial, Tenecteplase had a lower risk of ICH in the ≥75 years old population when compared to tPA [194]. The risk of stroke is further dependent on the adjunctive parenteral anticoagulant used with fibrinolytics. In the ASSENT 3 (Assessment of the Safety and Efficacy of a New Thrombolytic 3) trial, the use of unfractionated heparin was associated with a lower rate of ICH compared to enoxaparin (1.2% vs. 6.7%) [195]. The ExTRACT-TIMI-25 (Enoxaparin Versus Unfractionated Heparin With Fibrinolysis for ST-Elevation Myocardial Infarction) trial showed enoxaparin without bolus in the elderly (≥75 years) had a similar risk of bleeding and a nonsignificant reduction in death and MI when compared to unfractionated heparin [196]. The addition of dual antiplatelet with clopidogrel and aspirin in patients with fibrinolysis offers a further reduction in ischemic outcomes; however, the trials excluded patients ≥75 years old [197, 198]. The STREAM (Strategic Reperfusion Early after Myocardial Infarction) trial compared half dose tenecteplase with clopidogrel followed by coronary angiography with primary PCI in STEMI patients and found similar results in a composite of death, shock, and heart failure but with an increase in ICH. The trial protocol used a 300 mg loading dose of clopidogrel in the ≤75 years old while no loading dose was used in ≥75 years old; the outcomes were similar in both age groups [199]. Furthermore, a post-hoc analysis found a half dose of tenecteplase in the elderly (≥75 years old) was associated with a reduction in ICH compared to full dose tenecteplase without increased risk of ischemic outcomes [200]. Of the potent P2Y12 inhibitor, only ticagrelor had been directly compared with clopidogrel in patients receiving fibrinolytics. The TREAT (Ticagrelor in Patients With ST Elevation Myocardial Infarction Treated With Pharmacological Thrombolysis) trial found no additional benefit of ticagrelor over clopidogrel in patients undergoing fibrinolysis; further, there was an increased risk of minor bleeding [201]. The ongoing STREAM-2 trial in ≥60-year-old STEMI patients aims to compare the pharmaco-invasive strategy of immediate half dose tenecteplase followed by transfer to PCI center versus standard PCI therapy [202].

7.2 Role of Percutaneous Intervention

Revascularization guidelines in older patients with STEMI follow those of the general population, with immediate reperfusion being the primary goal [11, 115, 116]. Earlier trials comparing PCI versus fibrinolytic therapy had a low representation of older adults but showed consistent benefits of lower mortality and MI with PCI compared to fibrinolytic therapy [11, 121, 185–187]. In the PAMI (Primary Angioplasty in Myocardial Infarction) trial, PCI was compared with a tissue plasminogen activator [185]. Of the 395 patients included in this study, 38% were ≥65 years old; PCI, when compared with fibrinolytic therapy, was associated with a significant reduction in hospital mortality (5.7% vs. 15%), hospital death, MI, (8.6% vs. 20%) and in-hospital recurrent ischemic events (8.6% vs. 27.5%) in this age group [203, 204]. Similarly, results in subgroups of older adults in the GUSTO-IIb (Global Use of Strategies to Open Occluded Coronary Arteries in Acute Coronary Syndromes-IIb) and the DANAMI-2 (Danish Multicenter Randomized Study on Fibrinolytic Therapy Versus Acute Coronary Angioplasty in Acute Myocardial Infarction) trials found a significant reduction in 30-day mortality with PCI compared to thrombolytic therapy [11, 205, 206]. In one of the trials from the Netherlands, angioplasty was compared with streptokinase in 87 patients older than 75 years. Compared to streptokinase, PCI was significantly associated with a reduction in the 30-day composite of mortality, MI, and stroke (9% vs. 29%). The persistent mortality benefit was demonstrated in the PCI group (15% vs. 32%) at 2 years of follow-up [207]. In the Senior PAMI (Primary Angioplasty Versus Thrombolytic Therapy for Acute Myocardial Infarction in the Elderly study, NCT00136929), 483 ≥ 70 years old patients were randomized to PCI or to thrombolytic therapy; the trial was discontinued early because of slow recruitment. During the 30-day follow-up, both PCI and thrombolytic therapy were associated with a similar rate of mortality (10% vs. 13%), stroke (0.8% vs. 2.2%), and major bleeding (5.6% vs. 6.2%). However, reinfarction was significantly reduced in the PCI group compared to the thrombolytic group (1.6 vs. 5.4%) [208, 209]. In the TRIANA (TRatamiento del Infarto Agudo de miocardio eN Ancianos) trial, 266 ≥ 75 years old patients with STEMI were randomized to PCI or to fibrinolysis; the mean age was 81 years old. The trial found a numerical but importantly nonsignificant reduction in mortality, reinfarction, and disabling stroke, but recurrent ischemia was significantly reduced in the PCI group (0.8 vs. 9.7%). The authors of the TRIANA trial also reported a pooled analysis of 3 randomized trials and found a significant reduction in the composite of mortality, MI, and stroke (14.9% vs. 21.5%) with PCI compared to thrombolytic therapy; however, mortality was similar in both groups (10.7% vs. 13.8%) [210].

Overall, the use of PCI in older adults has steadily increased in recent years. In a retrospective analysis of the US national database, authors noted between 2004 to 2014, the use of PCI in patients 90 years older increased from 0.6% to 1.4% of all the PCI hospitalizations of which PCI for STEMI increased from 23.1% to 30.9% [211]. Similar trends from European and Asian registries suggest increasing use of PCI in older patients with STEMI [212–215]. Despite this increased rate of utilization, mortality in older patients with STEMI remains high. In a retrospective study from the Norwegian database, in-hospital mortality was 17% in ≥80 years old compared to only 4% in <80 years old. At the three years follow-up, survival further decreased to 52% in ≥80 years compared to 89% in <80 years old; in the PCI treated group of ≥80 years old, survival was slightly better (58%) [216]. Another study from the French registry reported an improvement in mortality with changes in management strategies over the year. With the increasing use of PCI, one-year STEMI mortality in ≥75 years decreased from 36.2% in 1995 to 21.1% in 2010; this improvement was also seen in the very elderly (≥85) [217]. Current guidelines recommend the use of PCI in STEMI patients without any limitation to life expectancy [115, 116]. However, the burden of geriatric syndromes remains a significant factor that influences the utilization of PCI in older patients with STEMI [214–216, 218].

7.3   Revascularization for NSTE-ACS/NSTEMI

Compared to the younger population, older patients who present with NSTE-ACS are less likely to undergo revascularization and usually have a worse prognosis [10]. Current guidelines support using an early invasive revascularization strategy in all age groups of patients with NSTE-ACS [13, 117]. The initial trials evaluating the use of an invasive strategy in NSTE-ACS were conducted when revascularization was performed without the use of stents or P2Y12 inhibitors. Later trials included percutaneous revascularization with glycoprotein IIb/IIIa inhibitor and long-term DAPT use. The TIMI IIIB (Thrombolysis in Myocardial Infarction IIIB) trial overall found better relief of angina, fewer rehospitalizations, and shorter lengths of stay with an invasive strategy but no differences in death and MI. Interestingly, in the subgroup of patients ≥65 years old, there was a significant reduction in death or MI at one year [219, 220]. However, the VANQWISH (Veterans Affairs Non-Q-Wave

Infarction Strategies in Hospital) study with 8% of the study population ≥75 years old found no difference in death or MI with an invasive strategy [221]. The FRISC II (FRagmin and Fast Revascularization during InStability in Coronary artery disease) was one of the initial trials to demonstrate a benefit of an invasive strategy in NSTEMI patients [222]. The RITA 3 (Randomized Intervention Trial of unstable Angina 3) trial found a significant reduction in mortality, MI, or refractory angina with an invasive, compared to a non-invasive, strategy (9.6% vs. 14.5%); however, the result was mainly driven by a reduction in refractory angina and overall there were no differences in death or MI between the two groups [223]. The ICTUS (Invasive versus Conservative Treatment in Unstable Coronary Syndromes) study failed to show any benefit of an early invasive compared to a conservative strategy, and even in the elderly subgroup (≥65 years old) there was no difference (23.6% vs. 24.4%) in death, MI, or rehospitalization for angina within one year [224]. A pooled analysis of three trials FRISC II, ICTUS, RITA-3 (FIR), in the ≥75-year age group found a significant reduction in cardiovascular mortality and MI with a routine invasive, compared with a selective invasive strategy involving medical management and angiography only in case of refractory angina, reinfarction, hemodynamic instability (26.1% vs. 34.9%) at five-year follow-up. The benefits were mainly attributable to a reduction in MI (15.2% vs. 24.7%), while mortality was similar though numerically less in the routine invasive arm (16.9% vs. 20.2%) during five-year follow-up [225]. The TACTICS–TIMI 18 (Treat Angina with Aggrastat and Determine Cost of Therapy with an Invasive or Conservative Strategy–Thrombolysis in Myocardial Infarction 18) compared early invasive and conservative strategies in patients who were treated with aspirin, heparin, and the glycoprotein IIb/IIIa inhibitor tirofiban. The trial showed a significant reduction in death and MI in the invasive group. Moreover, the benefit of the invasive strategy was higher in the older (≥75 years old) age group, with death or MI of 10.8% in the invasive arm and 21.6% in the conservative arm, but with a concomitant significant increased risk of bleeding in the invasive group (16.6% vs. 6.5%) [226].

More recently, five dedicated randomized controlled trials compared invasive and conservative strategies in the older population (Table 2) [227–231]. The Italian Elderly ACS trial was one of the first trials to investigate specifically the population ≥75 years of age to compare early invasive and conservative strategies. The trial enrolled 313 patients; the rate of revascularization was around 55% in the invasive group and 23% in the conservative group. The primary outcome of mortality, MI, stroke, repeat hospital admission, and severe bleeding was similar in both groups at one year follow-up (27.9% in the invasive vs. 34.6% in the conservative group). In a subgroup analysis, the authors observed that patients with elevated troponin who underwent an invasive strategy had a reduction in the primary outcome when compared with a conservative strategy, but a similar difference was not seen in the normal troponin group [227]. The After Eighty study enrolled >80 years old 457 patients and compared invasive strategy involving revascularization with medical management versus conservative strategy with only medical management. The primary outcome of mortality, MI, stroke, and urgent revascularization was

Table 2 Major randomized controlled trials comparing revascularization in older adults

Trial	N/Follow up/ mean age	Study design	Endpoints and major results
SENIOR PAMI (not published), 2005 [208]	483/12 M/78Y	STE-ACS, PCI vs. fibrinolysis	No difference in PE: Composite of death or stroke (11.3% vs. 13%, $p = 0.57$), reduction in SE of mortality, MI or stroke with PCI (11.6% vs. 18%, $p = 0.05$), no difference in major bleeding
TRIANA, 2011 [210]	266/1 M/81Y	STE-ACS, PCI vs. fibrinolysis	No difference in PE: Composite of mortality, MI, or stroke (18.9% vs. 25.4%, OR:0.69; $p = 0.21$), reduction in recurrent ischemia (0.8 vs. 9.7%, $p < 0.001$), no difference in major bleeding
TACTICS TIMI 18 (subgroup), 2001 [226]	278/6 M/≥75	NSTE-ACS, routine invasive vs. selective invasive	Significant reduction in PE: Composite of mortality MI, or re-hospitalization (10.8% vs. 21.6%; OR: 0.44; $p = 0.016$), significantly increased risk of major bleeding
Italian ACS Elderly, 2012 [227]	313/12 M/82Y	NSTE-ACS, routine invasive vs. selective invasive	No difference in PE: Composite of mortality, MI, stroke, or re-hospitalization (27.9% vs. 34.6%, HR: 0.80; $p = 0.26$), reduction in PE with invasive strategy in subgroup of + troponin, no difference in major bleeding
After Eighty, 2016 [228]	457/18 M/85Y	NSTE-ACS, invasive vs. optimal medical treatment	Significant reduction in PE: Composite of mortality, MI, revascularization, or stroke (40.6% vs. 61.4%, HR: 0·53; $p = 0·0001$), no difference in major bleeding
MOSCA, 2016 [229]	106/30 M/82Y	NSTE-ACS, routine invasive vs. selective invasive	No difference in PE: Composite of mortality, MI, revascularization, or rehospitalization (HR = 0.769 $p = 0.285$), no difference in major bleeding
80+, 2020 [230]	186/12 M/84Y	NSTE-ACS, routine invasive vs. optimal medical treatment	No difference in PE: Composite of mortality, MI, revascularization, stroke, or re-hospitalization (33.3% vs. 36.6%, HR:0.90; $p = 0.66$), reduction in urgent revascularization in invasive group, no difference in major bleeding
RINCAL, 2021 [231]	251/12 M/85Y	NSTE-ACS, routine invasive vs. optimal medical treatment	No difference in PE: Composite of mortality or MI (18.5% vs. 22.2%, HR: 0.79; $p = 0.39$), no difference in major bleeding
DEAR-OLD, ongoing [235]	696/12 M/≥75Y	NSTE-ACS, routine invasive vs. selective invasive	PE: Composite of mortality, MI, revascularization, or stroke

(continued)

Table 2 (continued)

Trial	N/Follow up/ mean age	Study design	Endpoints and major results
SENIOR-RITA, ongoing [236]	1668/60 M/≥75Y	NSTE-ACS, routine invasive vs. optimal medical treatment	PE: Composite of CV mortality or MI

CV cardiovascular, *MI* myocardial infarction, *M* months, *PE* primary endpoint, *SE* secondary endpoint, *Y* years. *SENIOR PAMI* primary angioplasty versus thrombolytic therapy for acute myocardial infarction in the elderly, *TRIANA* TRatamiento del Infarto Agudo de miocardio eN Ancianos, *TACTICS TIMI 18* treat angina with aggrastat and determine cost of therapy with an invasive or conservative strategy–thrombolysis in myocardial infarction 18, *MOSCA* coMOrbilidades en el Síndrome Coronario Agudo, *RINCAL* Revascularisation or medIcal therapy iN elderly patients with aCute anginAL syndromes

significantly reduced in the invasive arm compared to the conservative arm (40.6% vs. 61.4%); these results were mainly driven by the reduction in MI and urgent revascularization [228]. In another small trial of 106 patients (≥70 years old), comparing early invasive versus conservative strategies, the primary outcome of mortality, MI, and cardiac readmission was similar at the end of 2.5 years of follow-up. The authors did note that at three-month follow-up, mortality and recurrent MI were significantly less in the patients randomized to the early invasive strategy [229]. In a meta-analysis of randomized controlled trials involving subgroups of the TACTICS-TMI 18, FIR trials, Italian Elderly ACS, and After Eighty with a total of 1887 patients compared routine invasive strategy with a selective invasive strategy. The study reported a reduction in the composite of death or MI (20.8% vs. 28.4%), MI, and repeat revascularization in the routine invasive arm compared to the selective invasive arm. However, no difference was noted in overall mortality, CV mortality, or major bleeding [232]. The randomized 80+ study and the RINCAL trial were recently published; both trials, like the After Eighty study, compared an invasive strategy with revascularization and medical therapy versus medical therapy alone, and both were terminated early because of slow recruitment [230, 231]. The 80+ trial randomized 186 patients, and at 12-month follow-up, a similar rate of major adverse cardiovascular events was reported in both groups (33.3% vs. 36.6%). As expected, urgent revascularization was lower in the invasive arm, while other outcomes, including mortality, MI, stroke, and recurrent hospitalization, were similar in both groups [230]. The RINCAL (Revascularisation or medIcal therapy iN elderly patients with aCute anginAL syndromes) trial, randomized 251 patients ≥80 years old. The primary outcome of mortality or MI at the one year follow-up was similar in both strategies (18.5% vs. 22.2%). There was a numerical but nonsignificant reduction in urgent revascularization and MI in the invasive arm compared to the conservative arm [231]. Both trials reported similar risks of major bleeding in both strategies.

Retrospective data from US national inpatient sample database reported a significant increase in PCI for all the NSTE-ACS ≥90 years old patients from 5.4% in

2003 to 6.3% in 2014. Overall, of all the PCI performed in ≥90 years old, the percentage of NSTE-ACS increased from 49.6% to 52.6% in that same time frame. Additionally, PCI in NSTE-ACS patients was associated with a decrease in in-hospital mortality from 3.7% vs. 12.8% compared to patients without PCI, yet significant selection bias exists in observational studies [211]. A study from the UK database reported reduced five-year mortality in ≥80 years old NSTE-ACS patients managed with an invasive compared to conservative or medical management (36% vs. 55%) [233].

The current European and American guidelines for NSTE-ACS patients recommend similar invasive strategies in all age groups [13, 117]. Despite this, the use of invasive management strategies in patients with ACS continues to remain low in the very old, given their anatomic, pathophysiologic, and age-related complexities [234]. Currently, two large trials are actively recruiting patients to further evaluate the role of an invasive strategy in the elderly population. The SENIOR-RITA (British Heart Foundation SENIOR-RITA Trial) trial is a randomized open-label trial to compare the role of a routine invasive strategy compared with a conservative strategy in ≥75 years old NSTE-ACS patients [235]. The trial aims to enroll more than 1600 patients, and the primary outcome of the trial is death or MI. The DEAR-OLD trial is a randomized, open-label, noninferiority trial to compare a deferred invasive approach to an early invasive in ≥75 years old NSTEMI patients. The primary endpoint of this study is a composite of mortality, MI, stroke, and urgent revascularization at one year [236].

7.4   Role of Coronary Artery Bypass Grafting

Use of CABG in the older adult populations with ACS is often limited, which is driven by the increased perception of poor prognosis in this population with major surgery. Older patients usually have multivessel CAD, complex lesions, heart failure with low left ventricular function, and valvular disease [237]. Furthermore, multimorbidity, like diabetes mellitus, peripheral vascular disease, stroke, hypertension, and anemia, are commonly seen in the elderly, which increases their perioperative risk of worse outcomes with CABG. However, the data regarding the use of CABG in elderly patients with ACS is limited. While the use of CABG in very old patients >85 years old is overall decreasing, there have been improvements in patient selection over time [238, 239].

Older adults should be evaluated based on their functional status and other geriatric syndromes, followed by a shared decision with patient and care team rather than a "one size fits all" approach. The 2021, ACC/AHA/SCAI guideline for coronary artery revascularization recommendation does not mention any age limitation while considering revascularization in patients with ACS. However, the guideline identifies that the evidence for elderly patients (≥75 years old) is limited and recommends individualizing patient care based on patient preference, cognitive function, and life expectancy [120].

8 Conclusion

The older adult population is expanding rapidly and is disproportionality affected by a high burden of cardiovascular disease. The mortality and morbidity risks for older patients with acute coronary syndrome are increased by a multitude of factors, including the presence of geriatric syndromes, the pathophysiologic changes accompanying the normal aging process, a higher burden of multivessel coronary artery disease, decreased candidacy for invasive procedures because of frailty and/or comorbidities, and increased likelihood for adverse effects of pharmacologic therapies. The intensity and invasiveness of interventions are individually based, and shared decision-making has an important role in optimizing outcomes in the older ACS patient population.

Older adults undergoing invasive interventions have much higher risks when compared to younger patients. Older patients also have a higher burden of anatomic disease, including left main involvement, diffuse three-vessel disease, calcifications, and other anatomic complexities. Physiologic changes with advanced age and coexisting multimorbidity further amplify the risks of hemodynamic collapse. Age-related risks, including geriatric syndromes, introduce another layer of complexity in the diagnostic approach and management. Considerations in the management of ACS in older adults goes beyond a disease-centric approach and also involve considerations regarding geriatric syndromes and shared decision-making to improve health outcomes in older patients with ACS.

Acknowledgments None.
Conflict of InterestThe authors declare that they have no relevant interests.

Presentation None.

Funding and Financial Disclosure Dr. Damluji receives research funding from the Pepper Scholars Program of the Johns Hopkins University Claude D. Pepper Older Americans Independence Center funded by the National Institute on Aging P30-AG021334 and mentored patient-oriented research career development award from the National Heart, Lung, and Blood Institute K23-HL153771-01.

References

1. United Nations Global Issues: Ageing. https://www.un.org/en/global-issues/ageing. World Health organization https://www.who.int/news-room/fact-sheets/detail/ageing-and-health

2. United States Census Bureau, The Older Population in the United States: 2019. https://www.census.gov/data/tables/2019/demo/age-and-sex/2019-older-population.html.

3. Global Burden of Cardiovascular Diseases Collaboration. The burden of cardiovascular diseases among US states, 1990-2016. JAMA Cardiol. 2018;3(5):375–89. https://doi.org/10.1001/jamacardio.2018.0385.

4. Cardiovascular Disease: A Costly Burden for America. https://www.heart.org/en/get-involved/advocate/federal-priorities/cardiovascular-disease-burden-report.

5. Dunbar SB, Khavjou OA, Bakas T, Hunt G, Kirch RA, Leib AR, Morrison RS, Poehler DC, Roger VL, Whitsel LP, American Heart Association. Projected Costs of Informal Caregiving for Cardiovascular Disease: 2015 to 2035: A Policy Statement From the American Heart Association. Circulation. 2018;137:e558–77. https://doi.org/10.1161/CIR.0000000000000570.

6. Rodríguez-Queraltó O, Guerrero C, Formiga F, Calvo E, Lorente V, Sánchez-Salado JC, Llaó I, Mateus G, Alegre O, Ariza-Solé A. Geriatric assessment and in-hospital economic cost of elderly patients with acute coronary syndromes. Heart Lung Circ. 2021;30(12):1863–9.

7. The economic impact of acute coronary syndrome on length of stay: an analysis using the Healthcare Cost and Utilization Project (HCUP) databases. https://doi.org/10.3111/1369699 8.2014.885907.

8. Simpson J, Javanbakht M, Vale L. Early invasive strategy in senior patients with non-ST-segment elevation myocardial infarction: is it cost-effective? A decision-analytic model and value of information analysis. BMJ Open. 2019;9:e030678. https://doi.org/10.1136/bmjopen-2019-030678.

9. Forné C, Subirana I, Blanch J, et al. A cost-utility analysis of increasing percutaneous coronary intervention use in elderly patients with acute coronary syndromes in six European countries. Eur J Prev Cardiol. 2021;28(4):408–17. https://doi.org/10.1177/2047487320942644.

10. Alexander KP, Newby LK, Cannon CP, et al. American Heart Association Council on Clinical Cardiology, & Society of Geriatric Cardiology. Acute coronary care in the elderly, part I: non-ST-segment-elevation acute coronary syndromes: a scientific statement for healthcare professionals from the American Heart Association Council on Clinical Cardiology: in collaboration with the Society of Geriatric Cardiology. Circulation. 2007;115(19):2549–69.

11. Alexander KP, Newby LK, Armstrong PW, et al. Acute coronary care in the elderly, part II: ST-segment-elevation myocardial infarction: a scientific statement for healthcare professionals from the American Heart Association Council on Clinical Cardiology: in collaboration with the Society of Geriatric Cardiology. Circulation. 2007;115(19):2570–89.

12. Yancy CW, Jessup M, Bozkurt B, et al. 2013 ACCF/AHA guideline for the management of ST-elevation myocardial infarction: a report of the American College of Cardiology Foundation/American Heart Association Task Force on Practice Guidelines. J Am Coll Cardiol. 2013;61:e78–140.

13. Amsterdam EA, Wenger NK, Brindis RG, et al. 2014 AHA/ACC guideline for the management of patients with non–ST-elevation acute coronary syndromes: a report of the American College of Cardiology/American Heart Association Task Force on Practice Guidelines. J Am Coll Cardiol. 2014;64:e139–228.

14. McClelland RL, Chung H, Detrano R, Post W, Kronmal RA. Distribution of coronary artery calcium by race, gender, and age: results from the multi-ethnic study of atherosclerosis (MESA). Circulation. 2006;113(1):30–7. https://doi.org/10.1161/CIRCULATIONAHA.105.580696.

15. Batchelor WB, Anstrom KJ, Muhlbaier LH, Grosswald R, Weintraub WS, O'Neill WW, Peterson ED. Contemporary outcome trends in the elderly undergoing percutaneous coronary interventions: results in 7,472 octogenarians. National Cardiovascular Network Collaboration. J Am Coll Cardiol. 2000;36(3):723–30. https://doi.org/10.1016/s0735-1097(00)00777-4.).

16. Feldman DN, Gade CL, Slotwiner AJ, et al. Comparison of outcomes of percutaneous coronary interventions in patients of three age groups (<60, 60 to 80, and >80 years) (from the New York state angioplasty registry). Am J Cardiol. 2006;98(10):1334–9.

17. North BJ, Sinclair DA. The intersection between aging and cardiovascular disease. Circ Res. 2012;110(8):1097–108. https://doi.org/10.1161/CIRCRESAHA.111.246876.
18. Damluji A, Ramireddy A, Forman DE. Management and care of older cardiac patients https://doi.org/10.1016/b978-0-12-809657-4.64094-2.
19. O'Neill DE, Forman DE. Cardiovascular care of older adults. BMJ (Clinical research ed). 2021;374:n1593. https://doi.org/10.1136/bmj.n1593.
20. Lee BH. Oh, aging and arterial stiffness. Circ J. 2010;74:2257–62.
21. Scioli MG, Bielli A, Arcuri G, Ferlosio A, Orlandi A. Ageing and microvasculature. Vasc Cell. 2014;6:19Y.
22. Safar M. Arterial aging—hemodynamic changes and therapeutic options. Nat Rev Cardiol. 2010;7:442–9. https://doi.org/10.1038/nrcardio.2010.96.
23. American Heart Association, Inc. AHA Statistical Update. Heart Disease and stroke statistics—2021 Update: A report from the American Heart Association. Circulation. 2021;143:e254–743. https://doi.org/10.1161/CIR.0000000000000950e254.
24. Myerson M, Coady S, Taylor H, Rosamond WD, Goff DC Jr, ARIC Investigators. Declining severity of myocardial infarction from 1987 to 2002: the atherosclerosis risk in communities (ARIC) study. Circulation. 2009;119(4):503–14.
25. Rosengren A, Wallentin L, Simoons M, Gitt AK, Behar S, Battler A, Hasdai D. Age, clinical presentation, and outcome of acute coronary syndromes in the Euroheart acute coronary syndrome survey. Eur Heart J. 2006;27(7):789–95. https://doi.org/10.1093/eurheartj/ehi774.
26. Arnold AM, Psaty BM, Kuller LH, Burke GL, Manolio TA, Fried LP, Robbins JA, Kronmal RA. Incidence of cardiovascular disease in older Americans: the cardiovascular health study. J Am Geriatr Soc. 2005;53(2):211–8. https://doi.org/10.1111/j.1532-5415.2005.53105.x.
27. Dunlay SM, Chamberlain AM. Multimorbidity in older patients with cardiovascular Disease. Curr Cardiovasc Risk Rep. 2016;10:3. https://doi.org/10.1007/s12170-016-0491-8.
28. Feinstein AG. Clinical judgement. New York, NY: Williams & Wilkins; 1967.
29. Centers for Medicare & Medicaid Services. Chronic Conditions Overview. https://www.cms.gov/Research-Statistics-Data-and-Systems/Statistics-Trends-and-Reports/Chronic-Conditions/CC_Main.html. Accessed 25 Nov 2015.
30. Bell SP, Saraf AA. Epidemiology of multimorbidity in older adults with cardiovascular disease. Clin Geriatr Med. 2016;32(2):215–26. https://doi.org/10.1016/j.cger.2016.01.013.
31. Arnett DK, Goodman RA, Halperin JL, Anderson JL, Parekh AK, Zoghbi WA. AHA/ACC/HHS strategies to enhance application of clinical practice guidelines in patients with cardiovascular disease and comorbid conditions: from the American Heart Association, American College of Cardiology, and U.S. Department of Health and Human Services. J Am Coll Cardiol. 2014;64(17):1851–6.
32. Breen K, Finnegan L, Vuckovic K, et al. Multimorbidity in patients with acute coronary syndrome is associated with greater mortality, higher readmission rates, and increased length of stay: a systematic review. J Cardiovasc Nurs. 2020;35(6):E99–E110.
33. Forman DE, Maurer MS, Boyd C, et al. Multimorbidity in older adults with cardiovascular disease. J Am Coll Cardiol. 2018;71:2149–61.
34. Khezrian M, McNeil CJ, Murray AD, Myint PK. An overview of prevalence, determinants and health outcomes of polypharmacy. Ther Adv Drug Saf. 2020;11:2042098620933741.
35. Morin L, Johnell K, Laroche ML, Fastbom J, Wastesson JW. The epidemiology of polypharmacy in older adults: register-based prospective cohort study. Clin Epidemiol. 2018;10:289–98.
36. Walckiers D, Van der Heyden J, Tafforeau J. Factors associated with excessive polypharmacy in older people. Arch Public Health. 2015;73:50.
37. Young EH, Pan S, Yap AG, Reveles KR, Bhakta K. Polypharmacy prevalence in older adults seen in United States physician offices from 2009 to 2016. PLoS One. 2021;16(8):e0255642.
38. Maher RL, et al. Clinical consequences of polypharmacy in elderly. Expert Opin Drug Saf. 2014;13(1):57–65.

39. Gurwitz JH, Field TS, Harrold LR, Rothschild J, Debellis K, Seger AC, Cadoret C, Fish LS, Garber L, Kelleher M, Bates DW. Incidence and preventability of adverse drug events among older persons in the ambulatory setting. JAMA. 2003;289(9):1107–16.

40. Sheikh-Taha M, Asmar M. Polypharmacy and severe potential drug-drug interactions among older adults with cardiovascular disease in the United States. BMC Geriatr. 2021;21(1):233.

41. Krishnaswami A, Steinman MA, Goyal P, Zullo AR, Anderson TS, Birtcher KK, Goodlin SJ, Maurer MS, Alexander KP, Rich MW, Tjia J, Geriatric Cardiology Section Leadership Council, American College of Cardiology. Deprescribing in older adults with cardiovascular Disease. J Am Coll Cardiol. 2019;73(20):2584–95.

42. Petersen RC, Smith GE, Waring SC, Ivnik RJ, Tangalos EG, Kokmen E. Mild cognitive impairment: clinical characterization and outcome. Arch Neurol. 1999;56(3):303–8. https://doi.org/10.1001/archneur.56.3.303.

43. US Preventive Services Task Force. Screening for cognitive impairment in older adults: US preventive services task force recommendation statement. JAMA. 2020;323(8):757–63. https://doi.org/10.1001/jama.2020.0435.

44. Petersen RC, Lopez O, Armstrong MJ, Getchius TSD, Ganguli M, Gloss D, Gronseth GS, Marson D, Pringsheim T, Day GS, Sager M, Stevens J, Rae-Grant A. Practice guideline update summary: mild cognitive impairment: report of the guideline development, dissemination, and implementation Subcommittee of the American Academy of Neurology. Neurology. 2018;90:126–35.

45. Ward A, Tardiff S, Dye C, Arrighi HM. Rate of conversion from prodromal Alzheimer's disease to Alzheimer's dementia: a systematic review of the literature. Dement Geriatr Cogn Dis Extra. 2013;3(1):320–32. https://doi.org/10.1159/000354370.

46. Alzheimer's disease facts and figures. Alzheimers Dement. 2021;17(3):327–406. https://doi.org/10.1002/alz.12328. Epub 2021 Mar 23

47. Unverzagt FW, Gao S, Baiyewu O, et al. Prevalence of cognitive impairment: data from the Indianapolis study of health and aging. Neurology. 2001;57(9):1655–62.

48. Plassman BL, Langa KM, Fisher GG, Heeringa SG, Weir DR, Ofstedal MB, Burke JR, Hurd MD, Potter GG, Rodgers WL, Steffens DC, McArdle JJ, Willis RJ, Wallace RB. Prevalence of cognitive impairment without dementia in the United States. Ann Intern Med. 2008;148(6):427–34.

49. Newman AB, Fitzpatrick AL, Lopez O, Jackson S, Lyketsos C, Jagust W, Ives D, Dekosky ST, Kuller LH. Dementia and Alzheimer's disease incidence in relationship to cardiovascular disease in the Cardiovascular Health Study cohort. J Am Geriatr Soc. 2005;53(7):1101–7.

50. Deckers K, et al. Coronary heart disease and risk for cognitive impairment or dementia: Systematic review and meta-analysis. PLoS One. 2017;12(9):e0184244. https://doi.org/10.1371/journal.pone.0184244.

51. Kasprzak D, Rzeźniczak J, Ganowicz T, et al. A review of acute coronary syndrome and its potential impact on cognitive function. Glob Heart. 2021;16(1):53.

52. Roberts RO, Knopman DS, Geda YE, Cha RH, Roger VL, Petersen RC. Coronary heart disease is associated with non-amnestic mild cognitive impairment. Neurobiol Aging. 2010;31(11):1894–902.

53. Gu SZ, Beska B, Chan D, et al. Cognitive decline in older patients with non- ST elevation acute coronary syndrome. J Am Heart Assoc. 2019;8(4):e011218.

54. American Psychiatric Association DSM-5 Task Force. Diagnostic and statistical manual of mental disorders, 5th ed.: DSM-5. Washington, DC: American Psychiatric Association; 2013.

55. Watt D, Koziol K, Budding D. Delirium and confusional states. In: Noggle C, Dean R, editors. Disorders in neuropsychiatry. New York: Springer Publishing Company; 2012.

56. Leslie DL, Marcantonio ER, Zhang Y, Leo-Summers L, Inouye SK. One-year health care costs associated with delirium in the elderly population. Arch Intern Med. 2008;168(1):27–32.

57. Inouye SK, Westendorp RG, Saczynski JS. Delirium in elderly people. Lancet. 2014;383(9920):911–22.

58. Grotti S, Falsini G. Delirium in cardiac patients. Eur Heart J. 2017;38(29):2244.

59. McPherson JA, Wagner CE, Boehm LM, et al. Delirium in the cardiovascular ICU: exploring modifiable risk factors. Crit Care Med. 2013;41(2):405–13.
60. Vives-Borrás M, Martínez-Sellés M, Ariza-Solé A, et al. Clinical and prognostic implications of delirium in elderly patients with non-ST-segment elevation acute coronary syndromes. J Geriatr Cardiol. 2019;16(2):121–8.
61. Xue QL. The frailty syndrome: definition and natural history. Clin Geriatr Med. 2011;27(1):1–15.
62. Hoogendijk EO, Afilalo J, Ensrud KE, Kowal P, Onder G, Fried LP. Frailty: implications for clinical practice and public health. Lancet. 2019;394:1365–75.
63. Bandeen-Roche K, Seplaki CL, Huang J, Buta B, Kalyani RR, Varadhan R, Xue QL, Walston JD, Kasper JD. Frailty in older adults: a nationally representative profile in the United States. J Gerontol A Biol Sci Med Sci. 2015;70(11):1427–34.
64. Abdulla A, Damluji S-EC, Xue Q-L, Hasan RK, Moscucci M, Forman DE, Bandeen-Roche K, Batchelor W, Walston JD, Resar JR, Gerstenblith G. Frailty and cardiovascular outcomes in the National Health and aging trends study. Eur Heart J. 2021;42(37):1.
65. Fried LP, Tangen CM, Walston J, et al. Frailty in older adults: evidence for a phenotype. J Gerontol A Biol Sci Med Sci. 2001;56(3):M146–56.
66. Abellan van Kan G, Rolland Y, Bergman H, Morley JE, Kritchevsky SB, Vellas B. The I.A.N.A Task Force on frailty assessment of older people in clinical practice. J Nutr Health Aging. 2008;12(1):29–37.
67. Rockwood K, Song X, MacKnight C, Bergman H, Hogan DB, McDowell I, Mitnitski A. A global clinical measure of fitness and frailty in elderly people. CMAJ. 2005;173(5):489–95.
68. Rockwood K, Andrew M, Mitnitski A. A comparison of two approaches to measuring frailty in elderly people. J Gerontol A Biol Sci Med Sci. 2007;62(7):738–43.
69. Rolfson DB, Majumdar SR, Tsuyuki RT, et al. Validity and reliability of the Edmonton frail scale. Age Ageing. 2006;35:526–9.
70. Gobbens RJ, van Assen MA, Luijkx KG, et al. The Tilburg frailty indicator: psychometric properties. J Am Med Dir Assoc. 2010;11:344–55.
71. Gilbert T, Neuburger J, Kraindler J, et al. Development and validation of a hospital frailty risk score focusing on older people in acute care settings using electronic hospital records: an observational study. Lancet. 2018;391:1775–82.
72. Turner G, Clegg A. Best practice guidelines for the management of frailty: a British geriatrics society, age UK and Royal College of general practitioners report. Age Ageing. 2014;43:744–7.
73. Tonet E, Pavasini R, Biscaglia S, Campo G. Frailty in patients admitted to hospital for acute coronary syndrome: when, how and why? J Geriatr Cardiol. 2019;16:129–37.
74. Abellan van Kan G, Rolland Y, Andrieu S, et al. Gait speed at usual pace as a predictor of adverse outcomes in community-dwelling older people an international academy on nutrition and aging (IANA) task force. J Nutr Health Aging. 2009;13:881–9.
75. Dumurgier J, Elbaz A, Ducimetiere P, et al. Slow walking speed and cardiovascular death in well functioning older adults: prospective cohort study. BMJ. 2009;339:b4460.
76. Chung KJNC, Wilkinson C, Veerasamy M, Kunadian V. Frailty scores and their utility in older patients with cardiovascular disease. Interv Cardiol. 2021;16:e05.
77. Blanco S, Ferrières J, Bongard V, Toulza O, Sebai F, Billet S, Biendel C, Lairez O, Lhermusier T, Boudou N, Campelo-Parada F, Roncalli J, Galinier M, Carrié D, Elbaz M, Bouisset F. Prognosis impact of frailty assessed by the Edmonton frail scale in the setting of acute coronary syndrome in the elderly. Can J Cardiol. 2017;33(7):933–9.
78. Graham MM, Galbraith PD, O'Neill D, Rolfson DB, Dando C, Norris CM. Frailty and outcome in elderly patients with acute coronary syndrome. Can J Cardiol. 2013;29(12):1610–5.
79. White HD, Westerhout CM, Alexander KP, Roe MT, Winters KJ, Cyr DD, Fox KA, Prabhakaran D, Hochman JS, Armstrong PW, Ohman EM, TRILOGY ACS investigators. Frailty is associated with worse outcomes in non-ST-segment elevation acute coronary syndromes: insights from the TaRgeted platelet inhibition to cLarify the optimal strateGy to

medicallY manage acute coronary syndromes (TRILOGY ACS) trial. Eur Heart J Acute Cardiovasc Care. 2016;5(3):231–42.

80. Damluji AA, Huang J, Bandeen-Roche K, Forman DE, Gerstenblith G, Moscucci M, Resar JR, Varadhan R, Walston JD, Segal JB. Frailty among older adults with acute myocardial infarction and outcomes from percutaneous coronary interventions. J Am Heart Assoc. 2019;8(17):e013686.

81. Kwok CS, Lundberg G, Al-Faleh H, Sirker A, Van Spall HGC, Michos ED, Rashid M, Mohamed M, Bagur R, Mamas MA. Relation of frailty to outcomes in patients with acute coronary syndromes. Am J Cardiol. 2019;124(7):1002–11.

82. Dou Q, Wang W, Wang H, et al. Prognostic value of frailty in elderly patients with acute coronary syndrome: a systematic review and meta-analysis. BMC Geriatr. 2019;19:222.

83. Rodrigues MA, Facchini LA, Thumé E, Maia F. Gender and incidence of functional disability in the elderly: a systematic review. Cad Saude Publica. 2009;25(Suppl 3):S464–76.

84. Okoro CA, Hollis ND, Cyrus AC, Griffin-Blake S. Prevalence of disabilities and health care access by disability status and type among adults — United States, 2016. MMWR Morb Mortal Wkly Rep. 2018;67:882–7.

85. https://www.un.org/development/desa/disabilities/disability-and-ageing.html.

86. Spiers NA, Matthews RJ, Jagger C, Matthews FE, Boult C, Robinson TG, Brayne C. Diseases and impairments as risk factors for onset of disability in the older population in England and Wales: findings from the medical research council cognitive function and ageing study. J Gerontol Ser A. 2005;60(2):248–54.

87. Taş U, Verhagen AP, Bierma-Zeinstra SM, Hofman A, Odding E, Pols HA, Koes BW. Incidence and risk factors of disability in the elderly: the Rotterdam study. Prev Med. 2007;44(3):272–8.

88. Gill TM, Han L, Gahbauer EA, Leo-Summers L, Murphy TE. Risk factors and precipitants of severe disability among community-living older persons. JAMA Netw Open. 2020;3(6):e206021.

89. Cui K, Song R, Hui X, Shang Y, Qi X, Buchman AS, David A. Bennett and Weili Xu Association of cardiovascular risk burden with risk and progression of disability: mediating role of cardiovascular disease and cognitive decline. J Am Heart Assoc. 2020;9:e017346.

90. Chaudhry SI, McAvay G, Ning Y, Allore HG, Newman AB, Gill TM. Risk factors for onset of disability among older persons newly diagnosed with heart failure: the cardiovascular health study. J Card Fail. 2011;17(9):764–70.

91. Plichart M, Barberger-Gateau P, Tzourio C, et al. Disability and incident coronary heart disease in older community-dwelling adults: the Three-City study. J Am Geriatr Soc. 2010;58(4):636–42.

92. Afilalo J, Mottillo S, Eisenberg MJ, Alexander KP, Noiseux N, Perrault LP, Morin JF, Langlois Y, Ohayon SM, Monette J, Boivin JF, Shahian DM, Bergman H. Addition of frailty and disability to cardiac surgery risk scores identifies elderly patients at high risk of mortality or major morbidity. Circ Cardiovasc Qual Outcomes. 2012;5(2):222–8.

93. Mendes de Leon CF, Bang W, Bienias JL, Glass TA, Vaccarino V, Kasl SV. Changes in disability before and after myocardial infarction in older adults. Arch Intern Med. 2005;165(7):763–8.

94. Abdulaziz K, Perry JJ, Taljaard M, et al. National survey of geriatricians to define functional decline in elderly people with minor trauma. Can Geriatr J. 2016;19(1):2–8.

95. Dunlop DD, Semanik P, Song J, Manheim LM, Shih V, Chang RW. Risk factors for functional decline in older adults with arthritis. Arthritis Rheum. 2005;52(4):1274–82.

96. Njegovan V, Hing MM, Mitchell SL, Molnar FJ. The hierarchy of functional loss associated with cognitive decline in older persons. J Gerontol A Biol Sci Med Sci. 2001;56(10):M638–43.

97. Hajek A, Luck T, Brettschneider C, Posselt T, Lange C, Wiese B, Steinmann S, Weyerer S, Werle J, Pentzek M, Fuchs A, Stein J, Bickel H, Mösch E, Wagner M, Heser K, Maier W, Scherer JM, Riedel-Heller SG, König HH. Factors affecting functional impairment among elderly Germans - results of a longitudinal study. J Nutr Health Aging. 2017;21(3):299–306.

98. Hébert R, Brayne C, Spiegelhalter D. Factors associated with functional decline and improvement in a very elderly community-dwelling population. Am J Epidemiol. 1999;150(5):501–10.

99. Yaku H, Kato T, Morimoto T, et al. Risk factors and clinical outcomes of functional decline during hospitalisation in very old patients with acute decompensated heart failure: an observational study. BMJ Open. 2020;10(2):e032674.

100. Kamper AM, Stott DJ, Hyland M, Murray HM, Ford I. Predictors of functional decline in elderly people with vascular risk factors or disease. Age Ageing. 2005;34(5):450–5.

101. Levine D, Davydow D, Hough C, Langa K, Rogers M, Iwashyna T. Functional disability and cognitive impairment after hospitalization for myocardial infarction and stroke. Circ Cardiovasc Qual Outcomes. 2014:863–71.

102. Dodson JA, Arnold SA, Reid KJ, Gill TM, Rich MW, Masoudi FA, Spertus JA, Krumholz HM, Alexander KP. Physical function and independence one year following myocardial infarction: observations from the TRIUMPH registry. Am Heart J. 2012;163(5):790–6.

103. Hajduk AM, Dodson JA, Murphy TE, Tsang S, Geda M, Ouellet GM, Gill TM, Brush JE, Chaudhry SI. Risk model for decline in activities of daily living among older adults hospitalized with acute myocardial infarction: the SILVER-AMI study. J Am Heart Assoc. 2020;9(19):e015555.

104. Brieger D, Eagle KA, Goodman SG, Steg PG, Budaj A, White K, Montalescot G, GRACE Investigators. Acute coronary syndromes without chest pain, an underdiagnosed and undertreated high-risk group: insights from the global registry of acute coronary events. Chest. 2004;126(2):461–9.

105. Nanna MG, Hajduk AM, Krumholz HM, Murphy TE, Dreyer RP, Alexander KP, Geda M, Tsang S, Welty FK, Safdar B, Lakshminarayan DK, Chaudhry SI, Dodson JA. Sex-based differences in presentation, treatment, and complications among older adults hospitalized for acute myocardial infarction: the SILVER-AMI study. Circ Cardiovasc Qual Outcomes. 2019;12(10):e005691.

106. Ouellet GM, Geda M, Murphy TE, Tsang S, Tinetti ME, Chaudhry SI. Prehospital delay in older adults with acute myocardial infarction: the ComprehenSIVe evaluation of risk factors in older patients with acute myocardial infarction study. J Am Geriatr Soc. 2017;65:2391–6.

107. Silva M, Palhares D, Ribeiro L, Gomes P, Macfarlane P, Ribeiro A, Marcolino M. Prevalence of major and minor electrocardiographic abnormalities in one million primary care Latinos. J Electrocardiol. 2021;64:36–41. https://doi.org/10.1016/j.jelectrocard.2020.11.013. Epub 2020 Dec 2

108. Marcolino MS, Cury GA, Ribeiro AL. Electrocardiographic abnormalities in the elderly: a study in a large database of primary care patients. J Clin Exp Res Cardiol. 2017;3(2):204.

109. Molander U, Kumar Dey D, Sundh V, et al. ECG abnormalities in the elderly: prevalence, time and generation trends and association with mortality. Aging Clin Exp Res. 2003;15:488–93.

110. Gulati M, Levy P, et al. 2021 AHA/ACC/ASE/CHEST/SAEM/SCCT/SCMR guideline for the evaluation and diagnosis of CHEST pain. J Am Coll Cardiol. 2021;78(22):e187–285.

111. Eggers KM, Lind L, Venge P, Lindahl B. Factors influencing the 99th percentile of cardiac troponin I evaluated in community-dwelling individuals at 70 and 75 years of age. Clin Chem. 2013;59(7):1068–73.

112. He B, Wang K, Xu P, Zhou Q, Xu J. Determination of age- and sex-specific 99th percentile upper reference limits for high-sensitivity cardiac troponin I in healthy Chinese adults. Cardiology. 2022;147(3):261–70. https://doi.org/10.1159/000523721. Epub ahead of print

113. Welsh P, Preiss D, Shah ASV, McAllister D, Briggs A, Boachie C, McConnachie A, Hayward C, Padmanabhan S, Welsh C, Woodward M, Campbell A, Porteous D, Mills NL, Sattar N. Comparison between High-Sensitivity Cardiac Troponin T and Cardiac Troponin I in a Large General Population Cohort. Clin Chem. 2018;64(11):1607–16. https://doi.org/10.1373/clinchem.2018.292086. Epub 2018 Aug 20. PMID: 30126950; PMCID: PMC6398571

114. Gore MO, Seliger SL, Defilippi CR, Nambi V, Christenson RH, Hashim IA, Hoogeveen RC, Ayers CR, Sun W, McGuire DK, Ballantyne CM, de Lemos JA. Age- and sex-dependent

upper reference limits for the high-sensitivity cardiac troponin T assay. J Am Coll Cardiol. 2014;63(14):1441–8.

115. Yancy CW, Jessup M, Bozkurt B, et al. ACCF/AHA guideline for the management of ST-elevation myocardial infarction: a report of the American College of Cardiology Foundation/American Heart Association task force on practice guidelines. J Am Coll Cardiol. 2013;61(2013):e78–e140.

116. Ibanez B, James S, Agewall S, et al. 2017 ESC guidelines for the management of acute myocardial infarction in patients presenting with ST-segment elevation: the task force for the management of acute myocardial infarction in patients presenting with ST-segment elevation of the European Society of Cardiology (ESC). Eur Heart J. 2018;39:119–77.

117. Roffi M, Patrono C, Collet JP, et al. 2015 ESC guidelines for the management of acute coronary syndromes in patients presenting without persistent ST-segment elevation: task force for the Management of Acute Coronary Syndromes in patients presenting without persistent ST-segment elevation of the European Society of Cardiology (ESC). Eur Heart J. 2016;37(3):267–315.

118. 2016 ACC/AHA Guideline Focused Update on Duration of Dual Antiplatelet Therapy in Patients With Coronary Artery Disease: A Report of the American College of Cardiology/ American Heart Association Task Force on Clinical Practice Guidelines: An Update of the 2011 ACCF/AHA/SCAI Guideline for Percutaneous Coronary Intervention, 2011 ACCF/ AHA Guideline for Coronary Artery Bypass Graft Surgery, 2012 ACC/AHA/ACP/AATS/ PCNA/SCAI/STS Guideline for the Diagnosis and Management of Patients With Stable Ischemic Heart Disease, 2013 ACCF/AHA Guideline for the Management of ST-Elevation Myocardial Infarction, 2014 AHA/ACC Guideline for the Management of Patients With Non– ST-Elevation Acute Coronary Syndromes, and 2014 ACC/AHA Guideline on Perioperative Cardiovascular Evaluation and Management of Patients Undergoing Noncardiac Surgery.

119. Valgimigli M, Bueno H, Byrne RA, et al. 2017 ESC focused update on dual antiplatelet therapy in coronary artery disease developed in collaboration with EACTS: the task force for dual antiplatelet therapy in coronary artery disease of the European Society of Cardiology (ESC) and of the European Association for Cardio-Thoracic Surgery (EACTS). Eur Heart J. 2018;39(3):213–60.

120. Writing Committee Members, Lawton JS, Tamis-Holland JE, et al. 2021 ACC/AHA/SCAI Guideline for Coronary Artery Revascularization: A Report of the American College of Cardiology/American Heart Association Joint Committee on Clinical Practice Guidelines. J Am Coll Cardiol. 2022;79(2):e21–e129.

121. Randomised trial of intravenous streptokinase, oral aspirin, both, or neither among 17,187 cases of suspected acute myocardial infarction: ISIS-2. ISIS-2 (second international study of infarct survival) collaborative group. Lancet. 1988;2(8607):349–60.

122. Baigent C, Blackwell L, Collins R, et al., for the Antithrombotic Trialists' (ATT) CollaborationAspirin in the primary and secondary prevention of vascular disease: collaborative meta-analysis of individual participant data from randomised trials. Lancet. 2009;373:1849–60.

123. Krumholz HM, Radford MJ, Ellerbeck EF, Hennen J, Meehan TP, Petrillo M, Wang Y, Jencks SF. Aspirin for secondary prevention after acute myocardial infarction in the elderly: prescribed use and outcomes. Ann Intern Med. 1996;124(3):292–8.

124. Andreotti F, Rocca B, Husted S, et al. Antithrombotic therapy in the elderly: expert position paper of the European Society of Cardiology Working Group on thrombosis. Eur Heart J. 2015;36(46):3238–49. https://doi.org/10.1093/eurheartj/ehv304.

125. Coxib and traditional NSAID Trialists' (CNT) Collaboration, Bhala N, Emberson J, Merhi A, Abramson S, Arber N, Baron JA, Bombardier C, Cannon C, Farkouh ME, FitzGerald GA, Goss P, Halls H, Hawk E, Hawkey C, Hennekens C, Hochberg M, Holland LE, Kearney PM, Laine L, Lanas A, Lance P, Laupacis A, Oates J, Patrono C, Schnitzer TJ, Solomon S, Tugwell P, Wilson K, Wittes J, Baigent C. Vascular and upper gastrointestinal effects of non-steroidal

anti-inflammatory drugs: meta-analyses of individual participant data from randomised trials. Lancet. 2013;382(9894):769–79. https://doi.org/10.1016/S0140-6736(13)60900-9.

126. Wilson R, Gazzala J, House J. Aspirin in primary and secondary prevention in elderly adults revisited. South Med J. 2012;105(2):82–6.

127. Yusuf S, Zhao F, Mehta SR, Chrolavicius S, Tognoni G, Fox KK. Clopidogrel in Unstable Angina to Prevent Recurrent Events Trial Investigators. Effects of clopidogrel in addition to aspirin in patients with acute coronary syndromes without ST-segment elevation. N Engl J Med. 2001;345(7):494–502. https://doi.org/10.1056/NEJMoa010746.

128. Mehta SR, Yusuf S, Peters RJ, Bertrand ME, Lewis BS, Natarajan MK, Malmberg K, Rupprecht H, Zhao F, Chrolavicius S, Copland I, Fox KA, Clopidogrel in Unstable Angina to Prevent Recurrent Events Trial (CURE) Investigators. Effects of pretreatment with clopidogrel and aspirin followed by long-term therapy in patients undergoing percutaneous coronary intervention: the PCI-CURE study. Lancet. 2001;358:527–33.

129. Tantry US, Navarese EP, Bliden KP, Gurbel PA. Acetylsalicylic acid and clopidogrel hyporesponsiveness following acute coronary syndromes. Kardiol Pol. 2018;76(9):1312–9.

130. Wallentin L, Becker RC, Budaj A, et al. Ticagrelor versus clopidogrel in patients with acute coronary syndromes. N Engl J Med. 2009;361(11):1045–57. https://doi.org/10.1056/NEJMoa0904327.

131. Husted S, James S, Becker RC, et al. Ticagrelor versus clopidogrel in elderly patients with acute coronary syndromes: a substudy from the prospective randomized PLATelet inhibition and patient outcomes (PLATO) trial. Circ Cardiovasc Qual Outcomes. 2012;5(5):680–8. https://doi.org/10.1161/CIRCOUTCOMES.111.964395.

132. Wiviott SD, Braunwald E, McCabe CH, et al. Prasugrel versus clopidogrel in patients with acute coronary syndromes. N Engl J Med. 2007;357(20):2001–15. https://doi.org/10.1056/NEJMoa0706482.

133. Riesmeyer JS, Salazar DE, Weerakkody GJ, et al. Relationship between exposure to prasugrel active metabolite and clinical outcomes in the TRITON-TIMI 38 substudy. J Clin Pharmacol. 2012;52:789–97.

134. Cayla G, Cuisset T, Silvain J, et al. Platelet function monitoring to adjust antiplatelet therapy in elderly patients stented for an acute coronary syndrome (ANTARCTIC): an open-label, blinded-endpoint, randomised controlled superiority trial. Lancet. 2016;388(10055):2015–22. https://doi.org/10.1016/S0140-6736(16)31323-X.

135. Roe MT, Armstrong PW, Fox KA, et al. Prasugrel versus clopidogrel for acute coronary syndromes without revascularization. N Engl J Med. 2012;367(14):1297–309. https://doi.org/10.1056/NEJMoa1205512.

136. Roe MT, Goodman SG, Ohman EM, et al. Elderly patients with acute coronary syndromes managed without revascularization: insights into the safety of long-term dual antiplatelet therapy with reduced-dose prasugrel versus standard-dose clopidogrel. Circulation. 2013;128(8):823–33. https://doi.org/10.1161/CIRCULATIONAHA.113.002303.

137. Savonitto S, Ferri LA, Piatti L, et al. Comparison of reduced-dose prasugrel and standard-dose clopidogrel in elderly patients with acute coronary syndromes undergoing early percutaneous revascularization. Circulation. 2018;137(23):2435–45.

138. Yeh RW, Secemsky EA, Kereiakes DJ, et al. Development and validation of a prediction rule for benefit and harm of dual antiplatelet therapy beyond 1 year after percutaneous coronary intervention. JAMA. 2016;315:1735–49.

139. Schmucker J, Fach A, Mata Marin LA, et al. Efficacy and safety of ticagrelor in comparison to clopidogrel in elderly patients with ST-segment-elevation myocardial infarctions. J Am Heart Assoc. 2019;8:e012530.

140. Szummer K, Montez-Rath ME, Alfredsson J, et al. Comparison between ticagrelor and clopidogrel in elderly patients with an acute coronary syndrome—insights from the SWEDEHEART registry. Circulation. 2020;42:1700–8.

141. Avezum A, Makdisse M, Spencer F, Gore JM, Fox KA, Montalescot G, Eagle KA, White K, Mehta RH, Knobel E, Collet JP, GRACE Investigators. Impact of age on management and

outcome of acute coronary syndrome: observations from the global registry of acute coronary events (GRACE). Am Heart J. 2005;149:67–73.

142. Alexander KP, Roe MT, Chen AY, Lytle BL, Pollack CV Jr, Foody JM, Boden WE, Smith SC Jr, Gibler WB, Ohman EM, Peterson ED, CRUSADE Investigators. Evolution in cardiovascular care for elderly patients with non-ST–segment elevation acute coronary syndromes: results from the CRUSADE National Quality Improvement Initiative. J Am Coll Cardiol. 2005;46:1479–87.

143. Rogers WJ, Canto JG, Lambrew CT, Tiefenbrunn AJ, Kinkaid B, Shoultz DA, Frederick PD, Every N. Temporal trends in the treatment of over 1.5 million patients with myocardial infarction in the US from 1990 through 1999: the National Registry of Myocardial Infarction 1, 2 and 3. J Am Coll Cardiol. 2000, 36:2056–63.

144. Capranzano P, Angiolillo DJ. Antithrombotic Management of Elderly Patients with coronary artery disease. JACC Cardiovasc Interv. 2021;14(7):723–38.

145. Lee SY, Hong MK, Palmerini T, et al. Short-term versus long-term dual antiplatelet therapy after drug-eluting stent implantation in elderly patients: a meta-analysis of individual participant data from 6 randomized trials. JACC Cardiovasc Interv. 2018;11(5):435–43.

146. Theroux P, Ouimet H, McCans J, Latour JG, Joly P, Levy G, Pelletier E, Juneau M, Stasiak J, deGuise P, Walters DD. Aspirin, heparin, or both to treat acute unstable angina. N Engl J Med. 1988;319:1105–11.

147. The RISC Group. Risk of myocardial infarction and death during treatment with low dose aspirin and intravenous heparin in men with unstable coronary artery disease. Lancet. 1990;336:827–30.

148. Cohen M, Adams PC, Parry G, Xiong J, Chamberlain D, Wieczorek I, Fox KA, Chesebro JH, Strain J, Keller C, Kelly A, Lancaster G, Ali J, Kronmal R, Fuster V, Antithrombotic Therapy in Acute Coronary Syndromes Research Group. Combination antithrombotic therapy in unstable rest angina and non-Q-wave infarction in nonprior aspirin users: primary end points analysis from the ATACS trial. Circulation. 1994;89:81–8.

149. Gurfinkel EP, Manos EJ, Mejail RI, Cerda MA, Duronto EA, Garcia CN, Daroca AM, Mautner B. Low molecular weight heparin versus regular heparin or aspirin in the treatment of unstable angina and silent ischemia. J Am Coll Cardiol. 1995;26:313–8.

150. Fragmin during Instability in Coronary Artery Disease (FRISC) Study Group. Low-molecular-weight heparin during instability in coronary artery disease. Lancet. 1996;347:561–8.

151. The FRAX.I.S. Study Group. Comparison of two treatment durations (6 days and 14 days) of a low molecular weight heparin with a 6-day treatment of unfractionated heparin in the initial management of unstable angina or non-Q-wave myocardial infarction: FRAX.I.S. (FRAXiparine in Ischaemic syndrome). Eur Heart J. 1999;20:1553–62.

152. Blazing MA, de Lemos JA, White HD, Fox KA, Verheugt FW, Ardissino D, DiBattiste PM, Palmisano J, Bilheimer DW, Snapinn SM, Ramsey KE, Gardner LH, Hasselblad V, Pfeffer MA, Lewis EF, Braunwald E, Califf RM, A to Z Investigators. Safety and efficacy of enoxaparin vs unfractionated heparin in patients with non-ST-segment elevation acute coronary syndromes who receive tirofiban and aspirin: a randomized controlled trial. JAMA. 2004;292:55–64.

153. Ferguson JJ, Califf RM, Antman EM, Cohen M, Grines CL, Goodman S, Kereiakes DJ, Langer A, Mahaffey KW, Nessel CC, Armstrong PW, Avezum A, Aylward P, Becker RC, Biasucci L, Borzak S, Col J, Frey MJ, Fry E, Gulba DC, Guneri S, Gurfinkel E, Harrington R, Hochman JS, Kleiman NS, Leon MB, Lopez-Sendon JL, Pepine CJ, Ruzyllo W, Steinhubl SR, Teirstein PS, Toro-Figueroa L, White H, SYNERGY Trial Investigators. Enoxaparin vs unfractionated heparin in high-risk patients with non-ST-segment elevation acute coronary syndromes managed with an intended early invasive strategy: primary results of the SYNERGY randomized trial. JAMA. 2004;292:45–54.

154. Petersen JL, Mahaffey KW, Hasselblad V, Antman EM, Cohen M, Goodman SG, Langer A, Blazing MA, Le-Moigne-Amrani A, de Lemos JA, Nessel CC, Harrington RA, Ferguson JJ, Braunwald E, Califf RM. Efficacy and bleeding complications among patients randomized to

enoxaparin or unfractionated heparin for antithrombin therapy in non-ST-segment elevation acute coronary syndromes: a systematic overview. JAMA. 2004;292:89–96.

155. Lopes RD, Alexander KP, Marcucci G, White HD, Spinler S, Col J, Aylward PE, Califf RM, Mahaffey KW. Outcomes in elderly patients with acute coronary syndromes randomized to enoxaparin vs. unfractionated heparin: results from the SYNERGY trial. Eur Heart J. 2008;29:1827–33.

156. Campbell NR, Hull RD, Brant R, Hogan DB, Pineo GF, Raskob GE. Aging and heparin-related bleeding. Arch Intern Med. 1996;156:857–60.

157. Yusuf S, Mehta SR, Chrolavicius S, Afzal R, Pogue J, Granger CB, Budaj A, Peters RJ, Bassand JP, Wallentin L, Joyner C, Fox KA. Comparison of fondaparinux and enoxaparin in acute coronary syndromes. N Engl J Med. 2006;354:1464–76.

158. Schiele F. Fondaparinux and acute coronary syndromes: update on the OASIS 5–6 studies. Vasc Health Risk Manag. 2010;6:179–87.

159. Yusuf S, Mehta SR, Chrolavicius S, Afzal R, Pogue J, Granger CB, Budaj A, Peters RJ, Bassand JP, Wallentin L, Joyner C, Fox KA. Effects of fondaparinux on mortality and reinfarction in patients with acute ST-segment elevation myocardial infarction: the OASIS-6 randomized trial. JAMA. 2006;295:1519–30.

160. Antithrombotic therapy in the elderly: expert position paper of the European Society of Cardiology Working Group on Thrombosis.

161. Steg PG, van 't Hof A, Hamm CW, Clemmensen P, Lapostolle F, Coste P, Ten Berg J, Van Grunsven P, Eggink GJ, Nibbe L, Zeymer U, Campo dell' Orto M, Nef H

162. Steinmetz J, Soulat L, Huber K, Deliargyris EN, Bernstein D, Schuette D, Prats J, Clayton T, Pocock S, Hamon M, Goldstein P. Bivalirudin started during emergency transport for primary PCI. N Engl J Med. 2013;369(23):2207–17.

163. Shahzad A, Kemp I, Mars C, Wilson K, Roome C, Cooper R, Andron M, Appleby C, Fisher M, Khand A, Kunadian B, Mills JD, Morris JL, Morrison WL, Munir S, Palmer ND, Perry RA, Ramsdale DR, Velavan P, Stables RH. Unfractionated heparin versus bivalirudin in primary percutaneous coronary intervention (HEAT-PPCI): an open-label, single Centre, randomised controlled trial. Lancet. 2014;384:1849–58.

164. Lincoff AM, Bittl JA, Harrington RA, Feit F, Kleiman NS, Jackman JD, Sarembock IJ, Cohen DJ, Spriggs D, Ebrahimi R, Keren G, Carr J, Cohen EA, Betriu A, Desmet W, Kereiakes DJ, Rutsch W, Wilcox RG, de Feyter PJ, Vahanian A, Topol EJ. Bivalirudin and provisional glycoprotein IIb/IIIa blockade compared with heparin and planned glycoprotein IIb/IIIa blockade during percutaneous coronary intervention: REPLACE-2 randomized trial. JAMA. 2003;289(7):853–63.

165. Lopes RD, Alexander KP, Manoukian SV, Bertrand ME, Feit F, White HD, Pollack CV Jr, Hoekstra J, Gersh BJ, Stone GW, Ohman EM. Advanced age, antithrombotic strategy, and bleeding in non-ST-segment elevation acute coronary syndromes: results from the ACUITY (acute catheterization and urgent intervention triage strategy) trial. J Am Coll Cardiol. 2009;53(12):1021–30.

166. Navarese EP, Schulze V, Andreotti F, Kowalewski M, Kołodziejczak M, Kandzari DE, Rassaf T, Gorny B, Brockmeyer M, Meyer C, Berti S, Kubica J, Kelm M, Valgimigli M. Comprehensive meta-analysis of safety and efficacy of bivalirudin versus heparin with or without routine glycoprotein IIb/IIIa inhibitors in patients with acute coronary syndrome. JACC Cardiovasc Interv. 2015;8(1 Pt B):201–13. https://doi.org/10.1016/j.jcin.2014.10.003.

167. Hirsh J, Dalen JE, Anderson DR, Poller L, Bussey H, Ansell J, Deykin D, Brandt JT. Oral anticoagulants: mechanism of action, clinical effectiveness, and optimal therapeutic range. Chest. 1998;114(5 Suppl):445S–469S. https://doi.org/10.1378/chest.114.5_supplement.445s.

168. Wright IS. The use of the anticoagulants in the treatment of diseases of the heart and blood vessels. Ann Intern Med. 1949;30:80–91.

169. Rothberg MB, Celestin C, Fiore LD, et al. Warfarin plus aspirin after myocardial infarction or the acute coronary syndrome: meta-analysis with estimates of risk and benefit. Ann Intern Med. 2005;143:241–50.

170. Andreotti F, Testa L, Biondi-Zoccai GG, Crea F. Aspirin plus warfarin compared to aspirin alone after acute coronary syndromes: an updated and comprehensive meta-analysis of 25,307 patients. Eur Heart J. 2006;27:519–26.
171. Oldgren J, et al. Dabigatran vs. placebo in patients with acute coronary syndromes on dual antiplatelet therapy: a randomized, double-blind, phase II trial. Eur Heart J. 2011;32:2781–9.
172. Uchino K, Hernandez AV. Dabigatran association with higher risk of acute coronary events: meta-analysis of noninferiority randomized controlled trials. Arch Intern Med. 2012;172(5):397–402. https://doi.org/10.1001/archinternmed.2011.1666. Epub 2012 Jan 9
173. Alexander JH, et al. Apixaban, an oral, direct, selective factor Xa inhibitor, in combination with antiplatelet therapy after acute coronary syndrome: results of the apixaban for prevention of acute ischemic and safety events (APPRAISE) trial. Circulation. 2009;119:2877–85.
174. Alexander JH, Lopes RD, James S, et al. Apixaban with antiplatelet therapy after acute coronary syndrome (APPRAISE-2). N Engl J Med. 2011;365:699–708.
175. Mega JL, Braunwald E, Mohanavelu S, Burton P, Poulter R, Misselwitz F, Hricak V, Barnathan ES, Bordes P, Witkowski A, Markov V, Oppenheimer L, Gibson CM. ATLAS ACS-TIMI 46 study group. Rivaroxaban versus placebo in patients with acute coronary syndromes (ATLAS ACS-TIMI 46): a randomised, double-blind, phase II trial. Lancet. 2009;374(9683):29–38.
176. Mega JL, Braunwald E, Wiviott SD, Bassand JP, Bhatt DL, Bode C, Burton P, Cohen M, Cook-Bruns N, Fox KA, Goto S, Murphy SA, Plotnikov AN, Schneider D, Sun X, Verheugt FW, Gibson CM. Rivaroxaban in patients with a recent acute coronary syndrome. N Engl J Med. 2012;366(1):9–19.
177. http://www.ema.europa.eu/docs/en_GB/document_library/EPAR-Product_Information/human/000944/WC500057108.pdf.
178. Michniewicz E, Mlodawska E, Lopatowska P, et al. Patients with atrial fibrillation and coronary artery disease - double trouble. Adv Med Sci. 2018;63(1):30–5.
179. Dewilde WJ, Oirbans T, Verheugt FW, et al. Use of clopidogrel with or without aspirin in patients taking oral anticoagulant therapy and undergoing percutaneous coronary intervention: an open-label, randomised, controlled trial. Lancet. 2013;381(9872):1107–15. https://doi.org/10.1016/S0140-6736(12)62177-1.
180. Cannon CP, Bhatt DL, Oldgren J, Lip GYH, Ellis SG, Kimura T, Maeng M, Merkely B, Zeymer U, Gropper S, Nordaby M, Kleine E, Harper R, Manassie J, Januzzi JL, Ten Berg JM, Steg PG, Hohnloser SH, RE-DUAL PCI Steering Committee and Investigators. Dual antithrombotic therapy with dabigatran after PCI in atrial fibrillation. N Engl J Med. 2017;377(16):1513–24.
181. ten Berg JM, Steg PG, Bhatt DL, et al. Comparison of the effect of age (<75 versus ≥75) on the efficacy and safety of dual therapy (dabigatran + clopidogrel or ticagrelor) versus triple therapy (warfarin + aspirin + clopidogrel or ticagrelor) in patients with atrial fibrillation after percutaneous coronary intervention (from the RE-DUAL PCI trial). Am J Cardiol. 2020;125:735–43.
182. Lopes RD, Heizer G, Aronson R, Vora AN, Massaro T, Mehran R, Goodman SG, Windecker S, Darius H, Li J, Averkov O, Bahit MC, Berwanger O, Budaj A, Hijazi Z, Parkhomenko A, Sinnaeve P, Storey RF, Thiele H, Vinereanu D, Granger CB, Alexander JH, AUGUSTUS Investigators. Antithrombotic therapy after acute coronary syndrome or PCI in atrial fibrillation. N Engl J Med. 2019;380(16):1509–24.
183. Gibson CM, Mehran R, Bode C, Halperin J, Verheugt FW, Wildgoose P, Birmingham M, Ianus J, Burton P, van Eickels M, Korjian S, Daaboul Y, Lip GY, Cohen M, Husted S, Peterson ED, Fox KA. Prevention of bleeding in patients with atrial fibrillation undergoing PCI. N Engl J Med. 2016;375(25):2423–34.
184. Vranckx P, Valgimigli M, Eckardt L, et al. Edoxaban-based versus vitamin K antagonist-based antithrombotic regimen after successful coronary stenting in patients with atrial fibrillation (ENTRUST-AF PCI): a randomised, open-label, phase 3b trial. Lancet. 2019;394(10206):1335–43. https://doi.org/10.1016/S0140-6736(19)31872-0.

185. Effectiveness of intravenous thrombolytic treatment in acute myocardial infarction. Gruppo Italiano per lo studio della Streptochinasi nell'Infarto Miocardico (GISSI). Lancet. 1986;1(8478):397–402.
186. Indications for fibrinolytic therapy in suspected acute myocardial infarction: collaborative overview of early mortality and major morbidity results from all randomised trials of more than 1000 patients. fibrinolytic therapy trialists' (FTT) collaborative group. Lancet. 1994;343(8893):311–22.
187. White HD. Thrombolytic therapy in the elderly. Lancet. 2000;356:2028–30.
188. Thiemann DR, Coresh J, Schulman SP, et al. Lack of benefit for intravenous thrombolysis in patients with myocardial infarction who are older than 75 years. Circulation. 2000;101(19):2239.
189. Berger AK, Radford MJ, Wang Y, Krumholz HM. Thrombolytic therapy in older patients. J Am Coll Cardiol. 2000;36(2):366.
190. Stenestrand U, Wallentin L. Register of information and knowledge about Swedish heart intensive care admissions (RISK-HIA). Fibrinolytic therapy in patients 75 years and older with ST-segment-elevation myocardial infarction: one-year follow-up of a large prospective cohort. Arch Intern Med. 2003;163(8):965–71.
191. White HD, Barbash GI, Califf RM, et al. Age and outcome with contemporary thrombolytic therapy. Results from the GUSTO-I trial. Global utilization of streptokinase and TPA for occluded coronary arteries trial. Circulation. 1996;94(8):1826–33. https://doi.org/10.1161/01.cir.94.8.1826.
192. Longstreth WT Jr, Litwin PE, Weaver WD. Myocardial infarction, thrombolytic therapy, and stroke. A community-based study. The MITI project group. Stroke. 1993;24(4):587–90. https://doi.org/10.1161/01.str.24.4.587.
193. Gurwitz JH, Gore JM, Goldberg RJ, et al. Risk for intracranial hemorrhage after tissue plasminogen activator treatment for acute myocardial infarction participants in the National Registry of myocardial infarction 2. Ann Intern Med. 1998;129(8):597.
194. Assessment of the Safety and Efficacy of a New Thrombolytic (ASSENT-2) Investigators, Van De Werf F, Adgey J, et al. Single-bolus tenecteplase compared with front-loaded alteplase in acute myocardial infarction: the ASSENT-2 double-blind randomised trial. Lancet. 1999;354(9180):716–22.
195. Assessment of the Safety and Efficacy of a New Thrombolytic Regimen (ASSENT)-3 Investigators. Efficacy and safety of tenecteplase in combination with enoxaparin, abciximab, or unfractionated heparin: the ASSENT-3 randomised trial in acute myocardial infarction. Lancet. 2001;358(9282):605–13.
196. Antman EM, Morrow DA, McCabe CH, et al. Enoxaparin versus unfractionated heparin with fibrinolysis for ST-elevation myocardial infarction. N Engl J Med. 2006;354(14):1477–88.
197. Chen ZM, Jiang LX, Chen YP, et al. Addition of clopidogrel to aspirin in 45,852 patients with acute myocardial infarction: randomised placebo-controlled trial. Lancet. 2005;366(9497):1607–21.
198. Sabatine MS, Cannon CP, Gibson CM, et al. Addition of clopidogrel to aspirin and fibrinolytic therapy for myocardial infarction with ST-segment elevation. N Engl J Med. 2005;352(12):1179–89.
199. Armstrong PW, Gershlick AH, Goldstein P, et al. STREAM Investigative Team. Fibrinolysis or primary PCI in ST-segment elevation myocardial infarction. N Engl J Med. 2013;368(15):1379–87.
200. Armstrong PW, Zheng Y, Westerhout CM, et al. Reduced dose tenecteplase and outcomes in elderly ST-segment elevation myocardial infarction patients: insights from the strategic reperfusion early after myocardial infarction trial. Am Heart J. 2015;169(6):890–898 e1.
201. Berwanger O, Nicolau JC, Carvalho AC, et al. Ticagrelor vs clopidogrel after fibrinolytic therapy in patients with ST-elevation myocardial infarction: a randomized clinical Trial. JAMA Cardiol. 2018;3(5):391–9.

202. Armstrong PW, Bogaerts K, Welsh R, et al. The second strategic reperfusion early after myocardial infarction (STREAM-2) study optimizing pharmacoinvasive reperfusion strategy in older ST-elevation myocardial infarction patients. Am Heart J. 2020;226:140–6.
203. Grines CL, Browne KF, Marco J, Rothbaum D, Stone GW, O'Keefe J, Overlie P, Donohue B, Chelliah N, Timmis GC, et al. The Primary Angioplasty in Myocardial Infarction Study Group. A comparison of immediate angioplasty with thrombolytic therapy for acute myocardial infarction. N Engl J Med. 1993;328:673–9.
204. Stone GW, Grines CL, Browne KF, Marco J, Rothbaum D, O'Keefe J, Hartzler GO, Overlie P, Donohue B, Chelliah N, et al. Predictors of in-hospital and 6-month outcome after acute myocardial infarction in the reperfusion era: the primary angioplasty in myocardial infarction (PAMI) trial. J Am Coll Cardiol. 1995;25:370–7.
205. The Global Use of Strategies to Open Occluded Coronary Arteries in Acute Coronary Syndromes (GUSTO IIb) Angioplasty Substudy Investigators. A clinical trial comparing primary coronary angioplasty with tissue plasminogen activator for acute myocardial infarction. N Engl J Med. 1997;336:1621–8.
206. Andersen HR, Nielsen TT, Rasmussen K, Thuesen L, Kelbaek H, Thayssen P, Abildgaard U, Pedersen F, Madsen JK, Grande P, Villadsen AB, Krusell LR, Haghfelt T, Lomholt P, Husted SE, Vigholt E, Kjaergard HK, Mortensen LS, DANAMI-2 Investigators. A comparison of coronary angioplasty with fibrinolytic therapy in acute myocardial infarction. N Engl J Med. 2003;349:733–42.
207. de Boer MJ, Ottervanger JP, van't Hof AW, Hoorntje JC, Suryapranata H, Zijlstra F, Zwolle Myocardial Infarction Study Group. Reperfusion therapy in elderly patients with acute myocardial infarction: a randomized comparison of primary angioplasty and thrombolytic therapy. J Am Coll Cardiol. 2002;39:1723–8.
208. Grines C. Senior PAMI: a prospective randomized trial of primary angioplasty and thrombolytic therapy in elderly patients with acute myocardial infarction. Presented at Transcatheter Cardiovascular Therapeutics; Washington, D; October 16–21, 2005.
209. https://www.acc.org/latest-in-cardiology/clinical-trials/2010/02/23/19/21/senior-pami.
210. Bueno H, Betriu A, Heras M, et al. Primaryangioplasty vs. fibrinolysis in very old patientswith acute myocardial infarction: TRIANA (TRatamiento del Infarto Agudo de miocardio eN Ancianos) randomized trial and pooled analysis with previous studies. Eur Heart J. 2011;32:51–60.
211. Goel K, Gupta T, Gulati R, et al. Temporal trends and outcomes of percutaneous coronary interventions in nonagenarians: a National Perspective. JACC Cardiovasc Interv. 2018;11(18):1872–82. https://doi.org/10.1016/j.jcin.2018.06.026.
212. Fach A, Bünger S, Zabrocki R, et al. Comparison of outcomes of patients with STsegment elevation myocardial infarction treated by primary percutaneous coronary intervention analyzed by age groups (<75, 75 to 85, and >85 years);(results from the Bremen STEMI Registry). Am J Cardiol. 2015;116:1802–9.
213. Zuhdi ASM, Ahmad WAW, Zaki RA, et al. Acute coronary syndrome in the elderly: the Malaysian National Cardiovascular Disease Database-Acute Coronary Syndrome registry. Singap Med J. 2016;57:191–7.
214. Pek PP, Zheng H, Ho AFW, et al. Comparison of epidemiology, treatments and outcomes of ST segment elevation myocardial infarction between young and elderly patients. Emerg Med J. 2018;35(5):289–96. https://doi.org/10.1136/emermed-2017-206754.
215. Albert Ariza-Solé A, Alegre O, Elola FJ, et al. Management of myocardial infarction in the elderly. Insights from Spanish minimum basic data set. Eur Heart J Acute Cardiovasc Care. 2019;8:242–51.
216. Kvakkestad KM, Abdelnoor M, Claussen PA, Eritsland J, Fossum E, Halvorsen S. Long-term survival in octogenarians and older patients with ST-elevation myocardial infarction in the era of primary angioplasty: a prospective cohort study. Eur Heart J Acute Cardiovasc Care. 2016;5(3):243–52. https://doi.org/10.1177/2048872615574706.

217. Puymirat E, Aissaoui N, Cayla G, et al. Changes in one-year mortality in elderly patients admitted with acute myocardial infarction in relation with early management. Am J Med. 2017;130(5):555–63. https://doi.org/10.1016/j.amjmed.2016.12.005.
218. Rivero F, Bastante T, Cuesta J, Benedicto A, Salamanca J, Restrepo JA, Aguilar R, Gordo F, Batlle M, Alfonso F. Factors associated with delays in seeking medical attention in patients with ST-segment elevation acute coronary syndrome. Rev Esp Cardiol. 2016;69:279–85.
219. The TIMI IIIB Investigators. Effects of tissue plasminogen activator and a comparison of early invasive and conservative strategies in unstable angina and non–Q-wave myocardial infarction: results from the TIMI IIIB Trial. Circulation. 1994;89:1545–56.
220. Anderson HV, Cannon CP, Stone PH, Williams DO, McCabe CH, Knatterud GL, Thompson B, Willerson JT, Braunwald E. One-year results of the thrombolysis in myocardial infarction (TIMI) IIIB clinical trial: a randomized comparison of tissue-type plasminogen activator versus placebo and early invasive versus early conservative strategies in unstable angina and non-Q-wave myocardial infarction. J Am Coll Cardiol. 1995;26:1643–50.
221. Boden WE, O'Rourke RA, Crawford MH, Blaustein AS, Deedwania PC, Zoble RG, Wexler LF, Kleiger RE, Pepine CJ, Ferry DR, Chow BK, Lavori PW, Veterans Affairs Non-Q-Wave Infarction Strategies in Hospital (VANQWISH) Trial Investigators. Outcomes in patients with acute non-Q-wave myocardial infarction randomly assigned to an invasive as compared with a conservative management strategy. N Engl J Med. 1998;338:1785–92.
222. FRagmin and Fast Revascularisation during InStability in Coronary artery disease (FRISC II) Investigators. Invasive compared with noninvasive treatment in unstable coronary-artery disease: FRISC II prospective randomised multicentre study. Lancet. 1999;354:708–15.
223. Fox KA, Poole-Wilson PA, Henderson RA, Clayton TC, Chamberlain DA, Shaw TR, Wheatley DJ, Pocock SJ, Randomized Intervention Trial of unstable Angina Investigators. Interventional versus conservative treatment for patients with unstable angina or non-ST-elevation myocardial infarction: the British Heart Foundation RITA 3 randomised trial: randomised intervention Trial of unstable angina. Lancet. 2002;360:743–51.
224. de Winter RJ, Windhausen F, Cornel JH, Dunselman PH, Janus CL, Bendermacher PE, Michels HR, Sanders GT, Tijssen JG, Verheugt FW, Invasive versus Conservative Treatment in Unstable Coronary Syndromes (ICTUS) Investigators. Early invasive versus selectively invasive management for acute coronary syndromes. N Engl J Med. 2005;353:1095–104.
225. Damman P, Clayton T, Wallentin L, et al. Effects of age on longterm outcomes after a routine invasive or selective invasivestrategy in patients presenting with non-ST segment elevationacute coronary syndromes: a collaborative analysis of individualdata from the FRISC II - ICTUS - RITA-3 (FIR) trials. Heart. 2012;98(3):207–13.
226. Cannon CP, Weintraub WS, Demopoulos LA, Vicari R, Frey MJ, Lakkis N, Neumann FJ, Robertson DH, DeLucca PT, DiBattiste PM, Gibson CM, Braunwald E, TACTICS (Treat Angina with Aggrastat and Determine Cost of Therapy with an Invasive or Conservative Strategy)–Thrombolysis in Myocardial Infarction 18 Investigators. Comparison of early invasive and conservative strategies in patients with unstable coronary syndromes treated with the glycoprotein IIb/IIIa inhibitor tirofiban. N Engl J Med. 2001;344:1879–87.
227. Savonitto S, Cavallini C, Petronio AS, et al. Italian Elderly ACS Trial Investigators. Early aggressive versus initially conservative treatment in elderly patients with non-ST-segment elevation acute coronary syndrome: a randomized controlled trial. JACC Cardiovasc Interv. 2012;5(9):906–16.
228. Tegn N, Abdelnoor M, Aaberge L, et al. After Eighty Study Investigators. Invasive versus conservative strategy in patients aged 80 years or older with non-ST-elevation myocardial infarction or unstable angina pectoris (after eighty study): an open-label randomised controlled trial. Lancet. 2016;387(10023):1057–65.
229. Sanchis J, Núñez E, Barrabés JA, Marín F, Consuegra-Sánchez L, Ventura S, Valero E, Roqué M, Bayés-Genís A, del Blanco BG, Dégano I, Núñez J. Randomized comparison between the invasive and conservative strategies in comorbid elderly patients with non-ST elevation myocardial infarction. Eur J Intern Med. 2016;35:89–94.

230. Hirlekar G, Libungan B, Karlsson T, Bäck M, Herlitz J, Albertsson P. Percutaneous coronary intervention in the very elderly with NSTE-ACS: the randomized 80+ study. Scand Cardiovasc J. 2020;54:315–21.
231. de Belder A, Myat A, Blaxill J, Haworth P, O'Kane P, Hatrick R, Aggarwal RK, Davie A, Smith W, Gerber R, Byrne J, Adamson D, Witherow F, Alsanjari O, Wright J, Robinson DR, Hildick-Smith D. Revascularisation or medical therapy in elderly patients with acute anginal syndromes: the RINCAL randomised trial. EuroIntervention. 2021;17:67–74.
232. Garg A, Garg L, Agarwal M, et al. Routine invasive versus selective invasive strategy in elderly patients older than 75 years with non-ST-segment elevation acute coronary syndrome: a systematic review and meta-analysis. Mayo Clin Proc. 2018;93(4):436–44. https://doi.org/10.1016/j.mayocp.2017.11.022.
233. Kaura A, Sterne JAC, Trickey A, et al. Invasive versus non-invasive management of older patients with non-ST elevation myocardial infarction (SENIOR-NSTEMI): a cohort study based on routine clinical data. Lancet. 2020;396(10251):623–34. https://doi.org/10.1016/S0140-6736(20)30930-2.
234. Zaman MJ, Stirling S, Shepstone L, et al. The association between older age and receipt of care and outcomes in patients with acute coronary syndromes: a cohort study of the myocardial Ischaemia National Audit Project (MINAP). Eur Heart J. 2014;35(23):1551–8. https://doi.org/10.1093/eurheartj/ehu039.
235. https://clinicaltrials.gov/ct2/show/NCT03052036
236. Leng WX, Yang J, Li W, Wang Y, Yang YJ, DEAR-OLD investigators. Rationale and design of the DEAR-OLD trial: randomized evaluation of routinely deferred versus EARly invasive strategy in elderly patients of 75 years or OLDer with non-ST-elevation myocardial infarction. Am Heart J. 2018;196:65–73. https://doi.org/10.1016/j.ahj.2017.10.022.
237. Madhavan MV, Gersh BJ, Alexander KP, Granger CB, Stone GW. Coronary artery disease in patients ≥80 years of age. J Am Coll Cardiol. 2018;71(18):2015–40.
238. Olufajo OA, Wilson A, Zeineddin A, Williams M, Aziz S. Coronary artery bypass grafting among older adults: patterns, outcomes, and trends. J Surg Res. 2021;258:345–51.
239. Alkhouli M, Alqahtani F, Kalra A, et al. Trends in characteristics and outcomes of patients undergoing coronary revascularization in the United States, 2003–2016. JAMA Netw Open. 2020;3(2):e1921326.

Index